S0-AYH-357

GERIATRICS *At Your* FINGERTIPS®

2008-2009, 10th EDITION

Distribution Compliments of the
Geriatric Education Center
of Michigan

GERIATRICS *At Your* FINGERTIPS®

2008-2009, 10th EDITION

AUTHORS

David B. Reuben, MD

Keela A. Herr, PhD, RN

James T. Pacala, MD, MS

Bruce G. Pollock, MD, PhD

Jane F. Potter, MD

Todd P. Semla, MS, PharmD

Geriatrics At Your Fingertips® is published by the American Geriatrics Society as a service to health care providers involved in the care of older adults.

Although *Geriatrics At Your Fingertips®* is distributed by various companies in the health care field, it is independently prepared and published. All decisions regarding its content are solely the responsibility of the authors. Their decisions are not subject to any form of approval by other interests or organizations.

Some recommendations in this publication suggest the use of agents for purposes or in dosages other than those recommended in product labeling. Such recommendations are based on reports in peer-reviewed publications and are not based on or influenced by any material or advice from pharmaceutical or health care product manufacturers.

No responsibility is assumed by the authors or the American Geriatrics Society for any injury or damage to persons or property, as a matter of product liability, negligence, warranty, or otherwise, arising out of the use or application of any methods, products, instructions, or ideas contained herein. No guarantee, endorsement, or warranty of any kind, express or implied (including specifically no warrant of merchantability or of fitness for a particular purpose) is given by the Society in connection with any information contained herein. Independent verification of any diagnosis, treatment, or drug use or dosage should be obtained. No test or procedure should be performed unless, in the judgment of an independent, qualified physician, it is justified in the light of the risk involved.

Citation: Reuben DB, Herr KA, Pacala JT, *et al. Geriatrics At Your Fingertips: 2008-2009, 10th Edition.* New York: The American Geriatrics Society; 2008.

Copyright © 2008 by the American Geriatrics Society.

All rights reserved. Except where authorized, no part of this publication may be reproduced, stored in a retrieval system, or transmitted in any form or by any means, electronic, mechanical, photocopying, recording, or otherwise without prior written permission of the American Geriatrics Society, Empire State Building, Suite 801, 350 Fifth Avenue, New York, NY 10118.

ISSN 1553-152X
ISBN 978-1-886775-21-3

TABLE OF CONTENTS

AUTHORS

David B. Reuben, MD
Director, Multicampus Program in Geriatric Medicine and Gerontology
Chief, Division of Geriatrics
Archstone Foundation Chair
Professor of Medicine
David Geffen School of Medicine at UCLA
Los Angeles, CA

Keela A. Herr, PhD, RN
Professor
Chair, Adult and Gerontology Nursing
College of Nursing
The University of Iowa
Iowa City, IA

James T. Pacala, MD, MS
Associate Professor
Distinguished University Teaching Professor
Department of Family Medicine and Community Health
University of Minnesota School of Medicine
Minneapolis, MN

Bruce G. Pollock, MD, PhD
VP of Research
Centre for Addiction and Mental Health
Sandra A. Rotman Chair in Neuropsychiatry
Professor and Head, Division of Geriatric Psychiatry
The Rotman Research Institute
Baycrest Centre for Geriatric Care
University of Toronto
Toronto, Ontario, Canada

Jane F. Potter, MD
Chief, Section of Geriatrics and Gerontology
Harris Professor of Geriatric Medicine
University of Nebraska Medical Center
Omaha, NE

Todd P. Semla, MS, PharmD
Clinical Pharmacy Specialist
Department of Veterans Affairs
Pharmacy Benefits Management
Associate Professor
The Feinberg School of Medicine
Northwestern University
Chicago, IL

AAA	abdominal aortic aneurysm
ABG	arterial blood gas
ABI	ankle-brachial index
ACC	American College of Cardiology
ACE	angiotensin-converting enzyme
ACEI	angiotensin-converting enzyme inhibitor
ACIP	Advisory Committee on Immunization Practices
ACOG	American College of Obstetrics and Gynecology
ACR	American College of Rheumatology
ACTH	adrenocorticotropic hormone
AD	Alzheimer's disease
ADA	American Diabetes Association
ADLs	activities of daily living
AFB	acid-fast bacillus
AGS	American Geriatrics Society
AHA	American Heart Association
AHRQ	Agency for Healthcare Research and Quality
AIDS	acquired immune deficiency syndrome
AIMS	Abnormal Involuntary Movement Scale
ALT	alanine aminotransferase
AMD	age-related macular degeneration
APAP	acetaminophen
ARB	angiotensin receptor blocker
AS	aortic stenosis
ASA	acetylsalicylic acid or aspirin
ASA class	American Society of Anesthesiologists grading scale for surgical patients
AST	aspartate aminotransferase
ATA	American Thyroid Association
ATS	American Thoracic Society
AUA	American Urological Association
BMD	bone mineral density
BMI	body mass index
BP	blood pressure
BPH	benign prostatic hyperplasia
BUN	blood urea nitrogen
C&S	culture and sensitivity
CABG	coronary artery bypass graft
CAD	coronary artery disease
CBC	complete blood cell count
cfu	colony-forming unit
CHD	coronary heart disease
CI	confidence interval
CMS	Centers for Medicare and Medicaid Services
CNS	central nervous system
COPD	chronic obstructive pulmonary disease
CPAP	continuous positive airway pressure
CPK	creatine phosphokinase

CPR	cardiopulmonary resuscitation
Cr	creatinine
CrCl	creatinine clearance
CT	computed tomography
CXR	chest x-ray
CYP	cytochrome P-450
D&C	dilation and curettage
D5W	dextrose 5% in water
DBP	diastolic blood pressure
D/C	discontinue
DHIC	detrusor hyperactivity with impaired contractility
DMARD	disease-modifying anti-rheumatoid drug
DSM-IV	*Diagnostic and Statistical Manual of Mental Disorders*, 4th ed. (Washington, DC: American Psychiatric Association; 1994)
DVT	deep-vein thrombosis
ECF	extracellular fluid
ECG	electrocardiogram, electrocardiography
EEG	electroencephalogram
EF	ejection fraction
EPS	extrapyramidal symptoms
ESR	erythrocyte sedimentation rate
FDA	Food and Drug Administration
FEV_1	forced expiratory volume in 1 sec
FI	fecal incontinence
FOBT	fecal occult blood test
FVC	forced vital capacity
GAD	generalized anxiety disorder
GDS	Geriatric Depression Scale
GERD	gastroesophageal reflux disease
GFR	glomerular filtration rate
GI	gastrointestinal
GnRH	gonadotropin-releasing hormone
GU	genitourinary
Hb	hemoglobin
HbA_{1c}	glycosylated hemoglobin
HCTZ	hydrochlorothiazide
HDL	high-density lipoprotein
HF	heart failure
HR	heart rate
HT	hormone therapy
HTN	hypertension
hx	history
IADLs	instrumental activities of daily living
IBS	irritable bowel syndrome
IBW	ideal body weight
ICD	implantable cardiac defibrillator
INH	isoniazid
INR	international normalized ratio
IOP	intraocular pressure
iPTH	intact parathyroid hormone

JNC 7	Seventh Joint National Committee on Prevention, Detection, Evaluation, and Treatment of High Blood Pressure
K^+	potassium ion
LBW	lean body weight
LDL	low-density lipoprotein
LFT	liver function test
LMWH	low-molecular-weight heparin
LVEF	left ventricular ejection fraction
LVH	left ventricular hypertrophy
MAOI	monoamine oxidase inhibitor
MCV	mean corpuscular volume
MDI	metered-dose inhaler
MI	myocardial infarction
MMA	methylmalonic acid
MMSE	Mini-Mental State Examination (Folstein's)
MRA	magnetic resonance angiography
MRI	magnetic resonance imaging
MSE	mental status examination
NG	nasogastric
NSAIDs	nonsteroidal anti-inflammatory drugs
NPH	neutral protamine Hagedorn (insulin)
OCD	obsessive-compulsive disorder
OGTT	oral glucose tolerance test
OT	occupational therapy
PAD	peripheral arterial disease
PAH	pulmonary arterial hypertension
PCA	patient-controlled analgesia
PE	pulmonary embolism
PEF	peak expiratory flow
PNS	peripheral nervous system
POMA	Performance-Oriented Mobility Assessment
PPD	purified protein derivative (of tuberculin)
PPI	proton-pump inhibitor
PSA	prostate-specific antigen
PT	prothrombin time *or* physical therapy
PTCA	percutaneous transluminal coronary angioplasty
PTH	parathyroid hormone
PTT	partial thromboplastin time
PUVA	psoralen plus ultraviolet light of A wavelength
QT_c	QT (cardiac output) corrected for heart rate
RA	rheumatoid arthritis
RBC	red blood cells *or* ranitidine bismuth citrate
RF	rheumatoid factor
sats	saturations
SBP	systolic blood pressure
SD	standard deviation
SIADH	syndrome of inappropriate secretion of antidiuretic hormone
SPEP	serum protein electrophoresis
SSRIs	selective serotonin-reuptake inhibitors
sTfR	soluble transferrin receptor

TCA	tricyclic antidepressant
TD	tardive dyskinesia
TDD	telephone device for the deaf
TG	triglycerides
TIA	transient ischemic attack
TIBC	total iron-binding capacity
TSG	thyroid-stimulating globulin
TSH	thyroid-stimulating hormone
TTP	thrombotic thrombocytopenic purpura
TUIP	transurethral incision of the prostate
TURP	transurethral resection of the prostate
U	unit(s)
UA	urinalysis
UFH	unfractionated heparin
UI	urinary incontinence
UTI	urinary tract infection
UV	ultraviolet
VF	ventricular fibrillation
VIN	vulvar intraepithelial neoplasia
VT	ventricular tachycardia
VTE	venous thromboembolism
WBC	white blood cell(s)
WHO	World Health Organization
wt	weight

Drug Prescribing and Elimination

Drugs are listed by generic names; trade names are in *italics*. Check marks (✔) indicate drugs preferred for treating older adults. Formulations in text are bracketed and expressed in milligrams (mg) unless otherwise specified. Abbreviations for dosing, formulations, and route of elimination are defined below.

ac	before meals	IV	intravenous(ly)
C	capsule, caplet	K	renal elimination
ChT	chewable tablet	L	hepatic elimination
conc	concentrate	lot	lotion
CR	controlled release	max	maximum
crm	cream	mcg	microgram(s)
d	day(s)	MDI	metered-dose inhaler
ER	extended release	min	minute(s)
F	fecal elimination	mo	month(s)
fl	fluid	npo	nothing by mouth
g	gram(s)	NS	normal saline
gran	granules	oint	ointment
gtt	drop(s)	OTC	over-the-counter
h	hour(s)	OU	both eyes
hs	at bedtime	pc	after meals
IM	intramuscular(ly)	pch	patch
inj	injectable(s)	pk	pack, packet
IT	intrathecal(ly)	po	by mouth

pr	per rectum
prn	as needed
pwd	powder
qam	every morning
qhs	each bedtime
S	liquid (includes concentrate, elixir, solution, suspension, syrup, tincture)
SC	subcutaneous(ly)
sec	second(s)
shp	shampoo
sl	sublingual
sol	solution
Sp	suppository
spr	spray(s)
SR	sustained release
sus	suspension
syr	syrup
T	tablet
tab(s)	tablet(s)
tbsp	tablespoon(s)
tinc	tincture
TR	timed release
tsp	teaspoon(s)
wk	week(s)
XR	extended release
yr	year(s)

INTRODUCTION

Providing high-quality medical care for older adults requires a special set of knowledge, clinical skills, and attitudes. Many resources contain current, accurate information on evaluation and management of the older patient. However, few are portable enough to be used in the examining room, on nursing home or hospital rounds, or when the clinician is on call outside the office.

In 1998, the American Geriatrics Society (AGS) first published *Geriatrics At Your Fingertips (GAYF)*, a pocket guide that provides immediate access to specific information needed to care for older adults in various health care settings. The response was extraordinary, and *GAYF* soon became the society's best-selling publication. As electronic media have increasingly expanded into clinical practice, the AGS has made *GAYF* available as a download for PDAs, and a number of assessment instruments and other selected *GAYF* materials are on the following web site: www.geriatricsatyourfingertips.org.

In this 10th edition, we have added new sections on pulmonary artery hypertension, adverse events of atypical antipsychotics, and treatment of intolerable vasomotor symptoms in older women. Throughout the text and tables, we have updated information including recommended diagnostic tests and management strategies. Among these are new endocarditis prophylaxis guidelines and management of myocardial infarction and acute coronary syndrome. Tables and lists of drugs are designed to facilitate appropriate prescribing. Generic and trade names are provided, as well as information on dosages, how the drugs are metabolized or excreted, and which formulations are available. Specific caveats and cautions to be observed when using the medication in older adults are also included. We have also added to the Appendix a list of medications that have recently become available as generic formulations and might be less expensive for patients. Finally, we have increased the size of both the pages and the type for improved readability. This also allowed us to reformat many of the tables to facilitate easier use.

The goal of *GAYF* is to reduce to a minimum the amount of time that a practicing clinician must spend searching for specific information that is needed immediately to make patient care decisions. Accordingly, *GAYF* does not attempt to explain in detail the rationale underlying the strategies presented. In many instances, these strategies have been derived from guidelines published by organizations such as the Agency for Healthcare Research and Quality, the American Geriatrics Society, the American Heart Association, and the American Diabetes Association. Many of the guidelines can be obtained from the National Guideline Clearinghouse (www.guideline.gov). When no such guidelines exist, the strategies recommended herein represent the best opinions of the authors and the experts they have asked to review the chapters. In an effort to be comprehensive yet concise, references have been provided sparingly, but many others that are relevant are available from the organizations mentioned or in the most recent edition of the AGS *Geriatrics Review Syllabus*.

The authors welcome comments about the format and content of this edition of *GAYF* that may guide the preparation of future editions. All comments should be addressed to the American Geriatrics Society, Empire State Building, 350 Fifth Avenue, Suite 801, New York, NY 10118.

The authors are particularly grateful to Nancy Lundebjerg and Elvy Ickowicz at the AGS, who have served a vital role in the development of this book and continue to expand its distibution and readership. We are also grateful to the John A. Hartford Foundation for generously supporting the initial development and distribution of *GAYF* and its PDA versions.

We would also like to thank the following people who have reviewed parts of this edition:

Catherine A. DuBeau, MD
Perry Fine, MD
Rita A. Frantz, PhD, RN
Gail Greendale, MD
Jerry C. Johnson, MD
James Judge, MD

Anne M. Kenny, MD
Eric J. Lenze, MD
Alison Moore, MD
Larissa Rodriguez, MD
Thomas T. Yoshikawa, MD

Guidelines of the following organizations are the basis of parts of specific chapters:

Advisory Committee on Immunization Practices
Agency for Healthcare Research and Quality
Alzheimer's Association
American Academy of Neurology
American Association for Geriatric Psychiatry
American College of Cardiology
American College of Chest Physicians
American College of Gastroenterology
American College of Obstetrics and Gynecology
American College of Rheumatology
American Diabetes Association
American Geriatrics Society
American Heart Association
American Lung Association
American Pain Society
American Psychiatric Association
American Society of Anesthesiologists
American Thyroid Association
American Urological Association
The Endocrine Society
Ethnogeriatrics Committee, American Geriatrics Society
National Cholesterol Education Program
National Heart, Lung, and Blood Institute
U.S. Preventive Services Task Force
World Health Organization

Editorial Staff
Susan E. Aiello, DVM, ELS, Medical Editor
Carol S. Goodwin, Managing Editor
Pilar Wyman, Medical Indexer

Technical development and production of print and electronic versions:
Fry Communications, Inc.
Melissa Durborow, Group Manager
Rhonda Liddick, Composition Manager
Lori Weld, Composition
Jason Hughes, Technical Services Manager
Julie Stevens, Account Administrator
Terry Plyler, Systems Architect/Engineer

U.S. Biomedical Information Systems, Inc. (USBMIS, Inc.)
Eric Poirier, Chief Operations Officer

FORMULAS AND REFERENCE INFORMATION

Table 1. Conversions

Temperature	Liquid	Weight
F = (1.8)C + 32	1 fl oz = 30 mL	1 lb = 0.453 kg
C = (F − 32) / (1.8)	1 tsp = 5 mL	1 kg = 2.2 lb
	1 tbsp = 15 mL	1 oz = 30 g

Alveolar-Arterial Oxygen Gradient
A − a = 148 − 1.2($Paco_2$) − Pao_2 [normal = 10−20 mmHg, breathing room air at sea level]

Calculated Osmolality
Osm = 2Na + glucose / 18 + BUN / 2.8   [normal = 280–295]

Golden Rules of Arterial Blood Gases
• Pco_2 change of 10 corresponds to a pH change of 0.08.
• pH change of 0.15 corresponds to base excess change of 10 mEq/L.

Creatinine Clearance
See Appropriate Prescribing, p 10.
For renally eliminated drugs, dosage adjustments may be necessary if CrCl <60 mL/min.
Cockcroft-Gault formula:

$$\frac{IBW(140 − age)\ (0.85\ if\ female)}{(72)\ (stable\ serum\ creatinine)}$$

Many laboratories are reporting an estimated GFR as a measure of renal function.
GFR should not be equated to CrCl. Only CrCl should be used to adjust drug dosages.

Erythrocyte Sedimentation Rate
Westergren: women = (age + 10) / 2
            men = age / 2

Ideal Body Weight
• Men = 50 kg + (2.3 kg) (each inch of height >5 feet)
• Women = 45.5 kg + (2.3 kg) (each inch of height >5 feet)

Lean Body Weight
IBW + 0.4 (actual body weight − IBW)

Body Mass Index

$$\frac{\text{weight in kg}}{(\text{height in meters})^2} \quad or \quad \frac{\text{weight in lb}}{(\text{height in inches})^2} \times 704.5$$

Partial Pressure of Oxygen, Arterial (Pao$_2$) While Breathing Room Air
$100 - (\text{age}/3)$ estimates decline

Table 2. Motor Function by Nerve Roots

Level	Motor Function	Level	Motor Function
C4	Spontaneous breathing	L1–L2	Hip flexion
C5	Shoulder shrug	L3	Hip adduction
C6	Elbow flexion	L4	Hip abduction
C7	Elbow extension	L5	Great toe dorsiflexion
C8/T1	Finger flexion	S1–S2	Foot plantar flexion
T1–T12	Intercostal abdominal muscles	S2–S4	Rectal tone

Table 3. Lumbosacral Nerve Root Compression

Root	Motor	Sensory	Reflex
L4	Quadriceps	Medial foot	Knee jerk
	Dorsiflexors	Dorsum of foot	Medial hamstring
L5	Dorsiflexors	Dorsum of foot	Medial hamstring
S1	Plantar flexors	Lateral foot	Ankle jerk

Figure 1. Dermatomes

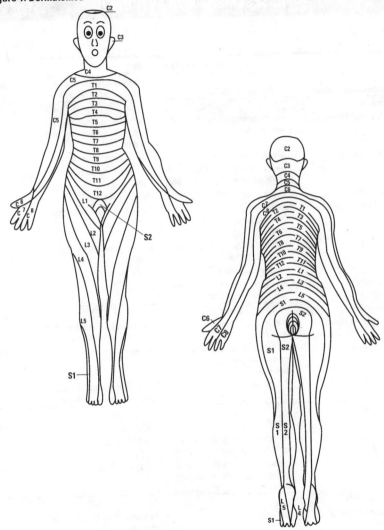

Source: *The Tarascon Pocket Pharmacopoeia*, 2008 classic shirt-pocket edition. Lompoc, CA: Tarascon Publishing, 2008:99. Reprinted with permission.

ASSESSMENT

Table 4. Assessing Older Adults*

Assessment Domain	Screening Methods	Further Assessment (if screen is positive)	See Page(s)
Medical			
Medical illnesses	Hx, screening physical examination	Additional targeted physical examination, laboratory and imaging tests	
Medications	Medications review	Pharmacy referral	10
Nutrition	Inquire about weight loss (>10 lbs in past 6 mo), calculate BMI	Dietary hx, malnutrition evaluation	139
Dentition	Oral examination	Dentistry referral	
Hearing	Handheld audioscope, Brief Hearing Loss Screener, whisper test	Ear examination, audiology referral	98
Vision	Inquire about vision changes, Snellen chart testing	Eye examination, ophthalmology referral	231
Pain	Inquire about pain	Pain inventory	170
Urinary incontinence	Inquire if patient has lost urine >5 times in past year	UI evaluation	107
Mental			
Cognitive status	3-item recall, Mini-Cog, MMSE	Mental status examination, dementia evaluation	244
Emotional status	GDS, PHQ-9, or other depression screen; inquire "Do you ever feel sad or blue?"	In-depth interview	247
Spiritual status	Spiritual hx	In-depth interview, chaplain or spiritual advisor referral	
Physical			
Functional status	ADLs, IADLs	PT/OT referral	245
Balance and gait	Observe patient getting up and walking, orthostatic BP and HR	POMA scale	
Falls	Inquire about falls in past year and difficulty with walking or balance	Falls evaluation	82
Environmental			
Social, financial status	Social hx	In-depth interview, social work referral	
Environmental hazards	Inquire about living situation, home safety checklist	Home evaluation	85

*See also Assessment Instruments, p 244.

SITES OF CARE FOR OLDER ADULTS

Table 5. Sites of Care

Site	Patient Needs and Services	Principal Funding Source
Home		
	ADL or IADL assistance	PP for informal caregiving
	Skilled nursing and/or rehabilitation services when patient can only occasionally leave the home at great effort	Medicare Part A for most nonphysician professional services (eg, nursing, OT, PT); PP for informal caregiving
Senior Citizen Housing	Housing	PP[a]
Assisted Living, Residential Care, Board-and-Care Facilities	IADL assistance, primarily with meals, housekeeping, and medication management	PP, Medicaid for some facilities
Hospital		
Acute Care	Acute hospital care	Medicare Part A
Chronic Care	Chronic skilled care (eg, chronic ventilator)	Medicare Part A, PP, Medicaid
Inpatient Rehabilitation	Intensive rehabilitation in which patient can tolerate 3 h of therapy/day	Medicare Part A[b]
Skilled Nursing Facility		
Transitional Care Unit	Intensive rehabilitation in which patient can tolerate 3 h of therapy/day	Medicare Part A[b]
Short Stay/ Rehabilitation	Skilled nursing care and/or rehabilitation in which patient cannot tolerate 3 h of therapy/day	Medicare Part A[b]
Long-term Care	ADL assistance and/or skilled nursing care	PP, Medicaid
Continuing Care Retirement Communities	Variety of living arrangements ranging from independent to skilled	PP
Hospice (home or facility-based)	Palliative/comfort care for life expectancy <6 mo	Medicare Part A

Note: PP = private pay
[a] May be subsidized for older adults spending over one-third of income for rent. Some facilities may have access to a social worker or informal caregiving services for hire.
[b] Medicare Part A pays for 20 days after a hospital stay of ≥3 days, patient pays $124/d (in 2007) for days 21–100 with Part A covering the rest; patient pays 100% after day 100.

SCHEDULED NURSING-HOME VISIT CHECKLIST
1. Evaluate patient for interval functional change
2. Check vital signs, weight, laboratory tests, consultant reports since last visit
3. Review medications (correlate to active diagnoses)
4. Sign orders
5. Address nursing staff concerns

6. Write a SOAP note (subjective data, objective data, assessment, plan)
7. Revise problem list as needed
8. Update advance directives at least yearly
9. Update resident; update family member(s) as needed

INFORMED DECISION MAKING

Physicians have no ethical obligation to offer care that is judged to be futile.

Three elements are needed for a patient's choices to be legally and ethically valid:

- A capable decision maker: Capacity is for the decision being made; patient may be capable of making some but not all decisions. If a person is sufficiently impaired, a surrogate decision maker must be involved. (See also **Figure 2**.)
- Patient's voluntary participation in the decision-making process.
- Sufficient information: Patient must be sufficiently informed; items to disclose in informed consent include:
  - Diagnosis
  - Nature, risks, costs, and benefits of possible interventions
  - Alternative treatments; relative benefits, risks, and costs
  - Likely results of no treatment
  - Likelihood of success
  - Advice or recommendation of the clinician

MISTREATMENT OF OLDER ADULTS

Risk Factors for Inadequate or Abusive Caregiving

- Cognitive impairment in patient, caregiver, or both
- Dependency (financial, psychological, etc) of caregiver on elderly patient, or vice versa
- Family conflict
- Family history of abusive behavior, alcohol or drug problems, mental illness, or mental retardation
- Financial stress
- Isolation of patient or caregiver, or both
- Depression or malnutrition in the patient
- Living arrangements inadequate for needs of the patient
- Stressful events in the family, such as death of a loved one or loss of employment

Source: Adapted from: Fulmer T. Elder mistreatment. In: Pompei P, Murphy JB, eds. *Geriatrics Review Syllabus: A Core Curriculum in Geriatric Medicine, 6th ed*. New York, NY: American Geriatrics Society; 2006:87. Reprinted with permission.

Figure 2. Informed Decision Making

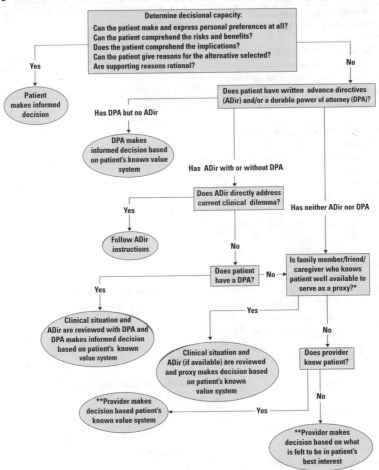

Determine decisional capacity:
Can the patient make and express personal preferences at all?
Can the patient comprehend the risks and benefits?
Does the patient comprehend the implications?
Can the patient give reasons for the alternative selected?
Are supporting reasons rational?

Yes → Patient makes informed decision

No → Does patient have written advance directives (ADir) and/or a durable power of attorney (DPA)?

Has DPA but no ADir → DPA makes informed decision based on patient's known value system

Has ADir with or without DPA → Does ADir directly address current clinical dilemma?

Yes → Follow ADir instructions

No → Does patient have a DPA?

Has neither ADir nor DPA → Is family member/friend/caregiver who knows patient well available to serve as a proxy?*

Does patient have a DPA? **No** → Is family member/friend/caregiver who knows patient well available to serve as a proxy?*

Yes → Clinical situation and ADir are reviewed with DPA and DPA makes informed decision based on patient's known value system

Is family member... **Yes** → Clinical situation and ADir (if available) are reviewed and proxy makes decision based on patient's known value system

Is family member... **No** → Does provider know patient?

Does provider know patient? **Yes** → **Provider makes decision based patient's known value system

Does provider know patient? **No** → **Provider makes decision based on what is felt to be in patient's best interest

* Most states have laws specifying who should serve as proxy when no ADir or DPA exists. For most of these states, the specified hierarchy of decision makers is (in order): legal guardian, spouse or domestic partner, adult children, parents, adult siblings, closest living relative, close friend.

** Or court-appointed decision maker; laws vary by state.

Table 6. Determining Suspicion and Clinical Signs of Possible Mistreatment of Older Adults

Abandonment

Question to Ask Patient: Is there anyone you can call to come and take care of you?
Clinical Signs:

- Evidence that patient is left alone unsafely
- Evidence of sudden withdrawal of care by caregiver
- Statements by patient about abandonment

Physical Abuse

Question to Ask Patient: Has anyone at home ever hit you or hurt you?
Clinical Signs:

- Anxiety, nervousness, especially toward caregiver
- Bruising, in various healing stages, especially bilateral or on inner arms or thighs
- Fractures, especially in various healing stages
- Lacerations
- Repeated emergency department visits
- Repeated falls
- Signs of sexual abuse
- Statements by patient about physical abuse

Exploitation

Question to Ask Patient: Has anyone taken your things?
Clinical Signs:

- Evidence of misuse of patient's assets
- Inability of patient to account for money and property or to pay for essential care
- Reports of demands for money or goods in exchange for caregiving or services
- Unexplained loss of Social Security or pension checks
- Statements by patient about exploitation

Neglect

Question to Ask Patient: Are you receiving enough care at home?
Clinical Signs:

- Contractures
- Dehydration
- Depression
- Diarrhea
- Fecal impaction
- Malnutrition
- Inappropriate use of medications
- Poor hygiene
- Pressure ulcers
- Repeated falls
- Repeated hospital admissions
- Urine burns
- Failure to respond to warning of obvious disease
- Statements by patient about neglect

Psychological Abuse

Questions to Ask Patient: Has anyone ever scolded or threatened you? Has anyone made fun of you?
Clinical Signs:

- Observed impatience, irritability, or demeaning behavior toward patient by caregiver
- Anxiety, fearfulness, ambivalence, or anger shown by patient about caregiver
- Statements by patient about psychological abuse

Assessment and Management
- Interview patient and caregiver separately.
- Ask patient some general screening questions, such as, "Are there any problems with family or household members that you would like to tell me about?" Follow up a positive response with more direct questions such as those suggested in **Table 6**.
- On physical examination, look for any unusual marks, signs of injury, or conditions listed in **Table 6**.
- If mistreatment is suspected, report case to Adult Protective Services (most states have mandatory reporting laws).
- If patient is in immediate danger of harm, create and implement plan to remove patient from danger (hospital admission, court protective order, placement in safe environment, etc).

CROSS-CULTURAL GERIATRICS

Clinicians should remember that:
- Individuals within every ethnic group can differ widely.
- Familiarity with a patient's background is useful only if his or her preferences are linked to the cultural heritage.
- Ethnic groups differ widely in
  ○ approach to decision making (eg, involvement of family and friends)
  ○ disclosure of medical information (eg, cancer diagnosis)
  ○ end-of-life care (eg, advance directives and resuscitation preferences)

In caring for older adults of any ethnicity:
- Use the patient's preferred terminology for his or her cultural identity in conversation and in health records.
- Determine whether interpretation services are needed; if possible, use professional interpreter rather than family member.
- Recognize that the patient may not conceive of illness in Western terms.
- Determine whether the patient is a refugee or survivor of violence or genocide.
- Explore early on the patient's preferences for disclosure of serious clinical findings, and reconfirm at intervals.
- Ask if the patient prefers to involve or defer to others in the decision-making process.
- Follow the patient's preferences regarding gender roles.

APPROPRIATE PRESCRIBING, DRUG INTERACTIONS, AND ADVERSE EVENTS

HOW TO PRESCRIBE APPROPRIATELY
- **Obtain a complete medication history.** Ask about previous treatments and responses as well as about other prescribers. Ask about allergies, OTC drugs, nutritional supplements, alternative medications, alcohol, tobacco, caffeine, and recreational drugs.
- **Avoid prescribing before a diagnosis is made.** Consider nondrug therapy.
- **Review medications regularly and before prescribing a new medication.** D/C medications that have not had the intended response, are no longer needed, or do not have a corresponding diagnosis.
- **Know the actions, adverse events, and toxicity profiles of prescribed medications.** Consider how new prescriptions might interact or complement current medications.
- **Consider the following for new medications:** Is the dosing regimen practical? Is the new medication the least expensive alternative if efficacy and safety are comparable to others in the drug class?
- **Start long-term medications at a low dose and titrate dose on the basis of tolerability and response.** Use drug concentration monitoring when available.
- **Attempt to reach a therapeutic dose before switching to or adding another medication.** Use combinations cautiously: titrate each medication to a therapeutic dose before switching to a combination product.
- **Educate patient and/or caregiver about each medication.** Include the regimen, therapeutic goal, cost, and potential adverse events or drug interactions. Provide written instructions.
- **Avoid using one medication to treat the adverse events caused by another.**
- **Attempt to use one medication to treat two or more conditions.**
- **Communicate with other prescribers.** Don't assume patients do, they assume you do!
- **Avoid using drugs from the same class or with similar actions** (eg, alprazolam and zolpidem).

WAYS TO REDUCE MEDICATION ERRORS
- Be knowledgeable about the medication's dose, adverse events, interactions, and monitoring.
- Write legibly to avoid misreading of the drug name (eg, *Celexa* versus *Celebrex*).
- Write out the directions, strength, route, quantity, and number of refills.
- Always precede a decimal expression of <1 with a zero (0); never use a zero after a decimal.
- Avoid abbreviations, especially easily confused ones (qd and qid).
- Do not use ambiguous directions, eg, as directed (ud) or as needed.
- Include the medication's purpose in the directions (eg, for high blood pressure).
- Write dosages for thyroid replacement therapy in mcg, not mg.
- Always re-read what you've written.
- For more information, see www.fda.gov/cder/drug/MedErrors/ or www.ismp.org/tools/abbreviations/

CRITERIA FOR MEDICATIONS OF CHOICE FOR OLDER ADULTS

- Established efficacy
- Compatible safety and adverse-event profile
- Low risk of drug or nutrient interactions
- Half-life <24 h with no active metabolites
- Elimination does not change with age, or there are known dosage adjustments for renal or hepatic function
- Convenient dosing—once or twice daily
- Strength and dosage forms match recommended dosages for older adults
- Affordable for the patient
- See also Medicare Part D Prescription Drug Plan, p 257.

PHARMACOLOGIC THERAPY AND AGE-ASSOCIATED CHANGES

Table 7. Age-associated Changes in Pharmacokinetics and Pharmacodynamics

Parameter	Age Effect	Disease, Factor Effect	Prescribing Implications
Absorption	Rate and extent are usually unaffected	Achlorhydria, concurrent medications, tube feedings	Drug-drug and drug-food interactions are more likely to alter absorption
Distribution	Increase in fat:water ratio; decreased plasma protein, particularly albumin	HF, ascites, and other conditions increase body water	Fat-soluble drugs have a larger volume of distribution; highly protein-bound drugs have a greater (active) free concentration
Metabolism	Decreases in liver mass and liver blood flow may decrease drug metabolism	Smoking, genotype, concurrent drug therapy, alcohol and caffeine intake may have more effect than aging	Lower dosages may be therapeutic
Elimination	Primarily renal; age-related decrease in GFR	Kidney impairment with acute and chronic diseases; decreased muscle mass results in less Cr production	Serum Cr not a reliable measure of kidney function; best to estimate CrCl using formula (see p 1)
Pharmaco-dynamics	Less predictable and often altered drug response at usual or lower concentrations	Drug-drug and drug-disease interactions may alter responses	Prolonged pain relief with opioids at lower dosages; increased sedation and postural instability to benzodiazepines; altered sensitivity to β-blockers

COMPLICATING FACTORS
Drug-Food or -Nutrient Interactions

Physical Interactions: Mg^{++}, Ca^{++}, Fe^{++}, Al^{++}, or zinc can lower oral absorption of levothyroxine and some quinolone antibiotics. Tube feedings decrease absorption of oral phenytoin and levothyroxine.

Decreased Drug Effect: Warfarin and vitamin K-containing foods (eg, green leafy vegetables, broccoli, brussels sprouts, greens, cabbage).

Decreased Oral Intake or Appetite: Medications can alter the taste of food (dysgeusia) or decrease saliva production (xerostomia), making mastication and swallowing difficult. Medications associated with dysgeusia include captopril and clarithromycin. Medications that can cause xerostomia include antihistamines, antidepressants, antipsychotics, clonidine, and diuretics.

Drug-Drug Interactions

A drug's effect can be increased or decreased by another drug because of impaired absorption (eg, sucralfate and ciprofloxacin), displacement from protein-binding sites (eg, warfarin and sulfonamides), inhibition or induction of metabolic enzymes (see **Table 8**), or because two or more drugs have a similar pharmacologic effect (eg, potassium-sparing diuretics, potassium supplements, and ACEIs).

Digoxin: Digoxin levels must be monitored with concomitant administration of many other medications.

The following **increase** digoxin concentration or effect, or both:

amiodarone	hydroxychloroquine	quinine
diltiazem	ibuprofen	spironolactone
erythromycin	indomethacin	tetracycline
esmolol	nifedipine	tolbutamide
flecainide	quinidine	verapamil

The following **decrease** digoxin concentration or effect, or both:

aminosalicylic acid	colestipol	psyllium
antacids	kaolin pectin	sulfasalazine
antineoplastics	metoclopramide	St. John's wort
cholestyramine		

Enzyme Inhibitors and Inducers: **Table 8** is a list of common drug-drug interactions via this mechanism.

Table 8. Selected CYP Isozyme Substrates, Inducers, and Inhibitors

Isozyme	Substrates[a]		Inducers[b]	Inhibitors[c]
CYP1A2				
	Amitriptyline	Naproxen	Carbamazepine	Amiodarone
	APAP	Nortriptyline	Cigarette smoke	Cimetidine
	Clozapine	Olanzapine	Omeprazole	Diltiazem
	Cyclobenzaprine	Riluzole	Phenobarbital	Estradiol
	Estradiol	Theophylline	Phenytoin	Fluoroquinolones
	Imipramine	Verapamil	Rifampin	Fluvoxamine
	Mexiletine	Warfarin-R[d]		Isoniazid
				Ketoconazole
				Ticlopidine

(cont.)

Table 8. Selected CYP Isozyme Substrates, Inducers, and Inhibitors (cont.)

Isozyme	Substrates[a]		Inducers[b]	Inhibitors[c]
CYP2C9				
	Celecoxib	Phenytoin	Carbamazepine	Amiodarone
	Diclofenac	Piroxicam	Phenobarbital	Cimetidine
	Fluvastatin	Sulfamethoxazole	Phenytoin	Fluconazole
	Glipizide	Tamoxifen	Rifampin	Fluvoxamine
	Ibuprofen	Tolbutamide	Secobarbital	Isoniazid
	Irbesartan	Warfarin		Omeprazole
	Losartan			Propoxyphene
				Ticlopidine
				Valproic acid
CYP2B6				
	Bupropion		Phenobarbital	Thiotepa
	Cyclophosphamide		Rifampin	Ticlopidine
	Efavirenz			
	Methadone			
CYP2C19				
	Amitriptyline	Pantoprazole	Aminoglutethimide	Fluoxetine
	Clomipramine	Phenobarbital	Carbamazepine	Fluvoxamine
	Cyclophosphamide	Phenytoin	Phenytoin	Ketoconazole
	Diazepam	Progesterone	Rifampin	Lansoprazole
	Lansoprazole	Rabeprazole		Omeprazole
	Omeprazole			Ticlopidine
CYP2D6				
	Amitriptyline	Imipramine		Amiodarone
	Aripiprazole	Metoprolol		Bupropion
	Codeine[d]	Mexiletine		Chlorpheniramine
	Clomipramine	Ondansetron		Cimetidine
	Desipramine	Paroxetine		Clomipramine
	Dextromethorphan	Propafenone		Darifenacin
	Donepezil	Risperidone		Diltiazem
	Duloxetine	Tamoxifen		Duloxetine
	Flecainide	Thioridazine		Fluoxetine
	Haloperidol	Timolol		Haloperidol
		Tramadol[e]		Methadone
		Venlafaxine		Mibefradil
				Paroxetine
				Propoxyphene
				Quinidine
				Valproic acid

(cont.)

Table 8. Selected CYP Isozyme Substrates, Inducers, and Inhibitors (cont.)

Isozyme	Substrates[a]		Inducers[b]	Inhibitors[c]
CYP3A4,5,7				
	Alprazolam	Lovastatin	Carbamazepine	Amiodarone
	Amiodarone	Methadone	Glucocorticoids	Cimetidine
	Amlodipine	Midazolam	Griseofulvin	Ciprofloxacin
	Aripiprazole	Nefazodone	Oxcarbazepine	Clarithromycin
	Astemizole	Nifedipine	Phenobarbital	Cyclosporine
	Atorvastatin	Nisoldipine	Phenytoin	Diltiazem
	Buspirone	Nitrendipine	Pioglitazone	Eplerenone
	Carbamazepine	Omeprazole	Rifabutin	Erythromycin
	Chlorpheniramine	Pioglitazone	Rifampin	Fluconazole
	Clarithromycin	Quetiapine	St. John's wort	Fluoxetine
	Clozapine	Quinidine	Troglitazone	Fluvoxamine
	Codeine	Quinine		Grapefruit juice
	Cyclosporine	Risperidone		Haloperidol
	Darifenacin	Sildenafil		Isoniazid
	Diazepam	Simvastatin		Itraconazole
	Dihydropyridine	Solifenacin		Ketoconazole
	calcium	Tacrolimus		Mibefradil
	channel	Tadalafil		Nefazodone
	blockers	Tamoxifen		Norfloxacin
	Diltiazem	Telithromycin		Propoxyphene
	Donepezil	Trazodone		Quinidine
	Erythromycin	Triazolam		Star fruit
	Estradiol	Vardenafil		Telithromycin
	Felodipine	Venlafaxine		Verapamil
	Fluoxetine	Verapamil		
	Gleevec	Vincristine		
	Haloperidol	Warfarin		
	Imatinib	Ziprasidone		
	Itraconazole	Zolpidem		
	Ketoconazole			

[a] Substrate: a drug metabolized by the isozyme.

[b] Inducer: a drug that increases the capacity of the isozyme to metabolize the substrate and potentially decreases the therapeutic effect of the substrate.

[c] Inhibitor: a drug that prevents the isozyme from metabolizing the substrate and increases the risk of toxicity of the substrate.

[d] R-isomer

[e] Analgesic effect decreased because of inhibition of substrate metabolism to its active metabolite by an inhibitor.

Note: The list of medications is not comprehensive but represents medications often prescribed for older adults or medications involved in very serious drug interactions (eg, cyclosporine). Some interactions in vivo or in vitro have been documented, whereas others are theoretical. For more information, consult a drug-drug interaction text or Internet resource, eg, http://medicine.iupui.edu/flockhart/.

COMMONLY USED HERBAL AND ALTERNATIVE MEDICATIONS

Note: Herbal and dietary supplements are not subject to the same regulatory process by the FDA that prescription and OTC medications are. Product and lot-to-lot variations can occur in composition and concentration of active ingredient(s), or be tainted with heavy metals or prescription medications (eg, sildenafil). Consumers are advised to purchase products by reputable manufacturers who follow good manufacturing procedures.

Chondroitin

Common Uses: Osteoarthritis

Adverse Events: Nausea, dyspepsia, changes in intraocular pressure

Comments: Ineffective in treatment of osteoarthritis; may be effective when combined with glucosamine, but this may be product dependent

Echinacea

Common Uses: Immune stimulant

Adverse Events: Hepatotoxicity

Drug Interactions: Immunosuppressants

Comments: D/C ≥2 wk before surgery; cross-sensitivity with chrysanthemum, ragweed, daisy, and aster allergies; kidney disease; immunosuppression; mixed results regarding effectiveness to shorten duration, reduce severity, or prevent colds; should not be taken for >10 d because of concern about immunosuppression

Feverfew

Common Uses: Anti-inflammatory, migraine prophylaxis

Adverse Events: Platelet inhibition, bleeding, GI upset

Drug Interactions: NSAIDs, antiplatelet agents, anticoagulants

Comments: D/C 7 d before surgery, active bleeding; cross-sensitivity with chrysanthemum and daisy; evidence lacking for either indication; minimum of 1-mo trial for migraine prophylaxis suggested

Garlic

Common Uses: HTN, hypercholesterolemia, platelet inhibitor

Adverse Events: Bleeding, GI upset, hypoglycemia

Drug Interactions: NSAIDs, antiplatelet agents, anticoagulants

Comments: D/C 7 d before surgery; effect on lipid lowering modest and of questionable clinical value

Ginger

Common Uses: Antiemetic, anti-inflammatory, dyspepsia

Adverse Events: Bleeding

Drug Interactions: NSAIDs, antiplatelet agents, anticoagulants

Comments: D/C 7 d before surgery; evidence lacking for antiemetic efficacy

Gingko biloba

Common Uses: Alzheimer's disease, memory, intermittent claudication, macular degeneration

Adverse Events: Bleeding, nausea, headache, GI upset, diarrhea, anxiety

Drug Interactions: MAOIs (increased effect and toxicity)

Comments: D/C 36 h before surgery; mixed results in dementia trials; recent trials tend to have negative results

Ginseng

Common Uses: Physical and mental performance enhancer

Adverse Events: HTN, tachycardia

Drug Interactions: Antiplatelet agents, anticoagulants, NSAIDs

Comments: D/C 7 d before surgery, kidney failure

Glucosamine

Common Uses: Osteoarthritis, rheumatoid arthritis

Adverse Events: GI distress, anorexia, insomnia, painful and itchy skin, peripheral edema, tachycardia

Comments: Allergy to shellfish; ineffective in treatment of osteoarthritis; may be effective when combined with chondroitin, but this may be product dependent

Kava kava

Common Uses: Anxiety, sedative

Adverse Events: Sedation, hepatotoxicity

Drug Interactions: Anticonvulsants (increased effect)

Comments: D/C 24 h before surgery; compared with placebo, kava has demonstrated antianxiety efficacy, but effect small and not robust

SAMe (S-adenosyl-methionine)

Common Uses: Depression, fibromyalgia, insomnia, osteoarthritis, rheumatoid arthritis

Adverse Events: GI distress, insomnia, dizziness, dry mouth, headache, restlessness

Drug Interactions: Antidepressants, St. John's wort, NSAIDs, antiplatelet agents, anticoagulants

Comments: Not effective for bipolar depression, hyperhomocysteinemia (theoretical), D/C $\geq$14 d before surgery

Saw palmetto

Common Uses: BPH

Adverse Events: Headache, nausea, GI distress, erectile dysfunction

Drug Interactions: Finasteride, a_1-adrenergic agonist properties in vitro may decrease efficacy

Comments: Efficacy in BPH did not differ from placebo in an adequately powered, randomized clinical trial

St. John's wort

Common Uses: Depression, anxiety

Adverse Events: Photosensitivity, hypomania

Drug Interactions: Potent CYP3A4 inducer (see **Table 8**), finasteride (decreased finasteride concentration and possible effectiveness)

Comments: Wear sunscreen with UVA and UVB coverage; avoid in fair-skinned patients; D/C 5 d before surgery; not effective in severe depression; effects reported to vary from those of conventional antidepressants, yet no more effective than placebo; evaluation of effectiveness may be complicated by product, extraction process, and composition

Valerian

Common Uses: Anxiety, insomnia

Adverse Events: Sedation, benzodiazepine-like withdrawal

Comments: Taper dose several weeks before surgery

ALCOHOL ABUSE
Definition
Possible Alcohol Dependence—DSM-IV: Three or more of the following:
- Tolerance, requiring more alcohol to get "high"
- Withdrawal, or drinking to relieve or prevent withdrawal
- Drinking in larger amounts or for a longer time than intended
- Persistent desire to drink or unsuccessful efforts to control drinking
- Spending a lot of time obtaining, using alcohol, or recovering from effects
- Giving up important occupational, social, or recreational activities because of drinking
- Drinking despite persistent or recurrent physical or psychologic problems caused or worsened by alcohol

Possible Alcohol Abuse—DSM-IV: Recurring problems with one or more of the following:
- Drinking resulting in the failure to fulfill major obligations at work or in the home
- Drinking in situations in which it is physically hazardous
- Alcohol-related legal problems
- Continued drinking despite social problems caused or worsened by alcohol

Hazardous Drinking: WHO definition—use of alcohol that places a person at risk of physical or psychologic complications. Increases risk of HTN, some cancers (eg, head and neck, esophagus, breast in women), and cirrhosis (higher in women). Possible increased risk of hip fracture and other injury.

Evaluation
Alcohol dependence or abuse is often missed in older adults because of reduced social and occupational functioning; signs more often are poor self-care, malnutrition, and medical illness.
Alcohol Misuse Screening: CAGE questionnaire has been validated in the older population.
C Have you ever felt you should **C**ut down?
A Does others' criticism of your drinking **A**nnoy you?
G Have you ever felt **G**uilty about drinking?
E Have you ever had an "**E**ye opener" to steady your nerves or get rid of a hangover?
(*Positive response to any suggests problem drinking.*)
Detecting Harmful Drinking ($\geq$2 drinks/d for women, $\geq$3 drinks/d for men is potentially harmful):
May be missed by CAGE; ask:
- How many days per week?
- How many drinks on those days?
- Maximal intake on any one day?
- What type (ie, beer, wine, or liquor)?
- What is in "a drink"?

Aggravating Factors
Alcohol and Aging: Higher blood concentrations per amount consumed due to decreased lean body mass and total body water; concomitant medications may interact with alcohol. No more than 1-2 drinks/d after age 65; abstain if cognitively impaired, on medications that interact, or comorbidities or disability are present.

Age-related Diseases: Cognitive impairment, HTN.
Medications: Many drug interactions, eg, APAP, antihypertensives, NSAIDs, sedatives, antidepressants.

Management of Alcohol Misuse/Abuse
Psychosocial Interventions:
- Problem drinking or alcohol misuse: Brief intervention; educate patient on effects of current drinking, point out current adverse events.
- Alcohol dependence or abuse: Self-help groups (eg, Alcoholics Anonymous); professional help (eg, psychodynamic, cognitive-behavioral, counseling, social support, family therapy, age-specific inpatient or outpatient).

Drug Therapy: Is useful only when used as an adjunct to psychosocial therapy.
- Naltrexone *(Depade, REVIA, Trexan)* 25 mg × 2 d, then 50 mg/d [T: 50]; 380 mg IM monthly; monitor LFTs, avoid in kidney failure and with opioid use; ~10% get nausea, headache (L, K).
- Acamprosate (*Campral*) 666 mg q 8 h, reduce dosage to 333 mg q 8 h if CrCl 30–50 mL/min or weight <132 lb (60 kg) [T: 333]; contraindicated if CrCl <30 mL/min; diarrhea is most common adverse drug event (K).

Acute Alcohol Withdrawal: See p 54.

SMOKING CESSATION
Nonpharmacologic Therapy
What Health Providers Should Do:
- **Ask** about tobacco use at every visit. **Advise** all users to quit. **Assess** willingness to quit. **Assist** the patient with a quit plan, education, pharmacotherapy.

Making the Decision to Quit:
Patients are more likely to stop smoking if they believe they could get a smoking-related disease and can make an honest attempt at quitting, that the benefits of quitting outweigh the benefits of continued smoking, or if they know someone who has had health problems as a result of smoking.

Setting a Quit Date and Deciding on a Plan:
Pick a specific day within the next month (gives time to develop a plan). Will nicotine replacement therapy be used? Will the patient attend a smoking cessation class? On quit day, get rid of all cigarettes and related items.

Managing Symptoms of Withdrawal:
- **Physical:** Pharmacotherapy (**Table 9**) helps physical symptoms.
  - Nicotine replacement improves quit rates.
    - Is contraindicated with recent MI, uncontrolled high BP, arrhythmias, severe angina, gastric ulcer
    - May not be needed if patient smokes fewer than 10 cigarettes/d; if used, recommend lower dosages
  - Other agents (bupropion, varenicline) may be used if nicotine contraindicated; use bupropion in combination with nicotine if prior failure using nicotine alone

- **Psychological:**
  - Avoid people and places where tempted to smoke.
  - Alter habits: 1) switch to juices or water instead of alcohol or coffee, 2) take a walk instead of a coffee break, 3) use oral substitutions, eg, sugarless gum or hard candy.
  - Three types of counseling and behavioral therapies are effective: 1) problem solving or skills training, 2) social support as part of treatment, and 3) social support outside of treatment.

Maintaining Smoking Cessation: Use the same methods that helped during withdrawal.
Adapted from www.goldcopd.org.

Table 9. Pharmacotherapy for Tobacco Abuse

Drug	Dosage	Formulations	Comments (Metabolism, Excretion)
Tobacco Abuse			
Bupropion (*Wellbutrin SR, Zyban*)	150 mg q 12 h × 7–12 wk	SR: 100, 150	Combined with nicotine replacement, doubles quit rate to 30% at 12 mo; contraindicated with seizure disorders (L)
Varenicline (*Chantix*[a])	0.5 mg × 3 d, 0.5 mg q 12 h × 4 d, then 1 mg q 12 h × 12–24 wk or longer	0.5, 1	Common adverse events: nausea, vivid dreams, constipation (L, K); reduce dosage if CrCl <30 mL/min
Nicotine Replacement			
Transdermal patches (eg, *Habitrol, NicoDerm*)	21 mg/d × 4–8 wk[b] 14 mg/d × 2–4 wk 7 mg/d × 2–4 wk	7, 14, 21	Apply to clean, nonhairy skin on upper torso, rotate sites; start 14 mg/d with cardiovascular disease or body wt <100 lb or if smoking <10 cigarettes/d (L)
(*Nicotrol*)	15 mg/d × 8 wk[b] 10 mg/d × 4–6 wk 5 mg/d × 4–6 wk	5, 10, 15	Gradually released over 16 h (L)
(*ProStep*)	22 mg/d × 4–8 wk[b] 11 mg/d × 4–8 wk	11, 22	People <100 lb start at lower dosage; reduce or D/C after 4–8 wk (L)
Polacrilex gum (*Nicorette*)	9–12 pieces/d	2, 4	Chew 1 piece when urge to smoke; usual 10–12/d, max 30/d; 4 mg if smoking >21 cigarettes/d (L)
Nasal spray[c] (*Nicotrol NS*)	1 spr each nostril q 30–60 min	0.5 mg/spr	Do not exceed 5 applications/h or 40 in 24 h (L)
Inhaler[c] (*Nicotrol Inhaler*)	6–16 cartridges/d	4 mg delivered/ cartridge	Max 16 cartridges/d with gradual reduction after 6–12 wk if needed (L)

(cont.)

Table 9. Pharmacotherapy for Tobacco Abuse (cont.)

Drug	Dosage	Formulations	Comments (Metabolism, Excretion)
Lozenge	1 po prn	2, 4	Do not exceed 20/d; do not bite or chew; wean over 12 wk
Lollipop	1 po prn	1, 2, 3, 4	Place in mouth when urge to smoke; remove when craving passes; gradually reduce dose over 4–8 wk; do not exceed 7/d

[a] Partial nicotine agonist that eases withdrawal and blocks effects of nicotine if patients resume smoking.
[b] The next lower dosage is less toxic and probably equally effective.
[c] Available by prescription only.

ANTICOAGULATION

WARFARIN THERAPY
Prescribing Warfarin

- For anticoagulation in nonacute conditions, initiate therapy by giving warfarin (*Coumadin, Carfin, Sofarin*) 2–5 mg/d as fixed dose [T: 1, 2, 2.5, 3, 4, 5, 6, 7.5, 10]; reduce dose if INR >2.5 on day 3.
- Half-life is 31–51 h; steady state is achieved on day 5–7 of fixed dose.
- Genetic factors can significantly affect appropriate dosing. Genetic testing is available to help guide proper prescribing in patients whose INR is difficult to stabilize.
- Warfarin therapy is implicated in **many** adverse drug-drug interactions.
- Some drugs that **increase** INR in conjunction with warfarin (type in *italics* = major interaction):
  - alcohol (with concurrent liver disease)
  - amiodarone
  - androgens
  - many antibiotics*
  - APAP (>1.3 g/d for >1 wk)
  - ASA (>3 g/d)
  - *celecoxib*
  - chloral hydrate
  - *cilostazol*
  - cimetidine
  - clofibrate
  - *duloxetine*
  - flu vaccine
  - isoniazid
  - *ketoprofen*
  - *naproxen*
  - propafenone
  - sulindac
  - *tamoxifen*
- Some drugs that **decrease** INR in conjunction with warfarin:
  - barbiturates
  - carbamazepine
  - cholestyramine
  - cyclosporine
  - dicloxacillin
  - griseofulvin
  - nafcillin
  - rifampin
  - sucralfate
  - vitamin K

* especially fluconazole, itraconazole, ketoconazole, miconazole, ciprofloxacin, erythromycin, *moxifloxacin*, metronidazole, *sulfamethoxazole*, *trimethoprim*

Table 10. Indications for Anticoagulation in the Absence of Active Bleeding or Severe Bleeding Risk

Condition	Target INR	Duration of Therapy
Hip fracture or replacement surgery	2–3	28–35 d
Major knee surgery	2–3	At least 10 d
Idiopathic venous thromboembolism (includes PE)	2–3	At least 6–12 mo[a]
Atrial fibrillation	2–3	Indefinitely
Mitral valvular heart disease with hx of systemic embolization or left atrial diameter >5.5 cm	2–3	Indefinitely
Cardiomyopathy with EF <25%	2–3	Indefinitely
Mechanical aortic valve with normal left atrial size and sinus rhythm	2–3[b]	Indefinitely
Mechanical aortic valve with enlarged left atrium and/or atrial fibrillation	2.5–3.5[b,c]	Indefinitely

(cont.)

Table 10. Indications for Anticoagulation in the Absence of Active Bleeding or Severe Bleeding Risk (cont.)

Condition	Target INR	Duration of Therapy
Mechanical mitral valve	2.5–3.5[b,c]	Indefinitely
Caged ball or caged disk valve	2.5–3.5[d]	Indefinitely
Bioprosthetic heart valve	2–3	3 mo
Acute MI complicated by severe left ventricular dysfunction, HF, previous emboli, mural thrombus on echocardiography	2–3	1–3 mo

[a] For first event of idiopathic DVT or PE, consider indefinite anticoagulation, particularly after cases of life-threatening embolism or in patients with thrombophilia such as Factor V Leiden mutation.

[b] If additional risk factors are present or if there is systemic embolism despite anticoagulation treatment, target INR is 2.5–3.5 and ASA 80–100 mg/d should be added.

[c] Alternative target INR 2.0–3.0 with addition of ASA 80–100 mg/d.

[d] With addition of ASA 80–100 mg/d.

Cessation of Anticoagulation Before Surgery

• If INR is between 2 and 3, hold warfarin 4 doses before surgery; longer if INR >3.

• If patient has recurrent thromboembolic disease or a mechanical valve, unfractionated heparin or LMWH at DVT/PE treatment dosages (see **Table 12**) should be started when the INR falls after warfarin is discontinued.

Table 11. Treatment of Warfarin Overdose

INR	Clinical Situation	Action
≥3.5 and <5	No significant bleeding	Omit next warfarin dose and/or lower dose
≥5 and <9	No significant bleeding	Omit next 1–2 doses of warfarin and restart therapy at lower dose; alternatively, omit 1 dose and give VK 1–2.5 mg po
≥9	No significant bleeding	D/C warfarin and give VK 3–10 mg po; give additional VK po if INR is not substantially reduced in 24–48 h. Restart warfarin at lower dose when INR is therapeutic.
Any elevation	Serious bleeding	D/C warfarin; give VK 10 mg by slow IV infusion, supplemented with fresh frozen plasma or prothrombin complex concentrate depending on urgency of situation; check INR q 6 h; repeat VK q 12 h as needed
Any elevation	Life-threatening bleeding	D/C warfarin; give VK 10 mg by slow IV infusion, supplemented with prothrombin complex concentrate; repeat this treatment as needed

Note: VK = vitamin K

Source: American College of Chest Physicians Consensus Panel on Antithrombotic Therapy: Ansell J, Hirsch J, Pollar L, et al. The pharmacology and management of the vitamin K antagonists. In: Seventh ACCP Conference on Antithrombotic and Thrombolytic Therapy. *Chest.* 2004; 126:204S–233S.

DVT/PE PROPHYLAXIS AND TREATMENT

• All surgical patients older than 60 yr are considered to be at high risk of postoperative DVT and should receive prophylaxis.

• See **Table 12** for DVT/PE prophylaxis dosages for specific surgeries.

- For surgeries not listed in **Table 12,** use unfractionated heparin, LMWH, or an intermittent pneumatic compression device for DVT prophylaxis.
- If warfarin is part of a long-term anticoagulation plan, it may be started the same day as acute anticoagulant. Specific conditions may require a period of overlap when both agents should be used (eg, for DVT or PE, heparin or similar products should be used a min of 5 d, including 1–3 d of overlap with therapeutic INR).

Table 12. Anticoagulants for DVT or PE Prophylaxis and Treatment			
Class, Agent	**DVT or PE Prophylaxis Dosage by Condition**	**DVT or PE Treatment Dosage**	**Comments**
Heparin			
Unfractionated heparin[a] (*Hep-Lock*)	General surgery: 5000 U SC 2 h before and q 12 h after surgery	5000 U IV bolus followed by 15 U/kg/h IV; **or** for outpatient treatment of DVT, 333 U/kg SC followed by 250 U/kg SC q 12 h	Bleeding, anemia, thrombocytopenia, hypertransaminasemia, urticaria (L, K)
LMWH			
Enoxaparin[a] (*Lovenox*)	THA, HFX: 30 mg SC q 12 h or 40 mg SC q 24 h KR: 30 mg SC q 12 h AS: 40 mg SC q 24 h	Outpatient treatment of DVT: 1 mg/kg SC q 12 h; inpatient treatment of DVT ± PE: 1 mg/kg SC q 12 h or 1.5 mg/kg SC q 24 h	Bleeding, spinal hematoma if spinal anesthesia, anemia, hyperkalemia, hyper-transaminasemia, thrombocytopenia, thrombocytosis, urticaria, angioedema; lower dosage in renal impairment
Dalteparin[a] (*Fragmin*)	Low-risk THA: 2500–5000 U SC before surgery, 5000 U SC q 24 h after surgery AS: 2500–5000 U SC before and after surgery	DVT: 100 U/kg SC q 12 h	Same (K)
Tinzaparin (*Innohep*)	NA	175 anti-Xa IU/kg SC q 24 h	Same (K)
Heparinoid			
Danaparoid (*Orgaran*)	THA, HFX, HIT: 750 anti-Xa U SC q 12 h	NA	Same as LMWH (K)
Factor Xa Inhibitor			
Fondaparinux[a] (*Arixtra*)	THA, HFX, KR: 2.5 mg/d SC beginning 6–8 h after surgery	Weight <50 kg: 5 mg/d SC; weight 50–100 kg: 7.5 mg/d SC; weight >100 kg: 10 mg/d SC	Lower dosage in renal impairment; contraindicated if CrCl <30 mL/min (K)

(cont.)

Table 12. Anticoagulants for DVT or PE Prophylaxis and Treatment (cont.)

Class, Agent	DVT or PE Prophylaxis Dosage by Condition	DVT or PE Treatment Dosage	Comments
Direct Thrombin Inhibitors			
Argatroban	HIT: 2 mcg/kg/min IV infusion	HIT: 2 mcg/kg/min IV infusion	↓ Dosage if hepatic impairment (L)
Lepirudin (*Refludan*)	HIT: 4 mcg/kg bolus, then 0.15 mg/kg/h	HIT: 4 mcg/kg bolus, then 0.15 mg/kg/h	↓ Bolus to 0.2 mg/kg if CrCl <60 mL/min
Thrombolytics			
Streptokinase (*Kabikinase, Streptase*)	NA	250,000 U IV over 30 min, then 100,000 U/h for 24 h[b]	Risk of hemorrhage ↑ with age and higher BMI; HTN, hallucination, agitation, confusion, serum sickness (L)

Note: THA = total hip arthroplasty (hip replacement); HFX = hip fracture surgery; AS= abdominal surgery; KR = knee replacement; HIT = heparin-induced thrombocytopenia; NA = not applicable
[a] Also indicated for anticoagulation in acute coronary syndrome (see **Table 14**).
[b] Dose in acute MI is 1.5 million U IV over 60 min.

DIAGNOSIS

Anxiety disorders as a whole are the most common mental disorders in older adults. Some anxiety disorders (panic attack, OCD) appear to be less prevalent in older than in younger adults. Generalized anxiety disorder (GAD) and new-onset anxiety in older adults are often secondary to physical illness, depression, or adverse events of or withdrawal from medications.

DSM-IV recognizes several anxiety disorders:
(*Italicized type indicates the most common anxiety disorders in older adults.*)
- Acute stress disorder
- Agoraphobia without a history of panic
- *Generalized anxiety disorder (GAD)*
- *Anxiety disorder due to a general medical condition*
- Obsessive-compulsive disorder (OCD)
- Panic disorder, with or without agoraphobia
- Post-traumatic stress disorder
- Social phobia (social anxiety disorder)
- Specific phobia
- Substance-induced anxiety disorder

DSM-IV Criteria for GAD
- Excessive anxiety and worry on more days than not for ≥6 mo, about a number of events or activities
- Difficulty controlling the worry
- Anxiety and worry associated with ≥3 of 6 symptoms:
  ○ restlessness or feeling keyed up or on edge
  ○ being easily fatigued
  ○ difficulty concentrating or mind going blank
  ○ irritability
  ○ muscle tension
  ○ sleep disturbance (difficulty falling or staying asleep, or restless unsatisfying sleep)
- Focus of anxiety and worry not confined to features of an Axis I disorder (primary psychiatric disorder); often, about routine life circumstances; may shift from one concern to another
- Anxiety, worry, or physical symptoms cause clinically significant distress or impairment in social, occupational, or other important areas of functioning
- Disturbance not due to the direct physiologic effects of a drug of abuse or a medication or to a medical condition; does not occur exclusively during a mood disorder, psychotic disorder, or a pervasive development disorder

DSM-IV Criteria for Panic Attack

Discrete period of intense fear or discomfort with ≥4 of the following (also, must peak within 10 min):

- Palpitations, rapid HR
- Sweating
- Feeling dizzy, unsteady, lightheaded, or faint
- Trembling or shaking
- Sensations of shortness of breath or smothering
- Choking feeling
- Chest pain or discomfort
- Nausea or abdominal distress
- Feelings of unreality or being detached from self
- Fear of losing control or going crazy
- Fear of dying
- Paresthesias
- Chills or hot flushes

Differential Diagnosis

- Panic disorder: recurrent, unexpected panic attacks
- Physical conditions producing anxiety
  - Cardiovascular: arrhythmias, angina, MI, HF
  - Endocrine: hyperthyroidism, hypoglycemia, pheochromocytoma
  - Neurologic: movement disorders, temporal lobe epilepsy, AD, stroke
  - Respiratory: COPD, asthma, pulmonary embolism
- Medications producing anxiety
  - Caffeine
  - Corticosteroids
  - Nicotine
  - Psychotropics: antidepressants, antipsychotics, stimulants
  - Sympathomimetics: pseudoephedrine, β-agonists
  - Thyroid hormones: overreplacement
- Withdrawal states: alcohol, sedatives, hypnotics, benzodiazepines, SSRIs
- Depression

EVALUATION

- Past psychiatric hx
- Drug review: prescribed, OTC, alcohol, caffeine
- Mental status evaluation
- Physical examination: Focus on signs and symptoms of anxiety (eg, tachycardia, hyperpnea, sweating, tremor).
- Laboratory tests: Consider CBC, blood glucose, TSH, B_{12}, ECG, oxygen saturation, drug and alcohol screening.

MANAGEMENT

Nonpharmacologic

- Cognitive-behavior therapy may be useful for GAD, panic disorder, and OCD.
- May be effective alone but mostly used in conjunction with pharmacotherapy.
- Requires a cognitively intact, motivated patient.

Pharmacologic (See **Table 29** for dosing of antidepressants.)
- Obsessive-compulsive: fluoxetine, fluvoxamine, paroxetine, sertraline; secondary choices include β-blockers and atypical antipsychotics
- Panic: sertraline, paroxetine; secondary choices include β-blockers and atypical antipsychotics
- Social phobia: paroxetine, sertraline, venlafaxine XR
- Generalized anxiety: duloxetine, escitalopram, paroxetine, sertraline, venlafaxine XR
- Post-traumatic stress: paroxetine, sertraline

Buspirone (BuSpar):
- Serotonin 1A partial agonist effective in GAD and anxiety symptoms accompanying general medical illness (although geriatric evidence is limited)
- Not effective for acute anxiety, panic, or OCD
- May take 2–4 wk for therapeutic response
- Recommended geriatric dosage: 7.5–10 mg q 12 h [T: 5, 10, 15, 30]
- No dependence, tolerance, withdrawal, CNS depression, or significant drug-drug interactions

Benzodiazepines:
- Most often used for acute anxiety, GAD, panic, OCD (**Table 13**)
- Preferred: intermediate–half-life drugs inactivated by direct conjugation in liver and therefore less affected by aging
- Avoid long-acting benzodiazepines (eg, flurazepam, diazepam, chlordiazepoxide)
- Linked to cognitive impairment, falls, sedation, psychomotor impairment
- Problems: dependence, tolerance, withdrawal, more so with short-acting benzodiazepines; seizure risk with alprazolam withdrawal
- Potentially fatal if combined with alcohol or other CNS depressants
- Only short-term (60–90 d) use recommended
- Not covered by Medicare Part D (see p 257)

Table 13. Benzodiazepines for Anxiety Recommended for Older Adults		
Drug	**Dosage**	**Formulations**
Lorazepam (*Ativan*)	0.5–2 mg in 2–3 divided doses	T: 0.5, 1, 2; S: 2 mg/mL; inj: 2 mg/mL
Oxazepam (*Serax*)	10–15 mg q 8–12 h	T: 10, 15, 30

Nonbenzodiazepine Hypnotics:
Zoldipem *(Ambien)*, zaleplon *(Sonata)*, eszopiclone *(Lunesta)*, and ramelteon *(Rozerem)* should not be used for treatment of anxiety disorders. See Sleep Disorders, **Table 97**.

CORONARY ARTERY DISEASE

Calculating Risk

- Risk factors:
  - Previous MI or angina
  - Age
  - Diabetes mellitus
  - Dyslipidemia
  - Family hx
  - HTN
  - Obesity
  - Sedentary lifestyle
  - Smoking
- To calculate 10-yr risk, see http://hp2010.nhlbihin.net/atpiii/calculator.asp?usertype=prof.
- If calculated 10-yr risk is 10%-20%, consider measurement of coronary artery calcification by CT or carotid intima-media thickness by ultrasonography to further clarify risk and direct treatment.

Diagnostic Cardiac Tests

- Cardiac catheterization is the gold standard.
- Stress testing: The heart is stressed either through exercise (treadmill, stationary bicycle) or, if the patient cannot exercise or the ECG is markedly abnormal, with pharmacologic agents (dipyridamole, adenosine, dobutamine). Exercise stress tests can be performed with or without cardiac imaging, while pharmacologic stress tests always include imaging. Imaging can be accomplished by echocardiography or single-photon-emission computed tomography (SPECT).

Acute Coronary Syndrome (ACS)

- ACS encompasses diagnoses of ST segment MI (STEMI), non-ST segment MI (NSTEMI), and unstable angina.
- Suspect ACS with anginal chest pain or anginal equivalent: arm, jaw, or abdominal pain (with or without nausea); acute functional decline.
- Diagnosis is based on symptoms along with cardiac serum markers and ECG findings:
  - STEMI: elevated serum markers, elevated ST segments
  - NSTEMI: elevated serum markers, depressed ST segments or inverted T-waves
  - Unstable angina: nonelevated serum markers, normal or depressed ST segments, normal or inverted T-waves
- Measuring cardiac serum markers:
  - Most protocols call for checking troponins T and I and creatine kinase MB isoenzymes (CK-MB) at presentation and 3, 6, 12, and 24 h later.
  - A single negative enzyme measurement, particularly within 6 h of symptom onset, does not exclude MI.
  - Elevated troponin in the face of normal CK-MB can indicate increased risk of MI in the ensuing 6 mo.
  - Troponins are not useful for detecting reinfarction within first wk of an MI. CK-MB is the preferred marker for early reinfarction.
  - Both CK-MB and cardiac troponins can have false-positive results due to subclinical ischemic myocardial injury or nonischemic myocardial injury.

Initial Management of ACS

- Bedrest with continuous ECG monitoring
- Oxygen to maintain saturation >90%
- ASA with or without clopidogrel (see **Table 14**)
- D/C NSAIDs
- If ischemia is ongoing (based on symptoms or ECG changes), give nitroglycerin 0.4 mg sl q 5 min for a total of 3 doses
- Nitroglycerin IV is indicated for persistent ischemia, HTN, large anterior infarction, or HF. Begin at 5-10 mcg/min IV and titrate to pain relief, SBP >90 mmHg, or resolution of ECG abnormalities.
- If chest pain persists on nitroglycerin therapy, give morphine sulfate 1–5 mg IV.
- Determine type of reperfusion strategy:
  ○ Thrombolytic therapy
    ▪ Indications: STEMI, presentation <3 h from symptom onset
    ▪ Absolute contraindications: prior hemorrhagic stroke, stroke or intracerebral event in past year, active internal bleeding, known intracranial malignant neoplasm, aortic dissection, structural cerebral vascular lesion, significant closed head trauma in previous 3 mo
    ▪ Relative contraindications: BP >180/110, stroke in previous 3 mo, dementia, INR ≥3, known bleeding diathesis, major surgery in previous 3 wk, prolonged (>10 min) or traumatic CPR, trauma or internal bleeding in previous 4 wk, noncompressible vascular puncture, active peptic ulcer, hx of severe and chronic HTN
  ○ Early invasive strategy with planned percutaneous cardiac intervention (angiography and PTCA with or without stent placement)
  Indications: STEMI, NSTEMI, unstable angina; preferred over thrombolytic or conservative therapy if:
    ▪ presentation >3h from symptom onset
    ▪ recurrent angina at rest or with low-level activity despite intensive medical therapy
    ▪ new ST segment depressions
    ▪ symptomatic HF or EF <40%
    ▪ new or worsening mitral regurgitation
    ▪ hemodynamic instability
    ▪ sustained VT
    ▪ PTCA in the previous 6 mo
    ▪ prior CABG
    ▪ high TIMI (see www.timi.org) or GRACE (see www.outcomes-umassmed.org/grace/acs_risk.cfm) score
  ○ Conservative therapy with medical management
  Indications: Low TIMI or GRACE score, lack of available cardiac catheterization facility, contraindication to thrombolytic therapy, patient or physician preference
  ○ Surgical reperfusion by CABG
  Indications: left main CAD, 3-vessel disease, failed PTCA, unsuitable for thrombolytic therapy or PTCA
- Administer antiplatelet agents, anticoagulants, and glycoprotein IIb/IIIa inhibitors according to reperfusion strategy (see **Table 14**):
  ○ Thrombolytic therapy: ASA and unfractionated heparin

Coronary Artery Disease – CARDIOVASCULAR 29

- Early invasive therapy with planned percutaneous cardiac intervention: ASA, clopidogrel, an anticoagulant, and a glycoprotein IIb/IIIa inhibitor
- Medical management: ASA, clopidogrel, and an anticoagulant; consider adding a glycoprotein IIb/IIIa inhibitor
- CABG: ASA and unfractionated heparin

Table 14. Antithrombotic Therapy in Acute Coronary Syndrome

Class, Agent	Dosage	Treatment Strategy			
		TT	PCI	MM	CABG
Antiplatelet Agents					
Aspirin	162–325 mg po initially, followed by 75–160 mg po q 24 h[a]	●	●	●	●
Clopidogrel (*Plavix*)	300 mg po initially, followed by 75 mg po q 24 h[b]		●	●	
Anticoagulants					
Bivalirudin (*Angiomax*)	0.1 mg/kg bolus, followed by 0.25 mg/kg/h IV		○		
Enoxaparin (*Lovenox*)	30 mg IV bolus, followed by 1 mg/kg SC q 12 h	○	●	●	
Dalteparin (*Fragmin*)	120 IU/kg SC q 12 h		○		
Fondaparinux (*Arixtra*)	2.5 mg/d SC		○	●	
Heparin (*Hep-Lock*)	60–70 U/kg (max 5000 U) IV bolus, followed by 12–15 U/kg/h IV	●	●	○	●
Glycoprotein IIb/IIIa Inhibitors					
Abciximab (*ReoPro*)	0.25 mg/kg IV bolus, followed by 0.125 mcg/kg/min (max 10 mcg/min)		●		
Eptifibatide (*Integrilin*)	180 mcg/kg IV bolus, followed by 2 mcg/kg/min IV		●	○	
Tirofiban (*Aggrastat*)	0.4 mcg/kg/min IV over 30 min, followed by 0.1 mcg/kg/min		●	○	

Note: TT = thrombolytic therapy; PCI = early invasive therapy with planned percutaneous cardiac intervention; CABG = acute coronary syndrome with emergent CABG a likely possibility; MM = conservative therapy with medical management

● = preferred or first-line treatment

○ = alternative or second-line treatment

[a] Use dose of 325 mg if patient is undergoing PCI and has not previously been on chronic ASA therapy; continue at same dose 1–6 mo after PCI before reducing dose. ASA therapy should be lifelong after ACS.

[b] Clopidogrel should also be used in MM if patient is allergic to ASA. In combination with ASA, clopidogrel causes increased risk of bleeding, so it should be used carefully. Clopidogrel should not be used if there is a reasonable possibility that patient will be undergoing CABG within the ensuing 5 days.

Ongoing Hospital Management of ACS

- An oral β-blocker should be started within 24 h of symptom onset and continued long term unless there is acute HF, evidence of a low-output state, pronounced bradycardia, or cardiogenic shock.

- An oral ACEI should be started within 24 h of symptom onset for patients with STEMI and for patients with NSTEMI or unstable angina who have clinical HF or EF <40% (see **Table 17**). If patient cannot tolerate ACEIs, give oral ARB.
- A statin should be started (if there are no contraindications) in all patients with NSTEMI or unstable angina regardless of baseline LDL, and should be strongly considered in all STEMI patients regardless of baseline LDL.
- Lipid-lowering therapy, preferably including the use of a statin, should be instituted with target levels of LDL cholesterol <70–100 mg/dL (see Dyslipidemia, p 35).
- Warfarin therapy is indicated in post-MI patients with AF, left ventricular thrombosis, or large anterior infarction (see **Table 10**).
- Patients with a hematocrit ≤30 and who are not in HF should receive a transfusion to increase hematocrit to >33.
- At time of discharge, prescribe rapid-acting nitrates prn: sublingual nitroglycerin or nitroglycerin spray q 5 min for max of 3 doses in 15 min. See **Table 15**.
- Longer-acting nitrates should be prescribed if symptomatic angina and treatment will be medical rather than surgical or angioplasty. May be combined with β-blockers or calcium channel blockers, or both. See **Table 15**.
- Calcium channel blockers should be used cautiously for management of angina only in non-Q-wave infarctions without systolic dysfunction and a contraindication to β-blockers.

Table 15. **Nitrate Dosages and Formulations**		
Medication	**Dosage**	**Formulations**
Oral		
Isosorbide dinitrate (*Isordil, Sorbitrate*)	10–40 mg 3 ×/d (6 h apart)	T: 5, 10, 20, 30, 40; ChT: 5, 10
Isosorbide dinitrate SR (*Isordil Tembids, Dilatrate SR*)	40–80 mg q 8–12 h	T: 40
Isosorbide mononitrate (*ISMO, Monoket*)	20 mg q 12 h (8 am and 3 pm)	T: 10, 20
Isosorbide mononitrate SR (*Imdur*)	start 30–60 mg/d; max 240 mg/d	T: 30, 60, 120
Nitroglycerin (*Nitro-Bid*)	2.5–9 mg q 8–12 h	T: 2.5, 6.5, 9
Sublingual		
Isosorbide dinitrate (*Isordil, Sorbitrate*)	1 tab prn	T: 2.5, 5, 10
Nitroglycerin (*Nitrostat*)	0.4 mg prn	T: 0.15, 0.3, 0.4, 0.6
Oral spray		
Nitroglycerin (*Nitrolingual, Nitromist*)	1–2 spr prn; max 3/15 min	0.4 mg/spr
Ointment		
Nitroglycerin 2% (*Nitro-Bid, Nitrol*)	start 0.5–4 inches q 4–8 h	2%

(cont.)

Table 15. Nitrate Dosages and Formulations (cont.)

Medication	Dosage	Formulations
Transdermal		
Nitroglycerin	1 pch 12–14 h/d	(all in mg/h)
(*Deponit*)		0.2, 0.4
(*Minitran*)		0.1, 0.2, 0.4, 0.6
(*Nitrek*)		0.2, 0.4, 0.6
(*Nitro-Dur*)		0.1, 0.2, 0.3, 0.4, 0.6, 0.8
(*Nitrodisc*)		0.2, 0.3, 0.4
(*Transderm-Nitro*)		0.1, 0.2, 0.4, 0.6, 0.8

POST-MI AND CHRONIC STABLE ANGINA CARE
- Unless contraindicated, all post-MI patients should be on ASA, a β-blocker, and an ACEI.
- Give clopidogrel for 9–12 mo after acute coronary syndrome and for 1 mo after acute MI. If patient received a drug-eluting stent, consider lifelong clopidogrel therapy.
- If β-blockers are contraindicated, use long-acting nitrates or long-acting calcium channel blockers for chronic angina.
- For refractory chronic angina despite treatment with β-blocker, calcium channel blocker, or nitrates, consider addition of ranolazine (*Ranexa*) 500–1,000 mg po q 12 h [T:500]; contraindicated in patients with QT prolongation or on QT-prolonging drugs, hepatic impairment, or on CYP3A inhibitors, including diltiazem (see p 14).
- Use sublingual or spray nitroglycerin for acute angina.
- Treat HTN (see p 37); goal of <140/90 or <130/80 if HF, diabetes mellitus, or kidney failure is present.
- Treat dyslipidemia (see p 35); goals of LDL <70–100 mg/dL and TG <150 mg/dL.
- Treat diabetes mellitus; see p 77 for target goals.
- Weight reduction in obese individuals; goal BMI (kg/m^2) <25.
- Aerobic exercise; goal 30 min at least 3 times/wk.
- Smoking cessation.
- Use folic acid 1 mg/d po to treat homocysteinemia; goal homocysteine <10 μmoles/L.
- Increase consumption of oily fish (eg, white canned or fresh tuna, salmon, mackerel, herring) and foods rich in α-linolenic acid (eg, flax-seed, canola, and soybean oils; flax seed; walnuts). Consider supplementation with fish oil capsules to achieve omega-3 fatty acid intake of 1 g/d.
- Strongly consider placement of implantable cardiac defibrillator (see p 50) in patients with LVEF ≤30% at least 40 d after MI or 3 mo after CABG.
- Avoid NSAIDs, especially those with COX-2 inhibition (see **Table 57**).

HEART FAILURE (HF)
Evaluation and Assessment
- All patients initially presenting with HF should have an echocardiogram to evaluate left ventricular function. An ejection fraction (EF) of <40% indicates systolic dysfunction. HF with an EF ≥40% indicates HF with preserved systolic function (diastolic dysfunction).

- Other routine assessment tests: orthostatic blood pressures, height, weight, BMI calculation, ECG, CXR, CBC, electrolytes, creatinine, BUN, lipid profile, fasting glucose, LFTs, TSH, UA
- Measurement of plasma brain natriuretic peptide (BNP) can be helpful in diagnosing acute HF. A BNP >100 pg/mL strongly suggests decreased left ventricular function or acute HF in the absence of renal disease.
- Optional: Radionuclide ventriculography, which measures EF more precisely, provides a better evaluation of right ventricular function, and is more expensive than echocardiography.

Table 16. Heart Failure Staging and Management

Clinical Profile	ACC/AHA Staging	New York Heart Association Staging	Management[a]
Asymptomatic but at high risk of developing HF (eg, HTN, diabetes mellitus, CAD present)	Stage A	—	RFR, E
Asymptomatic with structural disease: LVH, low EF, prior MI, or valvular disease	Stage B	Class I	RFR, E, ACEI (or ARB if unable to tolerate ACEI), BB
Low EF[b]; currently asymptomatic but with hx of symptoms	Stage C	Class I	RFR, E, DW, SR, ACEI (or ARB if unable to tolerate ACEI), BB
Low EF[b]; patient comfortable at rest but symptomatic on normal physical activity	Stage C	Class II	RFR, E, DW, SR, drug therapy for symptomatic HF (below), consider placement of ICD
Low EF[b]; patient comfortable at rest but symptomatic on slight physical activity	Stage C	Class III	
Low EF[b]; patient symptomatic at rest	Stage C	Class IV	
Normal EF; current or prior symptoms	Stage C	Class I-IV	RFR, drug therapy for symptomatic HF, control of ventricular rate
Refractory symptoms at rest in hospitalized patient requiring specialized interventions (eg, transplant) or hospice care	Stage D	Class IV	Decide on care preference; above measures or hospice as appropriate

[a] RFR = cardiac risk factor reduction, E = exercise (regular walking or cycling), BB = β blocker, DW = measurement of daily weight, SR = salt restriction (≤3 g/d if severe HF)
[b] Low EF = EF <40%

Drug Therapy for Symptomatic HF (AHA Stage C and D, NYHA Class II–IV)

For information on drug dosages and adverse events not listed below, see **Table 20**. Efficacy of different medications may vary significantly across racial and ethnic groups; eg, blacks may require higher doses of ACEIs and β-blockers and may benefit from isosorbide dinitrate/hydralazine therapy.

- Systolic dysfunction (low EF):
  - Diuretics if volume overload
  - ACEIs to target doses (see **Table 17**)

- An angiotensin II receptor blocker is indicated in patients who cannot take ACEIs (see **Table 17**).
- β-blockers to target doses (see **Table 17**) once volume status is stabilized
- Add low-dose digoxin (*Lanoxin*) [T: 0.125, 0.25; S: 0.05 mg/mL]; (*Lanoxicaps*) [T: 0.05, 0.1, 0.2], 0.125–0.375 mg/d (target serum levels 0.5–0.8 mg/dL) if HF is not controlled on diuretics and ACEIs. Digoxin may be less effective and even harmful in women.
- Adding an aldosterone antagonist can reduce mortality. Use either spironolactone (*Aldactone*) 25 mg/d po [T: 25] in patients with NYHA Class III or IV failure or eplerenone (*Inspra*) 25–50 mg/d po [T: 25, 50, 100]. Monitor serum potassium carefully and avoid these drugs if Cr >2.5 mg/dL in men or >2 mg/dL in women.
- Adding a combination of isosorbide dinitrate and hydralazine (see **Table 15** and **Table 20**; also available as a single preparation: *BiDil* 1–2 tabs po q 8 h [T: 20/37.5]) can be helpful for patients with persistent symptoms.
- Some clinicians recommend anticoagulation in patients with EF <25% (see **Table 10**).
- Calcium channel blockers and Class I antiarrhythmics are not indicated.
- HF with preserved systolic function (diastolic dysfunction; normal EF):
  - Diuretics should be used judiciously and only if there is volume overload.
  - There is no agreed-upon primary treatment. β-Blockers, ACEIs, and/or nondihydropyridine calcium channel blockers may be of benefit.
- Avoid thiazolidinediones (see **Table 35**) if possible in patients with HF and diabetes mellitus.

Source: Hunt SA, Abraham WT, Chin MH, Feldman AM, Francis GS, Ganiats TG, Jessup M, Konstam MA, Mancini DM, Michl K, Oates JA, Rahko PS, Silver MA, Stevenson LW, Yancy CW. ACC/AHA 2005 guideline update for the diagnosis and management of chronic heart failure in the adult—summary article: a report of the American College of Cardiology/American Heart Association Task Force on Practice Guidelines (Writing Committee to Update the 2001 Guidelines for the Evaluation and Management of Heart Failure). *Circulation* 2005;112:1825–1852.

Table 17. Target Dosages of ACEIs, Angiotensin II Receptor Blockers, and β-Blockers in Patients with HF

Agent	Starting Dosage	Target Dosage
ACEIs		
Benazepril	2.5 mg/d	40 mg/d
Captopril	12.5 mg q 12 h	50 mg q 8 h
Enalapril	2.5 mg/d	10 mg q 12 h
Fosinopril	5 mg/d	40 mg/d
Lisinopril	2.5 mg/d	20 mg/d
Moexipril	3.75 mg/d	15 mg/d
Perindopril	4 mg/d	8 mg/d
Quinapril	5 mg/d	40 mg/d
Ramipril	1.25 mg/d	10 mg/d
Trandolapril	1 mg/d	4 mg/d

(cont.)

Table 17. Target Dosages of ACEIs, Angiotensin II Receptor Blockers, and β-Blockers in Patients with HF (cont.)

Agent	Starting Dosage	Target Dosage
Angiotensin II Receptor Blockers		
Candesartan	4 mg/d	32 mg/d
Eprosartan	400 mg/d	400 mg q 12 h
Irbesartan	75 mg/d	150 mg/d
Losartan	12.5 mg/d	50 mg q 12 h
Olmesartan	20 mg/d	40 mg/d
Telmisartan	20 mg/d	80 mg/d
Valsartan	40 mg/d	320 mg q 12 h
β-Blockers		
Bisoprolol	1.25 mg/d	5 mg/d
Carvedilol	3.125 mg q 12 h	25 mg q 12 h
Carvedilol ER	10 mg/d	80 mg/d
Metoprolol XL	12.5–25 mg/d	200 mg/d

DYSLIPIDEMIA

Table 18. Treatment Indications for Dyslipidemia

Risk Category	Conditions	LDL-Cholesterol Goal	Initiate Non-pharmacologic Management	Consider Drug Therapy (see Table 19)
Low	0 or 1 risk factor[a]	<160 mg/dL	≥160 mg/dL	≥190 mg/dL; optional: 160–189 mg/dL
Moderate	≥2 risk factors; 10-yr CAD risk <10%[b]	<130 mg/dL	≥130 mg/dL	≥160 mg/dL
Moderately high	≥2 risk factors; 10-yr CAD risk 10–20%[b]	<130 mg/dL	≥130 mg/dL	≥130 mg/dL; optional: 100–129 mg/dL
High	CVD[c], DM, or 10-yr CAD risk >20%[b]	<100 mg/dL	≥100 mg/dL	≥100 mg/dL
Very high	DM + CVD[c]; acute coronary syndrome; multiple severe or poorly controlled risk factors	<70 mg/dL	≥100 mg/dL	≥100 mg/dL; optional: 70–99 mg/dL

Note: CVD = cardiovascular disease; DM = diabetes mellitus.
[a] Risk factors are cigarette smoking, HTN, HDL <40 mg/dL, family history of premature CAD, male age ≥45 yr, female age ≥55 yr.
[b] Calculation of 10-yr risk of CAD is available at http://hp2010.nhlbihin.net/atpiii/calculator.asp?usertype=prof
[c] CVD refers to CAD, angina, PAD, TIA, stroke, abdominal aortic aneurysm, or 10-yr CAD risk >20%.

Management

Nonpharmacologic: A cholesterol-lowering diet should be considered initial therapy for dyslipidemia and should be used as follows:
- The patient should be at low risk of malnutrition.
- The diet should be nutritionally adequate, with sufficient total calories, protein, calcium, iron, and vitamins.
- The diet should be easily understood and affordable (a dietitian can be very helpful).
- Cholesterol-lowering margarines can lower LDL cholesterol by 10% to 15% (*Take Control* 1–2 tbsp/d; *Benecol* 3 servings of 1.5 tsp each/d).

Pharmacologic: Target drug treatment according to type of dyslipidemia (**Table 19**).

Table 19. Medication Regimens for Dyslipidemia			
Condition	**Medication**	**Dosage**	**Formulations**
Elevated LDL, normal TG	Statin (HMG-CoA reductase inhibitor)[a]		
	Atorvastatin (*Lipitor*)	10–80 mg/d	T: 10, 20, 40, 80
	Fluvastatin (*Lescol, Lescol XL*)	20–80 mg/d in PM, max 80 mg	C: 20, 40; T: ER 80
	Lovastatin (*Mevacor, Altoprev*)	10–40 mg/d in PM or q 12 h	T: 10, 20, 40; T: ER 10, 20, 40, 60
	Pravastatin (*Pravachol*)	10–40 mg/d	T: 10, 20, 40, 80
	Aspirin/pravastatin (*Pravigard PAC*)	1 tab/d	T: 81/20, 81/40, 81/80, 325/20, 325/40, 325/80
	Rosuvastatin (*Crestor*)	10–40 mg/d	T: 5, 10, 20, 40
	Simvastatin (*Zocor*)	5–80 mg/d in PM	T: 5, 10, 20, 40, 80
Elevated TG (>500 mg/dL)	Fenofibrate (*Tricor, Lofibra*)	48–200 mg/d	T: 48, 54, 145, 160 C: 67, 134, 200
	Gemfibrozil (*Lopid*)	300–600 mg po q 12 h	T: 600
	Omega-3-acid ethyl esters (*Omacor*)	4 g/d in single or divided doses	C: 1 g
Combined elevated LDL, low HDL, elevated TG	Fenofibrate, gemfibrozil, or HMG-CoA if TG <300 mg/dL	As above	As above
Alternative for any of above	Niacin[b]	100 mg q 8 h to start; increase to 500–1000 mg q 8 h; extended release 150 mg qhs to start, increase to 2000 mg qhs as needed	T: 25, 50, 100, 250, 500; ER 150, 250, 500, 750, 1000 C: TR 125, 250, 400, 500
	Niacin ER (*Niaspan*)	500–2000 mg/d	T: 500, 750, 1000

(cont.)

Table 19. Medication Regimens for Dyslipidemia (cont.)			
Condition	**Medication**	**Dosage**	**Formulations**
Elevated LDL or combined with inadequate response to one agent	Lovastatin/niacin combination[a,b] (*Advicor*)	20 mg/500 mg qhs to start; increase to 40 mg/2000 mg prn	T: 20/500, 20/750, 20/1000
	Colesevelam (*WelChol*)	Monotherapy: 1850 mg po q 12 h; combination therapy: 2500–3750 mg/d in single or divided doses	T: 625
	Ezetimibe (*Zetia*)	10 mg/d	T: 10
	Ezetimibe/simvastatin[a] combination (*Vytorin*)	1 tab/d	T: 10/10, 10/20, 10/40, 10/80

[a] Measure transaminases at baseline, at 3 mo, and then periodically. Watch for statin-induced myopathy, usually presenting as diffuse, symmetric myalgias. If myopathy is suspected (higher risk at higher statin doses or in combination with fenofibrate, gemfibrozil, or niacin), measure CPK and transaminases; CPK levels >10 times the upper limit of normal indicate serious myopathy/rhabdomyolysis. Even if CPK and transaminases are normal, myalgias still may be due to statin; if this is the case, myalgias should disappear within 1 wk of discontinuing statin.

[b] Monitor for flushing, pruritus, nausea, gastritis, ulcer. Dosage increases should be spaced 1 mo apart. ASA 325 mg po 30 min before first niacin dose of the day is effective in preventing adverse events.

HYPERTENSION (HTN)

Definition, Classification
JNC 7 defines HTN as SBP ≥140 or DBP ≥90. In older adults, base treatment decisions primarily on the SBP level.

Evaluation and Assessment
• Measure both standing and sitting BP after 5 min of rest.
• Base diagnosis on two or more readings at each of two or more visits. Once diagnosis is made, evaluation includes:
  ○ Assessment of cardiac risk factors: smoking, dyslipidemia, obesity, and diabetes mellitus are important in older adults.
  ○ Assessment of end-organ damage: LVH, angina, prior MI, prior coronary revascularization, HF, stroke or TIA, nephropathy, peripheral arterial disease, retinopathy.
  ○ Routine laboratory tests: CBC, UA, electrolytes, creatinine, fasting glucose, total cholesterol, HDL cholesterol, and ECG.
  ○ Consider renal artery stenosis if sudden onset of HTN, sudden rise in BP in previously well-controlled HTN, or HTN despite treatment with three antihypertensives.

Aggravating Factors
• Emotional stress
• Excessive alcohol intake
• Excessive salt intake
• Lack of aerobic exercise
• Low potassium intake
• Low calcium intake
• Nicotine
• Obesity

Management

JNC 7 recommendations: Target is <140/90 (130/80 in patients with diabetes mellitus or kidney disease). Lowering BP below 120/80 is not recommended. Particularly in patients with "white coat" HTN, home monitoring of BP with a properly calibrated machine can produce more readings than office-based measurements.

Nonpharmacologic:

• Adequate calcium and magnesium intake as well as a low-fat diet for optimizing general health.
• Adequate dietary potassium intake; fruits and vegetables are the best sources.
• Aerobic exercise—30–45 min most days of the week.
• Moderation of alcohol intake—limit to 1 oz of ethanol/d.
• Moderation of dietary sodium: watch for volume depletion with diuretic use. Goal: ≤2.4 g Na^+/d.
• Smoking cessation
• Weight reduction if obese: even a 10-lb weight loss can significantly lower BP. Goal: BMI (kg/m^2) <25.

Pharmacologic: Table 20 lists commonly used antihypertensives.

• Use antihypertensives carefully in patients with orthostatic BP drop.
• Base treatment decisions on standing BP.
• If no coexisting conditions, a thiazide diuretic, a β-blocker, or an ACEI can be used as a first-line drug.
• If coexisting conditions, therapy should be individualized (see **Table 21**).
• Combination drugs for hypertension are listed in **Table 22**.
• Available dose formulations of oral potassium supplements: [T: (mEq) 6, 7, 8, 10, 20; S: (mEq/15 mL) 20, 40; powders (mEq/pk) 15, 20, 25]
• Follow-up BP measurements monthly until target BP is attained; visits may be q 3–6 mo if BP is stable at target goal.

Hypertensive Emergencies and Urgencies:

• Elevated BP alone without symptoms or target end-organ damage does not require emergent BP lowering.
• Conditions requiring emergent BP lowering include hypertensive encephalopathy, intracranial hemorrhage, unstable angina, acute MI, acute left ventricular failure with pulmonary edema, dissecting aortic aneurysm.
• Most common initial treatment for emergent BP lowering is sodium nitroprusside (*Nipride*) 0.25–10 mg/kg/min as IV infusion.
• Nonemergent (ie, urgent) BP lowering is indicated only in cases in which BP needs to be lowered for procedural evaluation or treatment (such as β blockade before surgery, see p 187) or in asymptomatic people with SBP >210 or DBP >120.
  ○ Administer standard dose of a recommended antihypertensive orally (see **Table 20**) or an extra dose of patient's usual antihypertensive.
  ○ If the patient is npo, give **low** dose antihypertensive IV, titrating upward **slowly**. Options include β-blocker (eg, labetolol 20 mg), ACEI (eg, enalaprilat 0.625 mg over 5 min), or diuretic (eg, furosemide 10 mg).

Table 20. Oral Antihypertensive Agents

Class, Medication	Geriatric Dosage Range, Total mg/d (times/d)	Formulations	Comments (Metabolism, Excretion)
Diuretics			↓ potassium, Na, magnesium levels; ↑ uric acid, calcium, cholesterol (mild), and glucose (mild) levels
Thiazides			
✔ Chlorothiazide (*Diuril*)	125–500 (1)	T: 250, 500	
✔ Chlorthalidone (*Hygroton*)	12.5–25 (1)	T: 15, 25, 50, 100	↑ adverse events at >25 mg/d (L)
✔ HCTZ (*Esidrix, HydroDIURIL, Oretic*)	12.5–25 (1)	T: 25, 50, 100; S: 50 mg/mL; C: 12.5	↑ adverse events at >25 mg/d (L)
✔ Indapamide (*Lozol*)	0.625–2.5 (1)	T: 1.25, 2.5	Less or no hypercholesterolemia (L)
✔ Metolazone (*Mykrox*)	0.25–0.5 (1)	T rapid: 0.5	Monitor electrolytes carefully (L)
✔ Metolazone (*Zaroxolyn*)	2.5–5 (1)	T: 2.5, 5, 10	Monitor electrolytes carefully (L)
✔ Polythiazide (*Renese*)	1–4 (1)	T: 1, 2, 4	
Loop diuretics			
♥ Bumetanide (*Bumex*)	0.5–4 (1–3)	T: 0.5, 1, 2	Short duration of action, no hypercalcemia (K)
♥ Furosemide (*Lasix*)	20–160 (1–2)	T: 20, 40, 80; S: 10, 40 mg/5 mL	Short duration of action, no hypercalcemia (K)
♥ Torsemide (*Demadex*)	2.5–50 (1–2)	T: 5, 10, 20, 100	Short duration of action, no hypercalcemia (K)
Potassium-sparing drugs			
Amiloride (*Midamor*)	2.5–10 (1)	T: 5	(L, K)
Triamterene (*Dyrenium*)	25–100 (1–2)	T: 50, 100	(L, K)
Aldosterone receptor-blockers			
♥ Eplerenone (*Inspra*)	25–100 (1)	T: 25, 50, 100	(L, K)
♥ Spironolactone (*Aldactone*)	12.5–50 (1–2)	T: 25, 50, 100	Gynecomastia (L, K)
Adrenergic Inhibitors			
α_1-Blockers			Avoid as primary therapy for HTN unless patient has BPH
Doxazosin (*Cardura*)	1–16 (1)	T: 1, 2, 4, 8	(L)
Prazosin (*Minipress*)	1–20 (2–3)	T: 1, 2, 5	(L)
Terazosin (*Hytrin*)	1–20 (1–2)	T: 1, 2, 5, 10; C: 1, 2, 5, 10	(L, K)

(cont.)

✔ = preferred for treating older adults; ♥ = useful in treating HF.

Note: Listing of adverse events is not exhaustive, and adverse events are for the drug class except when noted for individual drugs.

Table 20. Oral Antihypertensive Agents (cont.)

Class, Medication	Geriatric Dosage Range, Total mg/d (times/d)	Formulations	Comments (Metabolism, Excretion)
Central α_2-agonists and other centrally acting drugs			Sedation, dry mouth, bradycardia, withdrawal HTN
Clonidine (*Catapres, Catapres-TTS*)	0.1–1.2 (2–3) *or* 1 pch/wk	T: 0.1, 0.2, 0.3; pch: 0.1, 0.2, 0.3 mg/d	Continue oral for 1–2 d when converting to patch (L, K)
Guanfacine (*Tenex*)	0.5–2 (1)	T: 1, 2	(K)
Methyldopa (*Aldomet*)	250–2500 (2)	T: 125, 250, 500; S: 250 mg/5 mL	(L, K)
Reserpine (*Serpasil*)	0.05–0.25 (1) ✔	T: 0.1, 0.25	Depression, nasal congestion, activation of peptic ulcer (L, K)
β-Blockers			Bronchospasm, bradycardia, acute HF, may mask insulin-induced hypoglycemia; lipid solubility is a risk factor for delirium
✔ Acebutolol (*Sectral*)	200–800 (1)	C: 200, 400	β_1, low lipid solubility, intrinsic sympathomimetic activity (L, K)
✔ Atenolol (*Tenormin*)	12.5–100 (1)	T: 25, 50, 100	β_1, low lipid solubility (K)
✔ Betaxolol (*Kerlone*)	5–20 (1)	T: 10, 20	β_1, low lipid solubility (L, K)
✔ ♥ Bisoprolol (*Zebeta*)	2.5–10 (1)	T: 5, 10	β_1, low lipid solubility (L, K)
✔ Carteolol (*Cartrol*)	1.25–10 (1)	T: 2.5, 5	β_1, low lipid solubility, intrinsic sympathomimetic activity (K)
✔ Metoprolol (*Lopressor*)	25–400 (2)	T: 25, 50, 100	β_1, moderate lipid solubility (L)
✔ ♥ Long-acting (*Toprol XL*)	50–400 (1)	T: 25, 50, 100, 200	(L)
Nadolol (*Corgard*)	20–160 (1)	T: 20, 40, 80, 120, 160	β_1, β_2, low lipid solubility (K)
Penbutolol (*Levatol*)	10–40 (1)	T: 20	β_1, β_2, high lipid solubility, intrinsic sympathomimetic activity (L, K)
Pindolol (*Visken*)	5–40 (2)	T: 5, 10	β_1, β_2, moderate lipid solubility, intrinsic sympathomimetic activity (K)

(cont.)

✔ = preferred for treating older adults; ♥ = useful in treating HF.
Note: Listing of adverse events is not exhaustive, and adverse events are for the drug class except when noted for individual drugs.

Table 20. Oral Antihypertensive Agents (cont.)

Class, Medication	Geriatric Dosage Range, Total mg/d (times/d)	Formulations	Comments (Metabolism, Excretion)
Propranolol (*Inderal*)	20–160 (2)	T: 10, 20, 40, 60, 80, 90; S: 4 mg/mL, 8 mg/mL, 80 mg/mL	β_1, β_2, high lipid solubility (L)
Long-acting (*Inderal LA, InnoPran XL*)	60–180 (1)	C: 60, 80, 120, 160	β_1, β_2, high lipid solubility (L)
Timolol (*Blocadren*)	10–40 (2)	T: 5, 10, 20	β_1, β_2, low to moderate lipid solubility (L, K)
Combined α- and β-blockers			Postural hypotension, bronchospasm
✔ ♥ Carvedilol (*Coreg*)	3.125–25 (2)	T: 3.125, 6.25, 12.5, 25	β_1, β_2, high lipid solubility (L)
✔ ♥ Extended-release (*Coreg CR*)	10-80 (1)	C: 10, 20, 40, 80	Multiply regular daily dose of carvedilol by 1.6 to convert to CR dose; do not take within 2 h of alcohol ingestion
✔ Labetalol (*Normodyne, Trandate*)	100–600 (2)	T: 100, 200, 300	β_1, β_2, moderate lipid solubility (L, K)
Direct Vasodilators			Headaches, fluid retention, tachycardia
♥ Hydralazine (*Apresoline*)	25–100 (2–4)	T: 10, 25, 50, 100	Lupus syndrome; used in combination with isosorbide dinitrate for HF in blacks (L, K)
Minoxidil (*Loniten*)	2.5–50 (1)	T: 2.5, 10	Hirsutism (K)
Calcium Antagonists			
Nondihydropyridines			Conduction defects, worsening of systolic dysfunction, gingival hyperplasia
✔ Diltiazem SR (*Cardizem CD, Cardizem SR, Dilacor XR, Tiazac*)	120–360 (1–2), max 480	C: 1/d: 120, 180, 240, 300, 360, 420; 2/d: 60, 90, 120; T: 30, 60, 90, 120, ER: 120, 180, 240	Nausea, headache (L)

(cont.)

✔ = preferred for treating older adults; ♥ = useful in treating HF.

Note: Listing of adverse events is not exhaustive, and adverse events are for the drug class except when noted for individual drugs.

Table 20. Oral Antihypertensive Agents (cont.)

Class, Medication	Geriatric Dosage Range, Total mg/d (times/d)	Formulations	Comments (Metabolism, Excretion)
✔ Verapamil SR (*Calan SR, Covera-HS, Isoptin SR, Verelan*)	120–360 (1–2)	T: SR 120, 180, 240; C: SR 100, 120, 180, 200, 240, 300, 360; T: 40, 80, 120	Constipation, bradycardia (L)
Dihydropyridines			Ankle edema, flushing, headache, gingival hypertrophy
✔ Amlodipine (*Norvasc*)	2.5–10 (1)	T: 2.5, 5, 10	(L)
✔ Felodipine (*Plendil*)	2.5–20 (1)	T: 2.5, 5, 10	(L)
✔ Isradipine (*DynaCirc*)	2.5–20 (2)	T: 2.5, 5	(L)
✔ Sustained release (*DynaCirc CR*)	2.5–10 (1)	T: 5, 10	
✔ Nicardipine (*Cardene*)	60–120 (3)	C: 20, 30	(L)
✔ Sustained release (*Cardene SR*)	60–120 (2)	T: 30, 45, 60	(L)
✔ Nifedipine SR (*Adalat CC, Procardia XL*)	30–60 (1)	T: 30, 60, 90	(L)
✔ Nisoldipine (*Sular*)	10–40 (1)	T: ER 10, 20, 30, 40	(L)
ACEIs*			Cough (common), angioedema (rare), hyperkalemia, rash, loss of taste, leukopenia
✔ ♥ Benazepril (*Lotensin*)	2.5–40 (1–2)	T: 5, 10, 20, 40	(L, K)
✔ ♥ Captopril (*Capoten*)	12.5–150 (2–3)	T: 12.5, 25, 50, 100	(L, K)
✔ ♥ Enalapril (*Vasotec*)	2.5–40 (1–2)	T: 2.5, 5, 10, 20	(L, K)
✔ ♥ Fosinopril (*Monopril*)	5–40 (1–2)	T: 10, 20, 40	(L, K)
✔ ♥ Lisinopril (*Prinivil, Zestril*)	2.5–40 (1)	T: 2.5, 5, 10, 20, 30, 40	(K)
✔ ♥ Moexipril (*Univasc*)	3.75–30 (1)	T: 7.5, 15	(L, K)
✔ ♥ Perindopril (*Aceon*)	4–8 (1–2)	T: 2, 4, 8	(L, K)
✔ ♥ Quinapril (*Accupril*)	5–40 (1)	T: 5, 10, 20, 40	(L, K)
✔ ♥ Ramipril (*Altace*)	1.25–20 (1)	T: 1.25, 2.5, 5, 10	(L, K)
✔ ♥ Trandolapril (*Mavik*)	1–4 (1)	T: 1, 2, 4	(L, K)

(cont.

✔ = preferred for treating older adults; ♥ = useful in treating HF.
* See **Table 17** for target doses in treating HF.
Note: Listing of adverse events is not exhaustive, and adverse events are for the drug class except when noted for individual drugs.

Table 20. Oral Antihypertensive Agents (cont.)

Class, Medication	Geriatric Dosage Range, Total mg/d (times/d)	Formulations	Comments (Metabolism, Excretion)
Angiotensin II Receptor Blockers (ARBs)*			Angioedema (very rare), hyperkalemia
✔ ♥ Candesartan (*Atacand*)	4–32 (1)	T: 4, 8, 16, 32	(K)
✔ ♥ Eprosartan (*Teveten*)	400–800 (1–2)	T: 400, 600	(biliary, K)
✔ ♥ Irbesartan (*Avapro*)	75–300 (1)	T: 75, 150, 300	(L)
✔ ♥ Losartan (*Cozaar*)	12.5–100 (1–2)	T: 25, 50, 100	(L, K)
✔ ♥ Olmesartan (*Benicar*)	20–40 (1)	T: 5, 20, 40	(F, K)
✔ ♥ Telmisartan (*Micardis*)	20–80 (1)	T: 20, 40, 80	(L)
✔ ♥ Valsartan (*Diovan*)	40–320 (1)	T: 80, 160, 320; C: 80, 160	(L, K)
Renin Inhibitor			
Aliskiren (*Tekturna*)	150-300 (1)	T: 150, 300	Monitor electrolytes and kidney function carefully in diabetic patients also taking an ACEI

✔ = preferred for treating older adults; ♥ = useful in treating HF
* See **Table 17** for target doses in treating HF.
Note: Listing of adverse events is not exhaustive, and adverse events are for the drug class except when noted for individual drugs.
Source: Data in part from The seventh report of the Joint National Committee on Prevention, Detection, Evaluation, and Treatment of High Blood Pressure: The JNC 7 report. *JAMA* 2003;289:2560–2572.

Table 21. Choosing Antihypertensive Therapy on the Basis of Coexisting Conditions

Condition	Appropriate for Use	Avoid or Contraindicated
Angina	β, D, non-D	
Atrial tachycardia and fibrillation	β, non-D	
Bronchospasm		β, αβ
Diabetes mellitus	ACEI, ARB, β, T[a]	T[a]
Dyslipidemia		β, T[b]
Essential tremor	β	
HF	AA, ACEI, ARB, β, αβ, L	D, non-D[c]
Hyperthyroidism	β	
MI	β, AA, ACEI	non-D
Osteoporosis	T	
Prostatism (BPH)	α	
Renal insufficiency	AA, ACEI[d]	
Urge UI	D, non-D	L, T

Note: AA = aldosterone antagonist; α = α-blocker; β = β-blocker; αβ = combined α- and β-blocker; ARB = angiotensin receptor blocker; D = dihydropyridine calcium antagonist; non-D = nondihydropyridine calcium antagonist; L = loop diuretic; T = thiazide diuretic
[a] Low-dose diuretics probably beneficial in type 2 diabetes; high-dose diuretics relatively contraindicated in types 1 and 2.
[b] Low-dose diuretics have a minimal effect on lipids.
[c] May be beneficial in HF caused by diastolic dysfunction.
[d] Use with great caution in renovascular disease.

Table 22. Combination Medications Containing an Antihypertensive Agent

Combination Type	Fixed-dose Combination, mg*	Trade Name
ACEIs and calcium channel blockers	Amlodipine/benazepril hydrochloride (2.5/10, 5/10, 5/20, 10/20)	Lotrel
	Enalapril maleate/felodipine (5/2.5, 5/5)	Lexxel
	Trandolapril/verapamil (2/180, 1/240, 2/240, 4/240)	Tarka
ACEIs and diuretics	Benazepril/HCTZ (5/6.25, 10/12.5, 20/12.5, 20/25)	Lotensin HCT
	Captopril/HCTZ (25/15, 25/25, 50/15, 50/25)	Capozide
	Enalapril maleate/HCTZ (5/12.5, 10/25)	Vaseretic
	Lisinopril/HCTZ (10/12.5, 20/25)	Prinzide, Zestoretic
	Moexipril hydrochloride/HCTZ (7.5/12.5, 15/25)	Uniretic
	Quinapril hydrochloride/HCTZ (10/12.5, 20/12.5, 20/25)	Accuretic
Angiotensin-receptor blockers and calcium channel blockers	Amlodipine/valsartan (5/160, 10/160, 5/320, 10/320)	Exforge
	Amlodipine/olmesartan (5/20, 5/40, 10/20, 10/40)	Azor
Angiotensin-receptor blockers and diuretics	Candesartan cilexetil/HCTZ (16/12.5, 32/12.5)	Atacand HCT
	Eprosartan mesylate/HCTZ (600/12.5, 600/25)	Teveten HCT
	Irbesartan/HCTZ (75/12.5, 150/12.5, 300/12.5)	Avalide
	Losartan potassium/HCTZ (50/12.5, 100/25)	Hyzaar
	Olmesartan/HCTZ (20/12.5, 40/12.5, 40/25)	Benicar HCT
	Telmisartan/HCTZ (40/12.5, 80/12.5)	Micardis HCT
	Valsartan/HCTZ (80/12.5, 160/12.5)	Diovan HCT
β-Blockers and diuretics	Atenolol/chlorthalidone (50/25, 100/25)	Tenoretic
	Bisoprolol fumarate/HCTZ (2.5/6.25, 5/6.25, 10/6.25)	Ziac
	Propranolol LA/HCTZ (40/25, 80/25)	Inderide
	Metoprolol tartrate/HCTZ (50/25, 100/25)	Lopressor HCT
	Nadolol/bendroflumethiazide (40/5, 80/5)	Corzide
	Timolol maleate/HCTZ (10/25)	Timolide
Calcium channel blocker and statin	Amlodipine/atorvastatin (2.5/10, 2.5/20, 2.5/40, 5/10, 5/20, 5/40, 5/80, 10/10, 10/20, 10/40, 10/80)	Caduet
Centrally acting drug and diuretic	Methyldopa/HCTZ (250/15, 250/25, 500/30, 500/50)	Aldoril
	Reserpine/chlorothiazide (0.125/250, 0.25/500)	Diupres
	Reserpine/HCTZ (0.125/25, 0.125/50)	Hydropres
Direct vasodilator and nitrate	Isosorbide dinitrate/hydralazine (20/37.5)	BiDil
Diuretic and diuretic	Amiloride hydrochloride/HCTZ (5/50)	Moduretic
	Spironolactone/HCTZ (25/25, 50/50)	Aldactazide
	Triamterene/HCTZ (37.5/25, 50/25, 75/50)	Dyazide, Maxzide

*Some drug combinations are available in multiple fixed doses. Each drug dose is reported in mg.

PULMONARY ARTERIAL HYPERTENSION (PAH)
Evaluation and Assessment
- PAH can be primary (unexplained) or secondary to underlying conditions.
- Almost all cases in older adults are secondary, most commonly associated with chronic pulmonary and/or cardiac disease, including COPD, interstitial lung disease, obstructive sleep apnea, pulmonary emboli, HF, and mitral valvular disease.
- Early symptoms are often nonspecific and include dyspnea on exertion, fatigue, and vague chest discomfort.
- Late symptoms include severe dyspnea on exertion, cyanosis, syncope, chest pain, HF, arrhythmias.
- Physical examination findings relate to manifestations of the associated conditions mentioned above.
- Diagnostic tests:
  - ECG may show right-axis deviation, right atrial and ventricular hypertrophy, T-wave changes
  - CXR may show large right ventricle, dilated pulmonary arteries
  - Echocardiography estimates pulmonary arterial pressure and evaluates possible valvular disease
  - Right heart catheterization is gold standard, with PAH defined as mean pulmonary arterial pressure >25 mmHg at rest or >30 mmHg during exercise.
- Additional tests (eg, pulmonary function tests, sleep study) may clarify severity of coexisting conditions.

Management
- Correct/optimize underlying conditions.
- Supplemental oxygen for chronic hypoxemia
- Diuretics for volume overload from HF
- Avoid calcium channel blockers unless they have been shown to be of benefit from a right heart catheterization vasodilator challenge study.
- Other agents have been studied mainly in primary PAH and are of uncertain effectiveness and safety in secondary PAH:
  - Warfarin (see p 21)
  - Prostacyclins: epoprostenol (*Flolan*) by continuous IV infusion, treprostinil (*Remodulin*) by continuous subcutaneous infusion, iloprost (*Ventavis*) by inhalation
  - Endothelial receptor antagonists: bosentan (*Tracleer*) 62.5 mg q 12 h × 4 wk, then 125 mg q 12 h; ambrisentan (*Letairis*) 5–10 mg/d
  - Sildenafil (*Revatio*) po up to 20 mg q 8 h

ATRIAL FIBRILLATION (AF)
Evaluation and Assessment
Causes:
- Cardiac disease: cardiac surgery, cardiomyopathy, HF, hypertensive heart disease, ischemic disease, pericarditis, valvular disease
- Noncardiac disease: alcoholism, chronic pulmonary disease, infections, pulmonary emboli, thyrotoxicosis

Standard testing: ECG, CXR, CBC, electrolytes, creatinine, BUN, TSH, echocardiogram

Management

- Correct precipitating cause.
- For patients with minimal symptoms or in whom prolonged sinus rhythm cannot be easily achieved, rate control plus anticoagulation is the preferred treatment strategy.
  - Rate control (target <80 beats/min) can be achieved with atenolol, metoprolol, diltiazem, or verapamil, given IV (in cases of acute hemodynamic instability) or po.
  - Digoxin can be used as a second-line agent for rate control.
  - Anticoagulation to INR 2–3 should be achieved with oral warfarin (see p 21) and continued indefinitely.
  - If anticoagulation is contraindicated, use ASA 325 mg/d po and continue indefinitely.
- For patients with unpleasant symptoms or decreased exercise tolerance on rate control therapy, rhythm control via direct-current or pharmacologic cardioversion is the preferred treatment strategy.
  - For direct-current cardioversion, two methods may be used:
    - Early cardioversion (<48 h from onset): perform transesophageal echocardiography to exclude intracardiac thrombus; if no thrombus, begin anticoagulation and cardiovert.
    - Delayed cardioversion: anticoagulate for 3 wk before cardioversion.
  - For pharmacologic cardioversion and rhythm maintenance (recommended only if AF produces symptoms significantly impairing quality of life), rhythm control drugs may be tried (see **Table 23**).
  - Continue anticoagulation for 4 wk after cardioversion.
- Attempt direct-current cardioversion in patients with acute-onset AF and compromised cardiac output or angina.

Table 23. Selected Medications for Rhythm Control in AF

Medication	Dosage	Formulations	Comments (Metabolism)
Amiodarone (Cordarone, Pacerone)	100–400/d	T: 200, 400	Most effective antifibrillatory agent but numerous adverse events, including pulmonary and hepatic toxic effects, hypothyroidism, corneal deposits, warfarin interaction (L)
Propafenone (Rythmol)	150–300 q 8 h	T: 150, 225, 300	Contraindicated in patients with ischemic and structural heart disease; adverse events include VT and HF (L)
Sotalol (Betapace, Betapace AF, Sorine)	80–160 q 12 h	T: 80, 120, 160, 240	Prolongs QT interval; adverse events include torsades de pointes, HF, exacerbation of COPD/bronchospasm (K)

AORTIC STENOSIS (AS)
Evaluation and Assessment
- Presence of symptoms—angina, syncope, HF (frequently diastolic dysfunction)—indicates severe disease and a life expectancy without surgery of <2 yr.
- Echocardiography is essential to measure aortic jet velocity (AJV) and aortic valve area (AVA).
  - Moderate AS is indicated by an AJV of 3–4 meters/sec and by an AVA of 1–1.5 cm^2.
  - Severe AS is indicated by an AJV >4 meters/sec and by an AVA <1 cm^2.
- For asymptomatic cases, echocardiography should be repeated annually for moderate AS and q 6–12 mo for severe AS.
- ECG and CXR should be obtained initially to look for conduction defects, LVH, and pulmonary congestion.

Treatment
- Aortic valve replacement (AVR) surgery
  - Alleviates symptoms and improves ventricular functioning.
  - In most cases, perform AVR promptly *after* symptoms have appeared.
  - Consider risks and benefits of AVR on individual basis (see pp 186–188).
- Avoid vasodilators if possible.

ABDOMINAL AORTIC ANEURYSM (AAA)
- Ultrasound should be performed if aortic diameter is felt to be >3 cm on physical examination.
- Ultrasonographic screening for AAA is recommended once for men between age 65 and 75 if former or current smoker.
- Management is based on diameter of AAA
  - <4.5 cm: ultrasound q 12 mo
  - 4.5–5.4 cm: ultrasound q 3–6 mo
  - >5.4 cm: surgical referral
- Endovascular versus open surgical repair
  - Both methods have similar 30-day mortality and rate of rupture.
  - Endovascular repair has significantly less perioperative morbidity.
  - Long-term complication rate (leaking, rupture) is higher for endovascular repair.
  - Consider open repair for patients with low risk of perioperative mortality and remaining life expectancy >10 yr.
  - Endovascular repair is appropriate for patients with higher comorbidities and shorter life expectancy.

PERIPHERAL ARTERIAL DISEASE (PAD)
Evaluation
Hx should include inquiry regarding the following:
- Lower extremity exertional fatigue or pain, or pain at rest
- Poorly healing or nonhealing wounds
- Cardiac risk factors

Physical examination should include the following:
- Palpation of pulses (brachial, radial, ulnar, femoral, popliteal, posterior tibial, and dorsalis pedis)
- Auscultation for abdominal, flank, and femoral bruits
- Inspection of feet

Diagnosis established by ankle-brachial index <0.9 or other test (**Table 24**).

Table 24. Management of PAD

Signs and Symptoms	Useful Tests	Treatment (see below)
Asymptomatic; diminished or absent peripheral pulses	ABI[a]	Risk factor reduction
Atypical leg pain	ABI, EABI[b]	Risk factor reduction, antiplatelet therapy
Claudication: exertional fatigue, discomfort, pain relieved by rest	ABI, EABI, Doppler ultrasound, pulse volume recording, segmental pressure measurement	Risk factor reduction, antiplatelet therapy, claudication therapy; consider endovascular or surgical revascularization if symptoms persist
Rest pain, nonhealing wound (see also p 217), gangrene	ABI, Doppler ultrasound, angiography (MRI, CT, or contrast)	Risk factor reduction, antiplatelet therapy, claudication therapy, endovascular or surgical revascularization

[a] Abnormal is <0.9; <0.4 is critical.
[b] Exercise treadmill test with ABI measurement

Treatment
Risk Factor Reduction
- Smoking cessation
- Lipid-lowering therapy (goal LDL <100 mg/dL, <70/dL in those at very high risk; see **Table 19**)
- BP control (goal <140/90, <130/80 in those with diabetes)
- Diabetes treatment (good foot care, HbA_{1c} <7%)

Antiplatelet Therapy
- ASA 75–325 mg/d
- Clopidogrel (*Plavix*) 75 mg/d (T: 75) if no response or intolerant of ASA

Claudication Therapy
- Walking program (goal: 50 min of intermittent walking 3–5 ×/wk)
- Cilostazol (*Pletal*) 100 mg q 12 h, 1 h before or 2 h after meals (contraindicated in patients with HF); second-line alternative therapy is pentoxifylline (*Trental*) 400 mg q 8 h [T: 400]
- If ACEI not contraindicated, routine use is recommended to prevent adverse cardiovascular events in patients with claudication.

Table 25. Classification of Syncope

Cause	Frequency (%)	Features	Increased Risk of Death
Vasovagal	21	Preceded by lightheadedness, nausea, diaphoresis; recovery gradual, frequently with fatigue	No
Cardiac	10	Little or no warning before blackout, rapid and complete recovery	Yes
Orthostatic	9	Lightheaded prodrome after standing, recovery gradual	No
Medication-induced	7	Lightheaded prodrome, recovery gradual	No
Seizure	5	No warning, may have neurologic deficits, slow recovery	Yes
Stroke, TIA	4	Little or no warning, neurologic deficits	Yes
Other causes	8	Preceded by cough, micturition, or specific situation	No
Unknown	37	Any of the above	Yes

Source: Adapted from Soteriades ES, Evans JC, Larson MG, et al. Incidence and prognosis of syncope. *N Engl J Med* 2002;347:878–885.

Evaluation

- Focus hx on events before, during, and after loss of consciousness; hx of cardiac disease (significantly worsens prognosis of syncope of all causes); careful medication review.
- Focus on cardiovascular and neurologic systems in physical examination.
- ECG and orthostatic BP or pulse check for all patients.
- Additional testing as suggested by initial evaluation:
  - Ambulatory ECG monitoring for further evaluation of arrhythmia
  - Stress testing to investigate ischemic heart disease
  - Echocardiography to investigate structural heart disease
  - Electrophysiologic studies in patients with prior MI or structural heart disease
  - Tilt-table testing for suspected vasovagal cause
  - Head imaging, electroencephalogram for suspected neurologic cause
  - If suspected orthostatic cause, evaluation for Parkinson's disease, autonomic neuropathy, diabetes mellitus, hypovolemia

Management

- Patients with cardiac syncope require immediate hospitalization on telemetry; exclude MI and PE.
- Strongly consider hospital admission for patients with syncope due to neurologic or unknown causes, particularly if concurrent heart disease.
- Patients with syncope due to vasovagal, orthostatic, medication-induced, or other causes can usually be managed as outpatients, particularly if there is no hx of heart disease.
- Treatment is correction of underlying cause.

ORTHOSTATIC (POSTURAL) HYPOTENSION

See also **Table 37**.

Evaluation and Assessment

- Associated with following symptoms usually after standing: lightheadedness, dizziness, syncope, blurred vision, diaphoresis, head or neck pain, decreased hearing
- Diagnosis: ≥20 mmHg drop in SBP or ≥10 mmHg in DBP within 3 min of rising to more upright position
- Causes
  - Medications, including antihypertensives, phenothiazines, tricyclic antidepressants, monoamine oxidase inhibitors, anti-Parkinsonian drugs, PDE5 inhibitors (for erectile dysfunction)
  - Autonomic dysregulation (suggested by lack of compensatory rise in heart rate with postural hypotension): age-related decreased baroreceptor sensitivity, Parkinson's disease and related disorders, peripheral neuropathy, prolonged bed rest
  - Hypovolemia
  - Anemia

Management

- Correct underlying disorder, particularly by discontinuing medications that could exacerbate hypotension
- Alter movement behavior: educate patients to rise slowly, flex calf and forearm muscles when standing, stand with one foot in front of other, avoid straining, and elevate head of bed
- Dietary changes: avoid alcohol, maintain adequate fluid intake, increase salt and caffeine intake
- Above-the-knee compression stockings (at least medium strength, eg, Jobst)
- Pharmacologic interventions:
  - Fludrocortisone *(Florinef)*: 0.1 mg q 8–24 h [T: 0.1]; use with caution in patients with HF, cardiac disease, hypertension, renal disease, esophagitis, peptic ulcer disease, or ulcerative colitis
  - Midodrine *(ProAmantine)*: 2.5–5 mg q 8–24 h [T: 2.5, 5]; use with caution in patients with HTN, diabetes, urinary retention, renal disease, hepatic disease, glaucoma
  - Caffeine: 1 cup of caffeinated coffee q 8–12 h; alternatively, caffeine tabs 100–200 mg q 8–12 h; useful for postprandial hypotension when taken with meals
  - Erythropoietin (see **Table 44**) can be useful for hypotension secondary to anemia

IMPLANTABLE CARDIAC DEFIBRILLATOR (ICD) PLACEMENT

Indications (consider life expectancy and comorbidities)

- Established:
  - Cardiac arrest due to ventricular fibrillation (VF) or ventricular tachycardia (VT)
  - Spontaneous sustained VT with structural heart disease
  - Spontaneous sustained VT without structural heart disease not alleviated by other treatments
  - Unexplained syncope with hemodynamically significant VF or VT inducible by electrophysiologic study when drug therapy is ineffective, not tolerated, or not preferred

- Nonsustained VT, CAD, and inducible VF by electrophysiologic study that is not suppressed by Class I antiarrhythmic
- LVEF ≤30%, NYHA Class II or III HF, and CAD ≥40 d after MI
- ICD + biventricular pacing for advanced HF (NYHA Class III or IV), LVEF ≤35%, and QRS interval ≥120 millisec
- Less established: Nonischemic cardiomyopathy with LVEF ≤35% and either premature ventricular complexes or nonsustained VT

Contraindications
- Terminal illness with life expectancy <6 mo
- Unexplained syncope without inducible VT or VF and without structural heart disease
- VT or VF due to transient or easily reversible disorder
- End-stage HF (ACC/AHA Stage D) not awaiting cardiac transplant

Complications
- Surgical: infection (1%–2%), hematoma, pneumothorax
- Device-related: lead dislodgement or malfunction, connection problems, inadequate defibrillation threshold
- Therapy-related: frequent shocks (appropriate or inappropriate), acceleration of VT, anxiety and other psychological stress
- Change in patient preferences: Remember to turn off ICD if patient indicates a desire not to be resuscitated.

DELIRIUM

DIAGNOSIS
Diagnostic Criteria—Adapted from *DSM-IV*
- Disturbed consciousness (ie, decreased attention, environmental awareness)
- Cognitive change (eg, memory deficit, disorientation, language disturbance) or perceptual disturbance (eg, visual illusions, hallucinations)
- Rapid onset (hours to days) and fluctuating daily course
- Evidence of a causal physical condition

Risk Factors
- Dementia greatly increases risk of delirium.
- Advanced age, comorbid physical problems (especially sleep deprivation, immobility, dehydration, pain, sensory impairment).

Evaluation
- Assume reversibility unless proven otherwise.
- Thoroughly review prescription and OTC medications.
- Exclude infection and other medical causes.
- Laboratory studies may include CBC, electrolytes, LFTs, renal function tests, serum albumin, serum calcium, serum glucose, UA, oxygen saturation, CXR, and ECG.
- Confusion Assessment Method (CAM): **both** acute onset and fluctuating course **and** inattention **and either** disorganized thinking **or** altered level of consciousness (Inouye SK. *N Engl J Med.* 2006;354(11):1157–1165.

CAUSES
(Italicized type indicates the most common causes in older adults.)
Medications (see Table 26)
- *Anticholinergics* (eg, diphenhydramine), TCAs (eg, amitriptyline, imipramine), antipsychotics (eg, chlorpromazine, thioridazine)
- Anti-inflammatory agents, including prednisone
- Benzodiazepines or alcohol—acute toxicity or withdrawal
- Cardiovascular (eg, digitalis, antihypertensives)
- Diuretics
- Lithium
- GI (eg, cimetidine, ranitidine)
- Opioid analgesics (especially meperidine)

Table 26. Medication-induced Delirium

Medication type	Potentially Differentiating Features	
	Early	*Late*
Anticholinergic	Cognitive impairment, visual impairment, dry mouth, constipation, urinary retention	↑ HR, mydriasis, ↓ bowel sounds
Serotonin syndrome	Tremor, diarrhea	Hyperreflexia, ↑ bowel sounds, diaphoretic
Neuroleptic malignant syndrome	↑ EPS	Marked rigidity, hyperthermia

Infections
Respiratory, skin, urinary tract, others

Metabolic Disorders
Acute blood loss, *dehydration, electrolyte imbalance,* end-organ failure (hepatic, renal), hyperglycemia, *hypoglycemia, hypoxia*

Cardiovascular
Arrhythmia, *HF, MI,* shock

Neurologic
CNS infections, head trauma, seizures, stroke, subdural hematoma, TIAs, tumors

Miscellaneous
Fecal impaction, *postoperative state,* sleep deprivation, urinary retention

PREVENTIVE MEASURES (many also valuable for management)
- Identify and remove or treat underlying cause(s)
- Provide general supportive measures:
  - Modify environment
    - communication to reorient to new surroundings
    - objects that provide orientation (eg, calendar, clock)
    - quiet, well-lit surroundings
    - familiar faces (eg, family members) at bedside for reassurance
    - sitters
  - Engage in stimulating activities during daytime
    - cognitive activities (eg, current events discussion, word games)
    - ambulation, active range-of-motion exercises
  - Correct sensory deficits
    - eyeglasses
    - adequate lighting
    - magnifying lenses
    - cerumen removal
    - hearing aids
    - portable amplification device
  - Promote normal sleep
    - warm milk at bedtime
    - relaxation tapes
    - back massage
    - nighttime noise reduction
  - Prevent dehydration: oral or parenteral supplementation if BUN/creatinine ratio >18

MANAGEMENT

Nonpharmacologic
Use physical restraints only as last resort to maintain patient safety (eg, to prevent patient from pulling out tubes or catheters).

Pharmacologic
- For acute agitation or aggression accompanying delirium: If patient is able to take medications po, consider low dose of atypical antipsychotic (**Table 78**) or haloperidol (*Haldol*) 0.5–2 mg po [T: 0.5, 1, 2, 5, 10, 20; S: 2 mg/mL]. If patient is not able to take medications po, haloperidol IM [5 mg/mL (lactate)] (twice as potent as po, peak effect 20–40 min versus 4–6 h for po). Titrate upward as needed. May repeat po dose q 4 h prn. May repeat IM dose q 1 h prn. Maintain effective dose for 2–3 d. Reevaluate q 30–60 min. Observe for development of EPS, QT prolongation.

- Other IM antipsychotics are less valuable because of the following concerns:
  - Ziprasidone (*Geodon*): cardiac conduction delays
  - Risperidone IM (*Risperdal Consta*): not appropriate for acute treatment, because only a small amount of drug is initially released from IM formulation.
  - Olanzapine IM (*Zyprexa IntraMuscular*): anticholinergic and hypotensive effects
- Avoid low-potency antipsychotics such as chlorpromazine (*Thorazine*) or thioridazine (*Mellaril*) because of their anticholinergic and arrhythmogenic properties (torsades de pointes).
- If delirium is secondary to alcohol or benzodiazepine withdrawal, use a benzodiazepine such as lorazepam (*Ativan*) in dosages of 0.5–2 mg q 4–6 h. Because these agents themselves may cause delirium, gradual withdrawal and discontinuation are desirable. If delirium is secondary to alcohol, also use thiamine 100 mg/d (po, IM, or IV).

DEMENTIA

DEMENTIA SYNDROME

Definition

Chronic acquired decline in memory and in at least one other cognitive function (eg, language, visual-spatial, executive) sufficient to affect daily life.

Estimated Frequencies of Causes of Dementia

- AD: 60%–70%
- Other progressive disorders: 15%–30% (eg, vascular, Lewy body, frontotemporal)
- Completely reversible dementia (eg, drug toxicity, metabolic changes, thyroid disease, subdural hematoma, normal-pressure hydrocephalus): 2%–5%

DIAGNOSIS OF AD

- Dementia syndrome
- Gradual onset and continuing decline
- Not due to another physical, neurologic, or psychiatric condition or to medications
- Deficits not seen exclusively during delirium

PROGRESSION OF AD

Mild Cognitive Impairment (preclinical)

- Report by patient or caregiver of memory loss
- Objective signs of memory impairment
- No functional impairment
- Mild construction, language, or executive dysfunction
- 6%–15% annual conversion rate to dementia syndrome
- Some cases of mild cognitive impairment may not progress to AD

Early, Mild Impairment (yr 1–3 from onset of symptoms) MMSE: 22–28

- Disoriented to date
- Naming difficulties (anomia)
- Recent recall problems
- Mild difficulty copying figures
- Decreased insight
- Social withdrawal
- Irritability, mood change
- Problems managing finances

Middle, Moderate Impairment (yr 2–8) MMSE: 10–21

- Disoriented to date, place
- Comprehension difficulties (aphasia)
- Impaired new learning
- Getting lost in familiar areas
- Impaired calculating skills
- Delusions, agitation, aggression
- Not cooking, shopping, banking
- Restless, anxious, depressed
- Problems with dressing, grooming

Late, Severe Impairment (yr 6–12) MMSE: 0–9

- Nearly unintelligible verbal output
- Remote memory gone
- Unable to copy or write
- No longer grooming or dressing
- Incontinent
- Motor or verbal agitation

NONCOGNITIVE SYMPTOMS

Psychotic Symptoms (eg, delusions, hallucinations)
- Seen in about 20% of AD patients
- Delusions may be paranoid (eg, people stealing things, spouse unfaithful)
- Hallucinations (approximately 11% of patients) are more commonly visual

Depressive Symptoms
- Seen in up to 40% of AD patients; may precede onset of AD
- May cause acceleration of decline if untreated
- Suspect if patient stops eating or withdraws

Agitation or Aggression
- Seen in up to 80% of patients with AD
- A leading cause of nursing-home admission
- Consider superimposed delirium or pain as a trigger

RISK AND PROTECTIVE FACTORS FOR AD

Definite Risks	Possible Risks	Possible Protections
Age	Other genes	Antioxidants (eg, vitamin E, beta carotene)
Family history	Head trauma	
Down syndrome	Hypercholesterolemia	
APOE-E4 (whites)	Hypertension	
	Lower educational level	
	Depression	
	Postmenopausal hormone therapy	

EVALUATION

Although completely reversible dementia (eg, drug toxicity) is rare, identifying and treating secondary physical conditions may improve function.
- Hx: Obtain from family or other caregiver
- Physical and neurologic examination
- Assess functional status
- Evaluate mental status for attention, immediate and delayed recall, remote memory, executive function, and depression. Screening tests may include Mini-Cog (p 244), number of animals named in 1 min, MMSE, PHQ-9, GDS (p 247)

Clinical Features Distinguishing AD and Other Types of Dementia
- AD: Memory, language, visual-spatial disturbances, indifference, delusions, agitation
- Frontotemporal dementia: Personality change, executive dysfunction, hyperorality, relative preservation of visual-spatial skills
- Lewy body dementia: visual hallucinations, delusions, EPS, fluctuating mental status, sensitivity to antipsychotic medications
- Vascular dementia: abrupt onset, stepwise deterioration, prominent aphasia, motor signs

Laboratory Testing
CBC, TSH, B_{12}, folate, serum calcium, liver and kidney function tests, electrolytes, serologic test for syphilis (selectively); genetic testing and commercial "Alzheimer blood tests" are not currently recommended for clinical use.

Neuroimaging

The likelihood of detecting structural lesions is increased with:

- Onset age <60 yr
- Focal (unexplained) neurologic signs or symptoms
- Abrupt onset or rapid decline (weeks to months)
- Predisposing conditions (eg, metastatic cancer or anticoagulants)

Neuroimaging may detect the 5% of cases with clinically significant structural lesions that would otherwise be missed.

FDG-PET scans approved by Medicare for atypical presentation or course of AD in which frontotemporal dementia diagnosis is suspected. See www.petscaninfo.com/portals/pat/medicare_guidelines_alzheimers.

TREATMENT

Primary goals of treatment are to improve quality of life and maximize functional performance by enhancing cognition, mood, and behavior.

General Treatment Principles

- Identify and treat comorbid physical illnesses (eg, HTN, diabetes mellitus)
- Promote brain health by exercise, balanced diet, stress reduction
- Avoid anticholinergic medications, eg, benztropine, diphenhydramine, hydroxyzine, oxybutynin, TCAs, clozapine, thioridazine
- Set realistic goals
- Limit prn psychotropic medication use
- Specify and quantify target behaviors
- Maximize and maintain functioning
- Establish and maintain alliance with patient and family
- Assess and monitor psychiatric status
- Intervene to decrease hazards of wandering
- Advise patient and family concerning driving
- Advise family about sources of care and support, financial and legal issues

Nonpharmacologic Approaches

To improve function:

- Behavior modification, scheduled toileting, and prompted toileting (see p 109) for UI
- Graded assistance (as little help as possible to perform ADLs), practice, and positive reinforcement to increase independence

For problem behaviors:

- Music during meals, bathing
- Walking or light exercise
- Simulate family presence with video or audio tapes
- Pet therapy
- Speak at patient's comprehension level
- Bright light, "white" noise (ie, low-level, background noise)

Pharmacologic Treatment of Cognitive Dysfunction

- Patients with a diagnosis of mild or moderate AD should receive a cholinesterase inhibitor that will increase level of acetylcholine in brain; donepezil also approved for severe AD (see **Table 27**).

- Controlled data for cholinergic drugs compared with placebo for 1 yr show modest symptomatic benefit for cognition, mood, behavioral symptoms, and daily function; open trials demonstrate benefit for 3 yr.
- Only 10%–25% of patients taking cholinesterase inhibitors show clinical improvement, but 80% have less rapid decline.
- Initial studies show benefits of these drugs for patients with dementia associated with Parkinson's disease, Lewy body dementia, and vascular dementia.
- Cholinesterase inhibitors have not been convincingly demonstrated to slow progression of mild cognitive impairment to dementia, but early treatment may help maintain function at higher level for longer periods.
- Cholinesterase inhibitors may attenuate noncognitive symptoms and delay nursing-home placement.
- To evaluate response:
    - Elicit caregiver observations of patient's behavior (alertness, initiative) and follow functional status (ADLs [p 245] and IADLs [p 246]).
    - Follow cognitive status (eg, improved or stabilized) by caregiver's report or serial ratings of cognition (eg, Mini-Cog, see p 244; MMSE).
- Memantine (*Namenda*) demonstrated modest efficacy compared with placebo in moderate to severe AD as monotherapy and when combined with donepezil (*Aricept*).
- Vitamin E at 1000 IU q 12 h found to delay functional decline in AD (caution in those with cardiovascular disease because ≥400 IU may increase mortality).
- *Ginkgo biloba* is not generally recommended (see p 15).

Table 27. Cognitive Enhancers

Medication	Formulations	Dosing (Metabolism)
Donepezil (*Aricept*)[a,b]	T: 5, 10; ODT: 5, 10;[c] S: 5 mg/mL	Start at 5 mg/d, increase to 10 mg/d after 1 mo (CYP2D6, 3A4) (L)
Galantamine (*Razadyne*)[d]	T: 4, 8, 12; S 4 mg/mL	Start at 4 mg q 12 h, increase to 8 mg q 12 h after 4 wk; recommended dosage 8 or 12 mg q 12 h (CYP2D6, 3A4) (L)
(*Razadyne ER*)	C: 8, 16, 24	Start at 1 capsule daily, preferably with food; titrate as above
Rivastigmine (*Exelon*)[a]	T: 1.5, 3, 4.5, 6; S: 2 mg/mL; pch: 4.6, 9.5	Start at 1.5 mg q 12 h and gradually titrate up to minimally effective dosage of 3 mg q 12 h; continue up to 6 mg q 12 h as tolerated; for pch, start at 4.6 mg/d, may be increased after ≥ 4 wk to 9.5 mg/d (recommended effective dosage): retitrate if drug is stopped (K)
Memantine (*Namenda* [NMDA antagonist])[b]	T: 5, 10	Start at 5 mg/d, increase by 5 mg at weekly intervals to max of 10 mg q 12 h; reduce dosage if kidney function impaired (K)

[a] Cholinesterase inhibitors. Continue if improvement or stabilization occurs; stopping medications can lead to rapid decline. Adverse events increase with higher dosing. Possible adverse events include nausea, vomiting, diarrhea, dyspepsia, anorexia, weight loss, leg cramps, bradycardia, insomnia, and agitation.
[b] Approved by FDA for moderate to severe AD.
[c] ODT = oral disintegrating tablet
[d] Increased mortality found in controlled studies of mild cognitive impairment.

Treatment of Agitation

- First, identify and examine context of behavior (is it harmful to patient or others) and environmental triggers (eg, overstimulation, unfamiliar surroundings, frustrating interactions); exclude underlying physical discomfort (eg, illnesses or medication); consider nonpharmacologic strategies (see p 57).
- Cognitive enhancers may slow deterioration, and agitation may worsen if discontinued. Low doses of antipsychotic medications have limited role but may be necessary. Note this use is off-label and increases risk of death compared with placebo in patients with AD. CATIE-AD trial (*NEJM* 2006;355:1525–1538) showed modest treatment benefit compared with placebo for olanzapine and risperidone that was mitigated by greater EPS, sedation, and confusion. In this trial, quetiapine did not appear to be efficacious compared with placebo but caused greater sedation. See also **Table 78** and **Table 79**.

Symptom	Medication	Dosage	Formulations
Agitation in context of nonacute psychosis	Risperidone[a] (*Risperdal*)	0.25–1.5 mg/d	T: 0.25, 0.5, 1, 2, 3, 4; S: 1 mg/mL
	Olanzapine[a] (*Zyprexa*) (*Zydis*)	2.5–10 mg/d	T: 2.5, 5, 7.5, 10, 15, 20 T: oral disintegrating; 5, 10, 15, 20
	Quetiapine[a] (*Seroquel*)	25–400 mg/d	T: 25, 100, 200, 300
	Aripiprazole[a] (*Abilify*)	5–10 mg/d	T: 5, 10, 15, 20, 30
Agitation in context of acute psychosis if IM is needed	Haloperidol[a] (*Haldol*)	0.5–2 mg/d[b]	Inj: 5 mg/mL (lactate)
Agitation in context of depression	SSRI, eg, citalopram (*Celexa*)	10–30 mg/d	T: 20, 40; S: 2 mg/mL
Anxiety, mild to moderate irritability	Trazodone (*Desyrel*) Buspirone (*BuSpar*)	50–100 mg/d[c] 30–60 mg/d[d]	T: 50, 100, 150, 300 T: 5, 7.5, 10, 15, 30
As a possible second-line treatment for significant agitation or aggression	Divalproex sodium (*Depakote, Epival*)	500–1500 mg/d[e]	T: 125, 250, 500; S: syr 250 mg/mL; sprinkle capsule: 125
	Carbamazepine (*Tegretol*)	300–600 mg/d[f]	T: 200; ChT: 100; S: sus 100/5 mL
	Olanzapine (*Zyprexa IntraMuscular*)	2.5–5 mg IM	Inj

Table 28. Agitation Treatment Guidelines

(cont.)

Table 28. Agitation Treatment Guidelines (cont.)

Symptom	Medication	Dosage	Formulations
Sexual aggression, impulse-control symptoms in men	Atypical antipsychotic or divalproex	See dosages above	
	If no response, estrogen (*Premarin*) *or*	0.625–1.25 mg/d	T: 0.3, 0.625, 0.9, 1.25, 2.5
	medroxyprogesterone (*Depo-Provera*)	100 mg IM/wk	Inj

[a] Increased risk of mortality and cerebrovascular events compared with placebo; use with particular caution in patients with cerebrovascular disease or hypovolemia.

[b] May need to give higher dosages in emergency situations; should be used for only short periods of time.

[c] Small divided daytime dosage and larger bedtime dosage; watch for sedation and orthostasis.

[d] Can be given q 12 h; allow 2–4 wk for adequate trial.

[e] Can monitor serum levels; usually well tolerated; check CBC, platelets for agranulocytosis, thrombocytopenia risk in older adults.

[f] Monitor serum levels; periodic CBCs, platelet counts secondary to agranulocytosis risk. Beware of drug-drug interactions.

CAREGIVER ISSUES

- Over 50% develop depression.
- Physical illness, isolation, anxiety, and burnout are common.
- Intensive education and support of caregivers may delay institutionalization.
- Adult day care for patients and respite services may help.
- Alzheimer's Association offers support, education services (eg, Safe Return); chapters are located in major cities throughout US (see p 259 for telephone, Web site).
- Family Caregiver Alliance offers support, education, information for caregivers (see p 259 for telephone, Web site).

ADDITIONAL REFERENCES

Blennow K, deLeon MJ, Zetterberg H. Alzheimer's disease. *Lancet* 2006; 368(9533):387–403.

EVALUATION AND ASSESSMENT

Recognizing and diagnosing late-life depression can be difficult. Older adults may complain of lack of energy or other somatic symptoms, attribute symptoms to old age or other physical conditions, or neglect to mention them to a health care professional. Consider evaluation and follow-up with structured self-assessment scale such as the GDS (see p 247) or the PHQ-9 (www.phqscreeners.com).

Medical Evaluation

TSH, B₁₂, calcium, liver and kidney function tests, electrolytes, UA, CBC

DSM-IV Criteria for Major Depressive Episode (Abbreviated)

Five or more of the following symptoms have been present during the same 2-wk period and represent a change from previous functioning; at least one of the symptoms is either depressed mood *or* loss of interest or pleasure.

- Depressed mood
- Loss of interest or pleasure in activities
- Significant weight loss or gain (not intentional), or decrease or increase in appetite
- Insomnia or hypersomnia
- Psychomotor agitation or retardation
- Fatigue or loss of energy
- Feelings of worthlessness or excessive or inappropriate guilt
- Diminished ability to think or concentrate, or indecisiveness
- Recurrent thoughts of death; suicidal ideation, attempt, or plan

The *DSM-IV* criteria are not specific for older adults; cognitive symptoms may be more prominent.

MANAGEMENT

Treatment should be individualized on the basis of hx, past response, and severity of illness as well as concurrent illnesses.

Nonpharmacologic

For mild to moderate depression or in combination with pharmacotherapy: cognitive-behavioral therapy, interpersonal therapy, problem-solving therapy.
For severe or psychotic depression, consider ECT (see p 63).

Pharmacologic

For mild, moderate, or severe depression: the duration of therapy should be at least 6–12 mo after remission for patients experiencing their first depressive episode. Most older adults with major depression require maintenance antidepressant therapy. Ensure adequate initial trial of 4–6 wk after titrating up to therapeutic dosage; if inadequate response, consider switching to a different first-line agent or second-line therapy or psychiatric referral/consult. Combining antidepressants can lead to significant adverse effects.

Choosing an Antidepressant (see **Table 29** and list on p 63)

First-line Therapy: Consider an SSRI for most older adults, especially those with:

- Heart conduction defects, ischemic heart disease, or hypertension
- Prostatic hyperplasia
- Uncontrolled glaucoma

Second-line Therapy: Consider venlafaxine, duloxetine, mirtazapine, or bupropion.

Table 29. Antidepressants Used for Older Adults

Class, Medication	Initial Dosage	Usual Dosage	Formulations	Comments (Metabolism, Excretion)
SSRIs				Class adverse events (EPS, hyponatremia) (L, K [10%])
Citalopram (*Celexa*)	10–20 mg qam	20–30 mg/d	T: 20, 40, 60; S: 5 mg/10 mL	
Escitalopram (*Lexapro*)	10 mg/d	10–20 mg/d	T: 10, 20	
Fluoxetine (*Prozac*)	5 mg qam	5–60 mg/d	T: 10; C: 10, 20, 40; S: 20 mg/5 mL; C: SR 90 (weekly dose)	Long half-lives of parent and active metabolite may allow for less frequent dosing; may cause more insomnia than other SSRIs; CYP2D6, -2C9, -3A4 inhibitor (L)
Fluvoxamine (*Luvox*)	25 mg qhs	100–300 mg/d	T: 25, 50, 100	Not approved as an antidepressant in US; CYP1A2, -3A4 inhibitor (L)
Paroxetine (*Paxil*)	5 mg	10–40 mg/d	T: 10, 20, 30, 40	Helpful if anxiety symptoms are prominent; increased risk of withdrawal symptoms (dizziness); CYP2D6 inhibitor (L)
(*Paxil CR*)	12.5 mg/d	12.5–37.5 mg/d	T: ER 12.5, 25, 37.5; S: 10 mg/5 mL	Increase by 12.5 mg/d no faster than once a week (L)
Sertraline (*Zoloft*)	25 mg qam	50–200 mg/d	T: 25, 50, 100; S: 20 mg/mL	(L)
Additional Medications				
Bupropion (*Wellbutrin*)	37.5–50 mg q 12 h	75–150 mg q 12 h	T: 75, 100	Consider for SSRI, TCA nonresponders; safe in HF; may be stimulating; can lower seizure threshold (L)
(*Wellbutrin SR, Zyban*)	100 mg q 12 or q 24 h	100–150 mg q 12 h	T: 100, 150, 200	
(*Wellbutrin XL*)	150 mg/d	300 mg/d	T: 150, 300	
Methylphenidate (*Ritalin*)	2.5–5 mg at 7 AM and noon	5–10 mg at 7 AM and noon	T: 5, 10, 20	Short-term treatment of depression or apathy in physically ill older adults; used as an adjunct (L)

(cont.)

Table 29. Antidepressants Used for Older Adults (cont.)

Class, Medication	Initial Dosage	Usual Dosage	Formulations	Comments (Metabolism, Excretion)
Mirtazapine (*Remeron*)	15 mg qhs	15–45 mg/d	T: 15, 30, 45	May increase appetite; sedating; oral disintegrating tab (SolTab) available (L)
Tricyclic Antidepressants				
◆Desipramine (*Norpramin*)	10–25 mg qhs	50–150 mg/d	T: 10, 25, 50, 75, 100, 150	Therapeutic serum level >115 ng/mL (L)
◆Nortriptyline (*Aventyl, Pamelor*)	10–25 mg qhs	75–150 mg/d	C: 10, 25, 50, 75; S: 10 mg/5 mL	Therapeutic window (50–150 ng/mL) (L)
Serotonin/Norepinephrine-Reuptake Inhibitors				
◆Duloxetine (*Cymbalta*)	20 mg/d	20–30 mg q 12 h	C: 20, 30, 60	Most common side effects: nausea, dry mouth, constipation, diarrhea, urinary hesitancy (L)
Venlafaxine (*Effexor*)	25–50 mg q 12 h	75–225 mg/d in divided doses	T: 25, 37.5, 50, 75, 100	Low anticholinergic activity; minimal sedation and hypotension; may increase BP and QT$_C$; may be useful when somatic pain present; EPS, withdrawal symptoms, hyponatremia (L)
(*Effexor XR*)	75 mg qam	75–225 mg/d	C: 37.5, 75, 150	Same as above

◆ = Also has primary indication for neuropathic pain.

Antidepressants to Avoid in Older Adults

- Amitriptyline (eg, *Elavil*): anticholinergic, sedating, hypotensive
- Amoxapine (*Asendin*): anticholinergic, sedating, hypotensive; also associated with EPS, tardive dyskinesia, and neuroleptic malignant syndrome
- Doxepin (eg, *Sinequan*): anticholinergic, sedating, hypotensive
- Imipramine (*Tofranil*): anticholinergic, sedating, hypotensive
- Maprotiline (*Ludiomil*): seizures, rashes
- Protriptyline (*Vivactil*): very anticholinergic; can be stimulating
- St. John's wort (see p 16)
- Trimipramine (*Surmontil*): anticholinergic, sedating, hypotensive

Electroconvulsive Therapy (ECT)

Generally safe and very effective. Potential complications include temporary confusion, arrhythmias, aspiration, falls.

Indications: Severe depression when a rapid onset of response is necessary; when depression is resistant to drug therapy; for patients who are unable to tolerate antidepressants, have previous response to ECT, have psychotic depression, severe catatonia, or depression with Parkinson's disease.

Evaluation: Before ECT, perform CXR, ECG, serum electrolytes, and cardiac examination. Additional tests (eg, stress test, neuroimaging, EEG) are used selectively.

Contraindications:
- Increased intracranial pressure
- Intracranial tumor
- MI within 3 mo (relative)
- Stroke within 1 mo (relative)

BIPOLAR DISORDER
See **Table 30**.
- 5%–19% of mood disorders in older adults.
- Usually begins in early adulthood, family hx.
- 10% may develop after age 50.
- Distinct period of abnormally and persistently elevated, expansive, or irritable mood for longer than 1 wk.
- Symptoms may include racing thoughts, pressured speech, decreased need for sleep, distractibility, grandiose delusions.
- A single manic episode is sufficient for a diagnosis if secondary causes are excluded.
- Late-onset mania may be secondary to head trauma, stroke, delirium, other neurologic disorders, alcohol abuse, or medications (eg, corticosteroids, L-dopa, thyroxine).
- Use aripiprazole, olanzapine, quetiapine, risperidone, or ziprasidone for acute mania (see **Table 79**) and D/C antidepressants if taking.
- If depression emerges in bipolar disorder, lamotrigine may be helpful.
- Initiate long-term treatment (see **Table 31**) as soon as patient is able to comply with oral therapy.

Table 30. Medications for Management of Bipolar Disorders				
	Mania		**Depression**	
Medication	**Acute**	**Maintenance**	**Acute**	**Maintenance**
Atypical antipsychotics	All +	Aripiprazole + Olanzapine +/−	Quetiapine + Olanzapine +/−	Olanzapine +/−
Mood stabilizers				
Lithium	+	+	+	+
Valproate	+	+/−	−	+/−
Lamotrigine	−	+/−	+	+
Carbamazepine	+	+/−	?	+/−
Antidepressants				
SSRIs	Avoid	Avoid	+	+
TCAs	Avoid	Avoid	−	−

Note: + = evidence to support use; +/− = some evidence to support use; − = evidence does not support use; ? = has not been studied

Table 31. Long-term Treatment of Bipolar Disorders*

Medication	Initial Dosage	Usual Dosage	Formulation	Comments
Lithium (*Eskalith, Eskalith CR, Lithobid*)	150 mg/d	300–900 mg/d Levels 0.4–0.8 mEq/L	C, T, XR	Risk of CNS toxicity; cognitive impairment; hypothyroidism; interactions with diuretics, ACEIs, calcium channel blockers, NSAIDs
Carbamazepine (*Tegretol, Tegretol XR*)	100 mg q 12 h	800–1200 mg/d Levels 4–12 mcg/L	T	Many drug interactions; may cause SIADH; risk of leukopenia, neutropenia, agranulocytosis, thrombocytopenia; monitor CBC; drowsiness, dizziness
Valproic acid (*Depacon, Depakene, Depakote*)	125 mg q 12 h	750 mg/d in divided doses Levels 50–125 mcg/L	T	Can cause weight gain, tremor, several drug interactions; risk of hepatotoxicity, pancreatitis, neutropenia, thrombocytopenia; monitor LFTs and platelets
Lamotrigine (*Lamictal*)	25 mg/d	100–200 mg/d	T	D/C if rash; interaction with valproate (when used together, begin at 25 mg q 48 h, titrate to 25–100 mg q 12 h); prolongs PR interval; somnolence, headache common

*Limited evidence base in older adults. See www.dshs.state.tx.us/mhprograms/TIMA.shtm. (See also **Table 64**.)

DERMATOLOGIC CONDITIONS

DERMATOLOGIC CONDITIONS COMMON IN OLDER ADULTS
For numerous dermatologic images, see http://tray.dermatology.uiowa.edu.

Actinic Keratosis
Erythematous, flat, rough, scaly papules 2–6 mm; may be easier felt than seen; precancerous (can develop into squamous or basal cell carcinoma); cutaneous horn may develop; affects sun-exposed areas, including lips (actinic cheilitis)

Risk Factors: UV light exposure (amount and intensity), increased age, fair coloring, immunosuppression

Prevention: Limit UV light exposure, use sunscreen with UVA and UVB coverage, wear protective clothing

Treatment
- Cryosurgery
- Topical 5-fluorouracil (*Carac* crm 0.5% daily × 4 wk, *Efudex* crm 5% q 12 h × 2–4 wk, *Fluoroplex* crm 1% q 12 h × 2–6 wk) to entire area affected
- Aminolevulinic acid (*Levulan Kerastick* 20%) applied to lesions with blue light illumination after 14–18 h, repeat in 8 wk
- Curettage with or without electrosurgery
- Chemical peels, dermabrasion, laser treatments

Basal Cell Carcinoma
Can affect any body surface exposed to the sun, most often head and neck

Types
- Nodular: pearly papule or nodule over telangiectases with a rolled border; may contain melanin
- Superficial: scaly erythematous patch or plaque, may contain melanin
- Morpheaform: indurated, whitish, scar-like plaque with indistinct margins

Risk Factors
- Exposure to UV radiation, especially intense intermittent exposure during childhood or adolescence
- Physical factors: fair skin, light eye color, red or blonde hair
- Exposure to ionizing radiation, arsenic, psoralen, UV-A radiation, smoking
- Immunosuppression (eg, after solid-organ transplant)

Prevention: Avoid sun exposure, use sunscreen with UVA and UVB coverage, wear protective clothing

Treatment: (localized control)
- Surgical: Mohs micrographic surgery, cryosurgery, excision, curettage and electrodessication
- Nonsurgical: radiotherapy, imiquimod 5% crm (*Aldara*) applied daily 5 d/wk × 6 wk (not for use on face, hands, or feet); photodynamic therapy

Candidiasis
Erythema, pustules, or cheesy, whitish matter in body folds; satellite lesions
Treatment: See intertrigo; antifungal powders (see **Table 32**)

Cellulitis
Ill-defined erythema, pain, blisters and exudates; most often affects lower dermis and subcutaneous tissue, commonly the legs; group A streptococci and *Staphylococcus aureus* most frequent pathogens
Treatment
- Antistaphylococcal penicillin, amoxicillin-clavulanate × 10 d
- Macrolide (eg, erythromycin), 1st-generation cephalosporin (eg, cephalexin), or tetracycline if penicillin allergy

Erysipelas
Bright red, edematous, and tender with unilateral distribution; orange peel appearance; well-demarcated border with vesicles and bullae; affects lower dermis and subcutaneous tissue, face and legs
Treatment: Penicillin; erythromycin or cephalosporin if penicillin allergy

Folliculitis
Multiple small, erythematous papules and pustules surrounding a hair; most often affects areas with coarse, short hair, ie, neck, beard, buttocks, thighs
Treatment
- Mild localized cases—topical antibiotic: mupirocin 2% (*Bactroban*), erythromycin, or clindamycin
- Extensive or severe cases—oral antistaphylococcal penicillin, amoxicillin-clavulanate, or erythromycin

Impetigo
Very contagious; nonbullous and bullous variants; honey-colored crusts on face around nose and mouth
Treatment
- Small, localized lesions: topical mupirocin 2% (*Bactroban*) q 8 h × 7–10 d, topical retapamulin 1% oint (*Altabax*) q 12 h × 5 d
- Widespread: oral antistaphylococcal penicillin, erythromycin, or a cephalosporin × 10 d

Intertrigo
Moist, erythematous lesions with local superficial skin loss; satellite lesions caused by *Candida*; can affect any place two skin surfaces rest against one another (eg, under breasts, between toes)
Treatment
- Keep area dry.
- Topical antifungals, absorbent pwd, 1% hydrocortisone or 0.1% triamcinolone crm q 12 h × 1–2 d if inflamed

Neurodermatitis
Generalized or localized itching, redness, scaling; can affect any skin surface
Treatment: Mid- to higher-potency topical corticosteroids (**Table 33**); exclude other causes, eg, allergies, irritants, xerosis

Onychomycosis

Thickening and discoloration; affects nails (*Tinea unguium*)

Treatment: Obtain nail specimens for laboratory culture to confirm diagnosis before prescribing itraconazole or terbinafine.

- Itraconazole (*Sporanox* [C: 100; S: 100 mg/mL]), contraindicated in HF (L)
  - Toenails: 200 mg po q 24 h × 3 mo, or 200 mg po q 12 h × 1 wk/mo, or pulse 400 mg po q 24 h × 7 d of each of 4 mo
  - Fingernails: 200 mg po q 12 h × 1 wk/mo × 2 mo
- Fluconazole (*Diflucan* [T: 50, 100, 150, 200; S: 10, 40 mg/mL]) (L)
  - Toenails: 150 or 300 mg po/wk × 6–12 mo
  - Fingernails: 150 or 300 mg po/wk × 3–6 mo
- Terbinafine (*Lamisil* [T: 250]), avoid if CrCl <50 mL/min
  - Toenails: 250 mg po q 24 h × 12 wk
  - Fingernails: 250 mg po q 24 h × 6 wk
- Ciclopirox (*Loprox, Penlac*): Toenails and fingernails—apply lacquer q 12 h to nails and adjacent skin; remove with alcohol q 7 d

Psoriasis

Well-defined, erythematous plaques covered with silver scales; severity varies; can affect all skin areas, nails (pitting)

Treatment

- Topical corticosteroids, UV light, PUVA, methotrexate, cyclosporine, etretinate, sulfasalazine, anthralin preparations and tar + 1%–4% salicylic acid
- Calcipotriene for nonfacial areas

Rosacea

Vascular and follicular dilatation; mild to moderate; can accompany seborrhea; can affect face (nose, chin, cheeks, forehead) or eyes (dryness, blepharitis, conjunctivitis)

Prevention: Avoid triggers (stress, prolonged sun exposure and exercise, hot and humid environment, alcohol, hot drinks, spicy foods); may be worsened by vasodilators, niacin, or topical corticosteroids. Wear sunscreen with UVA and UVB coverage (SPF ≥15) or sunblock with titanium and zinc oxide. See www.rosacea.org.

Treatment

- Topical (for mild cases and maintenance)
  - Azelaic acid 15% gel (*Finacea*) q 12–24 h or 20% crm (*Azelex, Finevin*) q 12 h
  - Metronidazole 0.75% crm (*MetroCream*) q 12 h or 1% crm or gel (*Noritate, MetroGel*) q 24 h
  - Sodium sulfacetamide 10% + sulfa 5% (*Rosula* aqueous gel, *Clenia* crm, foaming wash) q 12–24 h, avoid if sulfa allergy or kidney disease (K)
  - Erythromycin 2% sol q 12 h
  - Tretinoin 0.025% crm or liq, 0.01% gel qhs

- Oral (for moderate to severe papular-pustular rosacea)
  - Tetracycline 500 mg q 8–12 h × 6–12 wk
  - Doxycycline 50–100 mg q 12–24 h × 6–12 wk
  - Minocycline 50–100 mg q 12 h × 6–12 wk
  - Clarithromycin 250–500 mg q 12 h × 6–12 wk
  - Metronidazole 200 mg q 12–24 h × 4–6 wk
  - Erythromycin 250–500 mg q 12–24 h × 6–12 wk
  - Azithromycin 250–500 mg q 24 h × 6–12 wk

Scabies
Burrows, erythematous papules or rash, dry or scaly skin, pruritus (worse at night); spread by close, skin-to-skin or sexual contact; can affect interdigital webs, flexor aspects of wrists, axillae, umbilicus, nipples, genitalia

Treatment
- Infestation can result in epidemics; treat all contacts and treat environment
- Oatmeal baths, topical corticosteroids, or emollient creams for symptom relief
- Apply topical products from head to toe:
  - Permethrin 5% crm (*Elimite*), wash off after 8–14 h, repeat in 7–10 d if symptomatic or if live mites were found.
  - Lindane 1% crm (*K-well, Scabene*), wash off after 8–12 h
  - Crotamiton 10% crm (*Eurax*), less effective, leave on 48 h, repeat in 7–10 d if necessary
  - Ivermectin (*Stromectol*) 200 mcg/kg po, may repeat once in 1 or 2 wk [T: 3, 6]

Seborrheic Dermatitis
Greasy, yellow scales with or without erythematous base; common in Parkinson's disease and in debilitated patients; can affect nasal labial folds, eyebrows, hairline, sideburns, posterior auriculare and midchest

Treatment
- Hydrocortisone 1% or 2% crm q 12 h or triamcinolone 0.1% oint q 12 h × 2 wk
- Scalp: shampoo containing selenium sulfide, zinc, or tar
- Ketoconazole 2% crm for severe conditions if *Pityrosporum orbiculare* infection suspected

Skin Maceration
Erythema; abraded, excoriated skin; blisters; white and silver patches; can affect any area constantly in contact with moisture, covered by occlusive dressing or bandage; skin folds, groin, buttocks

Prevention and Treatment
- Eliminate cause of moisture.
  - Toileting program for incontinence (p 109)
  - Condom catheter
  - Indwelling catheter (reserve for most intractable conditions)
  - Fecal incontinence collector
- Protect skin from moisture.
  - Clean gently with mild soap after each incontinent episode.
  - Apply moisture barrier (eg, *Vaseline, Proshield, Smooth and Cool, Calmoseptine*).
  - Use disposable briefs that wick moisture from the skin; use linen incontinence pads when disposable briefs worsen perineal dermatitis.

Urticaria
Hives
- Uniform, red edematous plaques surrounded by white halos, can affect any skin surface
- Treatment
  - Identify cause.
  - Oral H_1 antihistamines (see **Table 85**) or oral H_2 antihistamines (see **Table 38**)
  - Oral glucocorticoids (eg, prednisone 40 mg q 24 h)
  - Doxepin (po or topical *Zonalon* 5%) for refractory cases

Angioedema
- Larger, deeper than hives; can affect lips, eyelids, tongue, larynx, GI tract
- Treatment
  - Oral H_1 antihistamines (see **Table 85**)
  - Oral glucocorticoids
  - For severe reactions, epinephrine 0.3 mL of a 1:1000 dilution (*EpiPen*) SC

Cholinergic
- Round, red papular wheals; can affect any skin surface
- Treatment
  - Hot shower may relieve itching
  - Oral H_1 antihistamines (see **Table 85**) 1 h before exercise

Xerosis
Dull, rough, flaky, cracked; nummular; can affect all skin surfaces
Treatment
- Increase humidity
- Avoid excess bathing and use of bath oils, which can lead to falls from slippery feet
- Tepid water in baths or showers
- Oatmeal baths
- Apply emollient oint (eg, *Aquaphor*) or crm (eg, *Eucerin*) immediately after bathing
- Hydrocortisone 1% oint

Table 32. Topical Antifungal Medications

Medication	Formulation	Dermatologic Indications	Dosing Frequency
Ciclopirox (*Loprox, Penlac*)	0.77% crm, gel, lot, sus; 1% shp; 8% lacquer	*Tinea pedis, T cruris, T corpis, T versicolor;* candidiasis; scalp seborrhea; onychomycosis	q 12 h; shp 3 ×/wk; lacquer qhs
Clotrimazole* (*Cruex, Mycelex,* others)	1% crm, sol	Candidiasis; dermatophytoses; superficial mycoses	q 12 h
Econazole nitrate (*Spectazole*)	1% crm	Candidiasis; *Tinea cruris, T corpis, T versicolor*	q 24 h
Ketoconazole (*Nizoral, Nizoral A-D**)	2% crm, 1% shp	Candidiasis; seborrhea; *Tinea cruris, T corpis, T versicolor*	q 12–24 h; shp 2 ×/wk

*OTC

(cont.)

Table 32. Topical Antifungal Medications (cont.)

Medication	Formulation	Dermatologic Indications	Dosing Frequency
Miconazole* (eg, *Micatin, Monistat-Derm*)	2% crm, lot, pwd, spr, tinc	*Tinea cruris, T corpis, T pedis*	q 12 h
Naftifine (*Naftin*)	1% crm, gel	*Tinea cruris, T corpis, T pedis*	crm q 12 h; gel q 12 h
Nystatin (*Mycostatin, Nilstat, Nystex*)	100,000 units/g crm, oint, pwd	Mucocutaneous candidiasis	q 8–12 h
Terbinafine (*Lamisil, LamisilAT**)	1% crm, sol	*Tinea cruris, T corpis, T pedis, T versicolor*	q 12 h
Tolnaftate* (*Absorbine Jr. Antifungal, Tinactin*, others)	1% crm, gel, S, pwd, spr	*Tinea cruris, T corpis, T pedis*	q 12 h

*OTC

Table 33. Topical Corticosteroids

Medication	Strength and Formulations	Frequency of Application
Lowest Potency		
Hydrocortisone acetate (*Hytone, Cortaid**)	0.25%, 0.5%, 1%, 2.5% crm, oint	q 6–8 h
Low Potency		
Alclometasone dipropionate (*Aclovate*)	0.05% crm, oint	q 8–12 h
Desonide (*DesOwen, Tridesilon*)	0.05% crm, lot, oint	q 6–12 h
Fluocinolone acetonide (*Synalar*)	0.01% crm, sol	q 6–12 h
Mid-potency		
Betamethasone dipropionate (*Diprosone*)	0.05% lot	q 6–12 h
Betamethasone valerate (*Valisone*)	0.1% crm	q 6–12 h
Clocortolone pivalate (*Cloderm*)	0.1% crm	q 6–24 h
Desoximetasone (*Topicort*)	0.05% crm	q 12 h
Fluocinolone acetonide (*Synalar*)	0.025% crm, oint	q 6–12 h
Flurandrenolide (*Cordran*)	0.05% crm, oint, lot, tape	q 12–24 h
Fluticasone propionate (*Cutivate*)	0.05% crm, 0.005% oint	q 12 h
Hydrocortisone butyrate (*Locoid*)	0.1% oint	q 12–24 h
Hydrocortisone valerate (*Westcort*)	0.2% crm, oint	q 6–8 h
Mometasone furoate (*Elocon*)	0.1% crm, lot, oint	q 24 h
Prednicarbate (*Dermatop*)	0.1% crm, lot	q 12 h
Triamcinolone acetonide (*Aristocort, Kenalog*)	0.025%, 0.1% crm, oint, lot	q 8–12 h

* OTC

(cont.)

Table 33. Topical Corticosteroids (cont.)

Medication	Strength and Formulations	Frequency of Application
High Potency		
Betamethasone dipropionate (*Diprosone*)	0.05% crm	q 6–12 h
Mometasone furoate (*Elocon*)	0.1%, crm, oint, lot	q 24 h
Triamcinolone acetonide (*Aristocort, Kenalog*)	0.5% oint	q 8–12 h
Higher Potency		
Amcinonide (*Cyclocort*)	0.1%, crm, oint, lot	q 8–12 h
Betamethasone dipropionate (*Diprolene AF*)	0.05% augmented crm	q 6–12 h
Betamethasone dipropionate (*Diprosone*)	0.05%, crm, oint	q 6–12 h
Betamethasone valerate (*Valisone*)	0.1% oint	q 6–12 h
Desoximetasone (*Topicort*)	0.25% crm, oint; 0.05% gel	q 12 h
Diflorasone diacetate (*Florone, Maxiflor*)	0.05%, crm, oint	q 6–12 h
Fluocinonide (*Lidex*)	0.05% crm, oint, gel	q 6–12 h
Halcinonide (*Halog*)	0.1% crm, oint	q 8–24 h
Triamcinolone acetate	0.5% crm	q 8–12 h
Super Potency		
Betamethasone dipropionate (*Diprolene*)	0.05% oint, lot	q 6–12 h
Clobetasol propionate (*Temovate*)	0.05% crm, oint, lot, gel, shp	q 12 h
Diflorasone diacetate (*Psorcon*)	0.05% optimized oint	q 8–24 h
Halobetasol propionate (*Ultravate*)	0.05% crm, oint	q 12 h

ADRENAL INSUFFICIENCY
Common Causes
***Secondary* (more common)**
- Abrupt discontinuation of chronic glucocorticoid administration
- Megestrol acetate
- Brain irradiation
- Traumatic brain injury
- Pituitary tumors

***Primary* (less common)**
- Autoimmune
- Tuberculosis

Evaluation
- Basal plasma cortisol >18 mcg/dL excludes adrenal insufficiency, and <3 mcg/dL is diagnostic.
- ACTH stimulation test: tetracosactin (*Synacthen Depot*) 250 mcg IM or IV; peak value >18 mcg/dL is normal, <15 mcg/dL is diagnostic.
- ACTH if adrenal insufficiency is diagnosed. If >100 pg/mL, insufficiency is primary.

Pharmacologic Therapy
For corticosteroid dose equivalencies, see **Table 34**. Hydrocortisone preferred for adrenal insufficiency (10–12 mg/m^2/d) in 2 or 3 divided doses. If primary adrenal insufficiency, add fludrocortisone to glucocorticoids.

Management
Stress doses of corticosteroids for patients with severe illness, injury, or undergoing surgery: In emergency situations, do not wait for test results. Give hydrocortisone 50 mg IV q 8 h. For less severe stress, double usual oral replacement dosage and taper back to baseline as quickly as possible.

HYPOTHYROIDISM
Common Causes
- Autoimmune (primary thyroid failure)
- Following therapy for hyperthyroidism
- Pituitary or hypothalmic disorders (secondary thyroid failure)
- Medications, especially amiodarone (rare after first 18 mo of therapy) and lithium

Evaluation
TSH, free T_4

Table 34. Corticosteroids

Medication	Approx Equivalent Dose (mg)	Relative Anti-inflammatory Potency	Relative Mineralo-corticoid Potency	Biologic Half-life (h)	Formulations
Betamethasone (*Celestone*)	0.6–0.75	20–30	0	36–54	T: 0.6; S: 0.6 mg/5 mL
Cortisone (*Cortone*)	25	0.8	2	8–12	T: 5; S: 50 mg/mL
Dexamethasone (*Decadron, Dexone, Hexadrol*)	0.75	20–30	0	36–54	T: 0.25, 0.5, 0.75, 1, 1.5, 2, 4; S: elixir 0.5 mg/5 mL; inj
Fludrocortisone (*Florinef*)*	NA	10	4	12–36	T: 0.1
Hydrocortisone (*Cortef, Hydrocortone*)	20	1	2	8–12	T: 5, 10, 20; S: 10 mg/5 mL; inj
Methylprednisolone (eg, *Medrol, Solu-Medrol, Depo-Medrol*)	4	5	0	18–36	T: 2, 4, 8, 16, 24, 32; inj
Prednisolone (eg, *Delta-Cortef, Prelone Syrup, Pediapred*)	5	4	1	18–36	S: 5 mg/5 mL; syr 5, 15 mg/5 mL
Prednisone (*Deltasone, Liquid Pred, Meticorten, Orasone*)	5	4	1	18–36	T: 1, 2.5, 5, 10, 20, 50; S: 5 mg/5 mL
Triamcinolone (eg, *Aristocort, Kenacort, Kenalog*)	4	5	0	18–36	T: 1, 2, 4, 8; S: syr 4 mg/5 mL

Note: NA = not available

* Usually given for orthostatic hypotension at 0.1 mg q 8–24 h and at 0.05–0.2 mg/d for primary adrenal insufficiency.

Pharmacologic Therapy

- Treatment of subclinical hypothyroidism (TSH 5–10 mIU/L, normal free T_4 concentration, and no overt symptoms) is controversial.
- Thyroxine (T_4, levothyroxine [*Eltroxin, Levo-T, Levothroid, Levoxyl, Synthroid*]). Start at 25 mcg and increase by 12- to 25-mcg intervals q 3–6 wk until TSH is in normal range [T: 25, 50, 75, 88, 100, 112, 125, 137, 150, 175, 200, 300 mcg].
- For myxedema coma: Load T_4 400 mcg IV or 100 mcg q 6–8 h for 1 d, then 100 mcg/d IV (until patient can take orally) and give stress doses of corticosteroids (see p 73); then start usual replacement regimen.
- Thyroid USP is not recommended. To convert thyroid USP to thyroxine: 60 mg USP = 50 mcg thyroxine.

- If patients are npo and must receive IV thyroxine, dose should be half usual po dose.
- Monitor TSH level at least q 12 mo (ATA) in patients on chronic thyroid replacement therapy.

HYPERTHYROIDISM
Common Causes
- Graves' disease
- Toxic nodule
- Toxic multinodular goiter
- Medications, especially amiodarone (can occur any time during therapy) and lithium

Evaluation
TSH, free T_4
- If TSH is low and free T_4 is normal, recheck TSH in 4–6 wk; if TSH is still low, check free T_3.
- If TSH is low and free T_4 or free T_3 is high, check radioactive iodine uptake and thyroid scan.

Pharmacologic Therapy
- Radioactive iodine ablation is usual treatment of choice, but surgery or medical therapy are options.
- Propylthiouracil (PTU): Start 100 mg po q 8 h, then adjust up to 200 mg po q 8 h prn [T: 50].
- Methimazole (*Tapazole*): Start 5–20 mg po q 8 h, then adjust [T: 5, 10].
- When dose has stabilized, follow TSH per hypothyroid monitoring.
- Adjunctive therapy with β-blockers (see **Table 20**) or calcium antagonists (see **Table 20**) may improve symptoms.

EUTHYROID SICK SYNDROME
Definition
Abnormal thyroid function tests in nonthyroidal illness

Evaluation
- Do not assess thyroid function in acutely ill patients unless thyroid dysfunction is strongly suspected.
- Low T_3, high reverse T_3, low T_4, low or high TSH may be seen.
- If TSH is very low (<0.1 mIU/L in high sensitivity assays), then hyperthyroidism is likely.
- If TSH is very high (>20 mIU/L), then hypothyroidism is likely.
- If thyroid disease is not strongly suspected, recheck in 3–6 wk.

SOLITARY THYROID NODULE
Evaluation
If TSH is normal, do fine-needle aspirate.
If TSH is low, do radionuclide scan; if "cold," do fine-needle aspirate.

Management
- "Hot" nodules: radioactive iodine or surgery
- Malignant nodules: surgery
- Inconclusive biopsy of nodules: follow clinically and with ultrasound, and repeat fine-needle aspirate.

METABOLIC SYNDROME
Definition (Adult Treatment Panel III)
Increased risk of CAD, PAD, and type 2 diabetes
Presence of 3 or more of the following:
- Central obesity as measured by waist circumference: men >40 inches, women >35 inches
- Fasting blood triglycerides ≥150 mg/dL
- Blood HDL cholesterol: men <40 mg/dL, women <50 mg/dL
- BP ≥130/85 mmHg
- Fasting glucose ≥110 mg/dL

Management
- Weight loss if overweight (Mediterranean, DASH, and low-glycemic index food diets)
- Exercise
- Monitor and treat individual risk factors

DIABETES MELLITUS
Definition and Classification (ADA)
Diabetes mellitus is a group of metabolic diseases characterized by hyperglycemia resulting from defects in insulin secretion, insulin action, or both.
Type 1: Caused by an absolute deficiency of insulin secretion.
Type 2: Caused by a combination of resistance to insulin action and an inadequate compensatory insulin secretory response.
Criteria for Diagnosis—One or more of the following:
- Symptoms of diabetes (eg, polyuria, polydipsia, unexplained weight loss) plus casual plasma glucose concentration ≥200 mg/dL
- Fasting (no caloric intake for ≥8 h) plasma glucose ≥126 mg/dL
- 2 h Plasma glucose ≥200 mg/dL during an OGTT

Diagnosis should be confirmed by reevaluating on a subsequent day.
Pre-diabetes—Either of the following:
- Impaired fasting glucose: defined as fasting plasma glucose ≥100 and <126 mg/dL
- Impaired glucose tolerance: 2-h plasma glucose 140–199 mg/dL

Management
Prevention/Delay of Type 2 Diabetes in Patients with Impaired Glucose Tolerance
- Weight loss (5%–10%) if overweight
- Exercise (30 min daily)

Evaluate for Comorbid Conditions (AGS, ADA): Depression (see p 61), polypharmacy (see p 10), cognitive impairment (see p 244), urinary incontinence (see p 107), falls (see p 82), pain (see p 170) (AGS), PAD (claudication history and assessment of pedal pulses) (see p 47) (ADA), stress test if ≥2 additional CAD risk factors (see p 28).

Goals of Treatment (ADA, AGS):

- Outpatient: Average preprandial capillary blood glucose 80–120 mg/dL, average bedtime capillary blood glucose 100–140 mg/dL, and HbA_{1c} <7% (ADA) (<8% if frail; life expectancy <5 yr; or high risk of hypoglycemia, polypharmacy, or drug interaction) (AGS).
- Inpatient: ≤110 mg/dL in intensive-care units and preprandial in noncritical-care units; ≤180 mg/dL postprandial in noncritically ill patients.

Nonpharmacologic Interventions:

- Limit protein intake to ≤0.8 g/kg/d if any chronic kidney disease
- High-fiber diet (25 g insoluble and 25 g soluble/d)
- Lifestyle (eg, regular exercise, alcohol and smoking cessation)
- Patient and family education for self-management (reimbursed by Medicare)
- Self-monitoring of blood glucose

Pharmacologic Interventions for Type 2:

- Management of glycemia: stepped therapy* (ADA), see **Table 35**.

   Step 1: Metformin (unless CrCl <60 mL/min) beginning 500 mg q 12 or 24 h; can titrate up q 5–7 d to max of 2000 mg/d if no adverse events and blood glucose uncontrolled.

   Step 2: Add one of the following:
   - Basal insulin (intermediate at bedtime or long-acting at bedtime or morning) 10 U or 0.2 U/kg; can increase by 2-4 U q 3 d depending on fasting blood glucose. When fasting blood glucose is 70-130 mg/dL, check pre-lunch, dinner, and bedtime blood glucose concentrations and add rapid- or intermediate-acting insulin (see **Table 36**).
   - Sulfonylurea
   - Glitizone (thiazolidinedione)

   Step 3: Combine step 2 agents. Do not use sulfonylureas with rapid- or very rapid-acting insulins.

   Step 4: Other agents (**Table 35**) may be appropriate for selected patients.

*Reinforce lifestyle modifications at every visit.

- Management of treatment-associated hypoglycemia
   - Patients should have fast-acting carbohydrate (eg, glucose tabs, hard candy, paste (Instant Glucose), or instant fruit that provides 15–30 g
   - Effects may last only 15 min, so need to eat and recheck blood glucose
   - If hypoglycemia is severe (patient unconscious or cannot ingest carbohydrate), then glucagon 0.5–1 mg SC or IM
   - In medical settings, 25–50 g of D50 IV restores glucose quicker.
- Manage HTN (BP goal <130/80 mmHg; also see HTN, p 37).
- Treat lipid disorders (see p 35) as CHD risk equivalent with target LDL <70 mg/dL if other risk factors are present (NHLBI), HDL >40 mg/dL, TG <150 mg/dL, as appropriate. If total cholesterol ≥135 mg/dL and no overt heart disease, statin therapy to reduce LDL by 30%–40% regardless of baseline LDL (ADA) with goal of LDL <100 mg/dL; if overt heart disease, LDL goal of <70 mg/dL, using a high-dose statin, is an option. Statins should be used as primary prevention against macrovascular complications in patients with type 2 diabetes and other cardiovascular risk factors (ACP).

- ACEI or angiotensin II receptor blocker if albuminuria, HTN, or another cardiovascular risk factor. Check kidney function within 1–2 wk of initiation of therapy, with each dosage increase, and at least yearly.
- ASA 75–162 mg/d.

Table 35. Non-insulin Agents for Treating Diabetes Mellitus

Medication	Dosage	Formulations	Comments (Metabolism)
Oral Agents			
2nd-Generation Sulfonylureas			Increase insulin secretion; lower HbA$_{1c}$ by 1.0%–2.0%
Glimepiride (*Amaryl*)	4–8 mg once (begin 1–2 mg)	T: 1, 2, 4	Numerous drug interactions, long-acting (L, K)
Glipizide (generic or *Glucotrol*)	2.5–40 mg once or divided 5–20 mg once	T: 5, 10	Short-acting (L, K)
(*Glucotrol XL*)		T: ER 2.5, 5, 10	Long-acting (L, K)
Glyburide (generic or *DiaBeta, Micronase*)	1.25–20 mg once or divided	T: 1.25, 2.5, 5	Long-acting, risk of hypoglycemia (L, K)
Micronized glyburide (*Glynase*)	1.5–12 mg once	T: 1.5, 3, 4.5, 6	(L, K)
α-Glucosidase Inhibitors			Delay glucose absorption; lower HbA$_{1c}$ by 0.5%–1.0%
Acarbose (*Precose*)	50–100 mg q 8 h, just before meals; start with 25 mg/d	T: 25, 50, 100	GI adverse events common, avoid if Cr >2 mg/dL, monitor LFTs (gut, K)
Miglitol (*Glyset*)	25–100 mg q 8 h, with 1st bite of meal; start with 25 mg/d	T: 25, 50, 100	Same as acarbose but no need to monitor LFTs (L, K)
DPP–4 Enzyme Inhibitor			
Sitagliptin (*Januvia*)	100 mg once daily as monotherapy or in combination with metformin or a thiazolidinedione; 50 mg/d if CrCl 31–50 mL/min; 25 mg/d if CrCl <30 mL/min	T: 25, 50, 100	Protects and enhances endogenous incretin hormones; lowers HbA$_{1c}$ by 0.5%–1.0% (K)

(cont.)

Table 35. Non-insulin Agents for Treating Diabetes Mellitus (cont.)

Medication	Dosage	Formulations	Comments (Metabolism)
Biguanides			Decrease hepatic glucose production; lower HbA$_{1c}$ by 1.0%–2.0%
Metformin (*Glucophage*)	500–2550 mg divided	T: 500, 850, 1000	Avoid in patients >80 yr unless CrCl ≥ 60 mL/min, Cr >1.5 mg/dL in men,
(*Glucophage XR*)	1500–2000 mg/d	T: ER 500	Cr >1.4 mg/dL in women, HF, COPD, ↑ LFTs; hold before contrast radiologic studies; may cause weight loss (K)
Meglitinides			Increase insulin secretion; lower HbA$_{1c}$ by 1.0%–2.0%
Nateglinide (*Starlix*)	60–120 mg q 8 h	T: 60, 120	Give 30 min before meals
Repaglinide (*Prandin*)	0.5 mg q 6–12 h if HbA$_{1c}$ <8% or previously untreated; 1–2 mg q 6–12 h if HbA$_{1c}$ ≥8% or previously treated	T: 0.5, 1, 2	Give 30 min before meals, adjust dosage at weekly intervals, potential for drug interactions, caution in hepatic, renal insufficiency (L)
Thiazolidinediones			Insulin resistance reducers; lower HbA$_{1c}$ by 0.5%–1.5%; ↑ risk of HF; avoid if NYHA Class III or IV cardiac status; D/C if any decline in cardiac status
Pioglitazone (*Actos*)	15 or 30 mg/d; max 45 mg/d as monotherapy, 30 mg/d in combination therapy	T: 15, 30, 45	Check LFTs at start, q 2 mo during 1st yr, then periodically; avoid if clinical evidence of liver disease or if serum ALT levels >2.5 times upper limit of normal; may increase risk of fractures in women (L, K)
Rosiglitazone (*Avandia*)	4 mg q 12–24 h	T: 2, 4, 8	Check LFTs at start, q 2 mo during 1st yr, then periodically; avoid if clinical evidence of liver disease or if serum ALT levels >2.5 times upper limit of normal; may increase risk of fractures in women (L, K)

(cont.)

Table 35. Non-insulin Agents for Treating Diabetes Mellitus (cont.)

Medication	Dosage	Formulations	Comments (Metabolism)
Combinations			
Glipizide and metformin (*METAGLIP*)	2.5/250 mg once; 20/2000 in 2 divided doses	T: 2.5/250, 2.5/500, 5/500	Avoid in patients >80 yr, Cr >1.5 mg/dL in men, Cr >1.4 mg/dL in women; see individual drugs (L, K)
Glyburide and metformin (*Glucovance*)	1.25/250 mg initially if previously untreated; 2.5/500 mg or 5/500 mg q 12 h with meals; max 20/2000/d	T: 1.25/250, 2.5/500, 5/500	Starting dose should not exceed total daily dose of either drug; see individual drugs (L, K)
Pioglitazone and metformin (*ACTOplus met*)	15/850 mg q 12–24 h	T: 15/850	See individual drugs.
Rosiglitazone and glimepiride (*Avandaryl*)	1 or 2 tab/d; max 8 mg/4 mg	T: 4/1, 4/2, 4/4	See individual drugs.
Rosiglitazone and metformin (*Avandamet*)	4/1000– 8/2000 mg in 2 divided doses	T: 1/500, 2/500, 4/500, 2/1000, 4/1000	Avoid in patients >80 yr, Cr >1.5 mg/dL in men, Cr >1.4 mg/dL in women; see individual drugs (L, K)
Pioglitazone and glimepiride (*Duetact*)	30/2 mg initially; max 45/8 mg	T: 30/2, 30/4	See individual drugs.
Sitagliptin and metformin (*Janumet*)	Begin with current doses; max 50/1000 mg	T: 50/500, 50/1000	See individual drugs.
Injectable Agents			
Exenatide *(Byetta)*	5–10 mcg SC q 12 h	1.2-, 2.4-mL pre-filled syringes	Incretin mimetic; lowers HbA_{1c} by 0.4%–0.9%; nausea and hypoglycemia common; less weight gain than insulin; avoid if CrCl <30 mL/min (K)
Pramlintide *(Symlin)*	60 mcg SC immediately before meals	0.6 mg/mL in 5-mL vial	Amylin analog; lowers HbA_{1c} by 0.4%–0.7%; nausea and hypoglycemia common; reduce pre-meal dose of short-acting insulin by 50% (K)

Table 36. Insulin Preparations

Preparation	Onset	Peak	Duration	Number of Injections or Inhalations/d
Rapid-acting				
Insulin glulisine (*Apidra*)	20 min	0.5–1.5 h	3–4 h	3
Insulin lispro (*Humalog*)	15 min	0.5–1.5 h	3–4 h	3
Insulin aspart (*NovoLog*)	30 min	1–3 h	3–5 h	3
Insulin inhaled (*Exubera*)[a] (1 mg inhaled = approx 3 IU regular insulin SC)	10–20 min	2 h	6 h	3
Regular (eg, *Humulin, Novolin*)[b]	0.5–1 h	2–3 h	8–12 h	1–3
Intermediate or long-acting				
NPH (eg, *Humulin, Novolin*)[b]	1–1.5 h	4–12 h	24 h	1–2
Insulin, zinc (*Lente*)	1–2.5 h	8–12 h	18–24 h	1–2
Insulin detemir (*Levemir*)	3–4 h	6–8 h	6–24 h depending on dose	1–2
Long-acting (*Ultralente*)	4–8 h	16–18 h	>36 h	1
Insulin glargine (*Lantus*)[c]	1–2 h	—	24 h	1
Isophane insulin and regular insulin inj, premixed (*Novolin 70/30*)	30 min	2–12 h	24 h	1–2

[a] Pulmonary spirometry before beginning, at 6 mo, and annually thereafter. If decline in FEV_1 is ≥20%, repeat function tests; if confirmed, D/C. If decline in FEV_1 is <20%, monitor more frequently and consider D/C. Not recommended in patients with underlying lung disease (eg, asthma, COPD). Absorption 20% lower in mild asthma, 2 times higher in COPD. Cough is common. Do not use in patients who smoke or have quit smoking in the last 6 mo; if patient begins smoking, D/C immediately because of increased risk of hypoglycemia.
[b] Also available as mixtures of NPH and regular in 50:50 proportions.
[c] To convert from NPH dosing, give same number of units once a day. For patients taking NPH q 12 h, decrease the total daily units by 20%, and titrate on basis of response. Starting dosage in insulin-naive patients is 10 U once daily hs.

Monitoring (ADA)

- Weight, BP, and foot examination, including monofilament testing at 4 plantar sites (great toe and base of first, third, and fifth metatarsals), palpation, and inspection, each visit; insensate feet should be inspected q 3–6 mo; well-fitted walking or athletic shoes may be of benefit
- HbA_{1c} twice/yr in patients with stable glycemic control; quarterly, if poor control
- Annual comprehensive dilated eye and visual examinations by an ophthalmologist or optometrist who is experienced in management of diabetic retinopathy
- Lipid profiles q 1–2 yr depending on whether values are in normal range
- Annual (unless microalbuminuria has previously been demonstrated) test for microalbuminuria by measuring albumin:creatinine ratio in a random spot collection
- Annual serum creatinine

DEFINITION

An event that results in a person inadvertently coming to rest on the ground or lower level with or without loss of consciousness or injury. Excludes falls from major intrinsic event (eg, seizure, stroke, syncope) or overwhelming environmental hazard.

ETIOLOGY

Typically multifactorial. Composed of intrinsic (eg, poor balance, weakness, chronic illness, visual or cognitive impairment), extrinsic (eg, polypharmacy), and environmental (eg, poor lighting, no safety equipment, loose carpets) factors. Commonly a nonspecific sign for one of many acute illnesses in older adults.

EVALUATION

Exclude acute illness or underlying systemic or metabolic process (eg, infection, electrolyte imbalance as indicated by hx, examination, and laboratory studies).
See **Figure 3** for recommended assessment and management.

- Laboratory tests for people at risk: CBC, serum electrolytes, BUN, Cr, glucose, B_{12}, thyroid function
- Bone densitometry in women not receiving osteoporosis treatment and in men with additional risk factors for osteoporotic fracture (see p 166)
- Echocardiography for those with cardiac conditions impairing blood flow to brain
- Imaging: neuroimaging if head injury or new, focal neurologic findings on examination or if a CNS process is suspected; spinal imaging to exclude cervical spondylosis or lumbar stenosis in patients with abnormal gait, neurologic examination, or lower extremity spasticity or hyperreflexia
- Ambulatory cardiac monitoring rarely helpful
- Arrhythmic evaluation only if clinical evidence of this diagnosis (eg, hx of cardiac events or abnormal ECG)
- Drug concentrations for anticonvulsants, antiarrhythmics, TCAs, and high-dose aspirin

History

- Circumstances of fall (eg, activity at time of fall, location, time)
- Associated symptoms (eg, lightheadedness, vertigo, syncope, weakness, confusion, palpitations)
- Relevant comorbid conditions (eg, prior stroke, parkinsonism, cardiac disease, diabetes mellitus, seizure disorder, depression, anxiety, anemia, sensory deficit, osteoarthritis, osteoporosis, cognitive or visual impairment)
- Previous falls
- Medication review, including OTC medications and alcohol use; note recent changes in medications (see p 10)
- Ask about person's ability to complete ADLs: bathing, dressing, transferring, continence (see p 245)

Figure 3. Assessment and Management of Falls

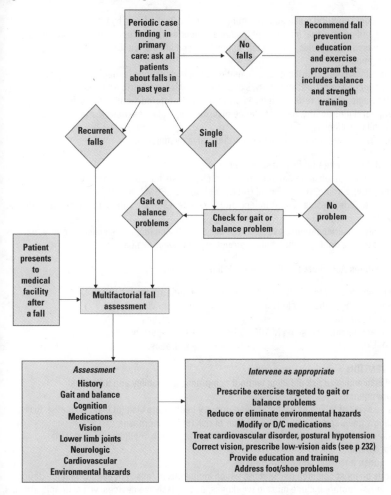

Sources: Adapted from American Geriatrics Society, British Geriatrics Society, and American Academy of Orthopaedic Surgeons Panel on Falls Prevention. Guideline for the prevention of falls in older persons. *J Amer Geriatr Soc*. 2001; 49(5):666; Tinetti M. Preventing falls in elderly persons. *N Engl J Med* 2003;348(1):42–49; and Ganz D, Bao Y, Shekelle P, Rubenstein L. Will my patient fall? *JAMA* 2007;207(1):77–86.

Physical Examination
Look for:
- Vital signs: postural pulse and BP changes at 1 and 2 min, fever, hypothermia
- Head and neck: visual impairment (especially poor acuity, reduced contrast sensitivity, decreased visual fields, cataracts), motion-induced imbalance (Dix-Hallpike test), bruit, nystagmus
- Musculoskeletal: arthritic changes, motion or joint limitations (especially lower extremity joint function), postural instability, skeletal deformities, podiatric problems
- Neurologic: slower reflexes, altered proprioception, altered mental status, focal deficits, peripheral neuropathy, gait or balance disorders, muscle weakness (especially leg), instability, tremor, rigidity
- Cardiovascular: heart arrhythmias, cardiac valve dysfunction

Gait, Balance, and Mobility Assessment
- Functional gait: observe patient rising from chair, walking (stride, length, velocity, symmetry), turning, sitting (Timed Get Up and Go test, POMA, p 244)
- Balance: Side-by-side, semi-tandem, and full tandem stance; Functional Reach test; POMA, p 244)
- Mobility: observe patient's use and fit of assistive device (eg, cane, walker) or personal assistance, extent of ambulation, restraint use, footwear evaluation

Medications Associated with Increased Risk of Falling

- Antipsychotics (especially phenothiazines)
- Sedatives, hypnotics (including benzodiazepines)
- Antidepressants (including MAOIs, SSRIs, TCAs)
- Antiarrhythmics (Class 1A)
- Anticonvulsants
- Anxiolytics
- Antihypertensives
- Diuretics

PREVENTION
Goal is to minimize risk of falling without compromising mobility and functional independence.
- Assess risk of falling as part of routine primary health care visit (at least annually). Risk of falling significantly increases as number of risk factors increases.
- Assess for risk factors using a multidisciplinary approach, including PT and OT if appropriate.
- Diagnose and treat underlying cause.
- Focus on most common risk factors, which include hx of falls, gait deficit, balance deficit. Other risk factors include muscle weakness, use of assistive devices, visual deficit, arthritis, impaired ADLs, depression, cognitive impairment, age >80 yr old.
- Begin fall prevention program targeting interventions for risk factors (see **Table 37**).
  - Evidence regarding use of hip protectors, as currently designed, does not support their effectiveness in preventing hip fractures in nursing home residents.
  - Recommend daily supplementation of calcium carbonate (1200 mg) and vitamin D (800 IU).

- Exercise program to include combination of resistance (strength) training, gait, balance, and coordination training
  - medical assessment before starting
  - tailor to individual capabilities
  - prescribed by qualified healthcare provider
  - regular review and progression

Table 37. Preventing Falls: Selected Risk Factors and Suggested Interventions

Factors	Suggested Interventions
Medication-related Factors	
Use of benzodiazepines, sedative-hypnotics, antidepressants, or antipsychotics	Consider agents with less risk of falls
	Taper and D/C medications, as possible
	Address sleep problems with nonpharmacologic interventions (see p 226)
	Educate regarding appropriate use of medications and monitoring for adverse events
Recent change in dosage or number of prescription medications *or* use of ≥4 prescription medications *or* use of other medications associated with fall risk	Review medication profile and reduce number and dosage of all medications, as possible
	Monitor response to medications and to dosage changes
Mobility-related Factors	
Presence of environmental hazards (eg, improper bed height, cluttered walking surfaces, lack of railings, poor lighting)	Improve lighting, especially at night
	Remove floor barriers (eg, loose carpeting)
	Replace existing furniture with safer furniture (eg, correct height, more stable)
	Install support structures, especially in bathroom (eg, railings, grab bars, elevated toilet seats)
	Use nonslip bathmats
Impaired gait, balance, or transfer skills	Refer to PT for comprehensive evaluation and rehabilitation and for training in use of assistive devices
	Gait training
	Balance or strengthening exercises (see also p 191)
	If able to perform tandem stance, refer for Tai Chi, dance, yoga, or postural awareness
	Provide training in transfer skills
	Prescribe appropriate assistive devices
	Recommend protective hip padding
	Recommend appropriate footwear (eg, good fit, non-slip, low heel height, large surface contact area)

(cont.)

Table 37. Preventing Falls: Selected Risk Factors and Suggested Interventions (cont.)

Factors	Suggested Interventions
Impaired leg or arm strength or range of motion, or proprioception	Strengthening exercises (eg, use of resistive rubber bands, putty)
	Resistance training 2–3 ×/wk to 10 repetitions with full range of motion, then increase resistance
	Tai Chi
	Physical therapy
Medical Factors	
Parkinson's disease, osteoarthritis, depressive symptoms, impaired cognition, carotid sinus hypersensitivity, other conditions associated with increased falls	Optimize medical therapy
	Monitor for disease progression and impact on mobility and impairments
	Determine need for assistive devices
	Use bedside commode if frequent nighttime urination
	Cardiac pacing in patients with carotid sinus hypersensitivity who experience falls due to syncope
Postural hypotension: drop in SBP ≥20 mmHg (or ≥20%) with or without symptoms, either immediately or within 3 min of standing (see also orthostatic postural hypotension, p 50)	Review medications potentially contributing and adjust dosing or switch to less hypotensive agents; avoid vasodilators and diuretics if possible
	Educate on activities to decrease effect (eg, slow rising, ankle pumps, hand clenching, elevation of head of bed) and to slow rising from recumbent or seated position, grab bars by toilet and bath
	Prescribe pressure stockings (eg, Jobst)
	Liberalize salt intake, if appropriate
	Caffeinated coffee (1 cup) or caffeine 100 mg with meals for postprandial hypotension
	Consider medication to increase BP (if HTN, HF, and hypokalemia not serious): -midodrine (*ProAmatine*) 2.5–5 mg q 8 h [T: 2.5, 5] -fludrocortisone (*Florinef*) 0.1 mg q 8–24 h [T: 0.1]
Visual or hearing impairment (see Visual Impairment, p 231; Hearing Impairment, p 98)	Refraction
	Cataract extraction
	Good lighting
	Home safety evaluation
	Mobility training for visually impaired
	Cerumen removal
	Audiological evaluation with hearing aid, if appropriate

DYSPHAGIA
See also p 183.

Presentation/Patient Complaints
Structural:
- Pocketing of food in cheeks, on hard palate, or under tongue
- Food gets stuck after swallowing
- Speech abnormalities: slurring, gurgly voice
- Orofacial changes: facial weakness, abnormal tongue movements

Functional:
- Inability to initiate a swallow
- Impaired ability to transfer food from mouth to esophagus
- Nasal regurgitation
- Coughing (aspiration)
- Drooling or excessive secretions
- Reluctance to eat specific foods or foods of certain consistency, or to eat at all

Common Causes
- Cerebrovascular accident/stroke
- Parkinson's disease
- Oropharyngeal tumors
- Zenker's diverticulum
- Cervical osteophytes
- GERD
- Multifactorial (eg, transfer dysphagia)

Evaluation
- Physical examination
  - Oral cavity, head, neck, and supraclavicular region
  - All cranial nerves with emphasis on nerves V, VII, IX, X, XI, XII
- Review medications for those that can decrease saliva production (eg, anticholinergics)
- Referral to speech-language pathologists
- Diagnostic tests
  - Modified barium swallow or videofluoroscopy to assess swallowing mechanism; may document aspiration
  - Upper endoscopy
  - Fiberoptic nasopharyngeal laryngoscopy provides detailed evaluation of lesions in oropharynx, hypopharynx, larynx, and proximal esophagus; also visualizes pooled secretions or food
  - Esophageal manometry often used in combination with barium radiography; more useful for assessment of esophageal dysphagia

Treatment
- Identify and treat underlying cause (eg, endoscopic dilation, cricopharyngeal myotomy, botulinum toxin injection in cricopharyngeal muscle)
- Dietary modifications based on recommendation of speech pathologist, occupational therapist, or dietitian

- Swallowing rehabilitation, eg, multiple swallows, tilt head back and place bolus on strong side, chin tuck
- Elevate head of the bed
- Review medications and administration for unsafe practices, eg, crushing enteric-coated or ER formulations

Food Consistencies
- Pureed: thick, homogenous textures; pudding-like
- Ground/minced: easily chewed without coarse texture; excludes most raw foods except mashed bananas
- Soft or easy to chew: soft foods prepared without a blender; tender meats cut to ≤1-cm pieces; excludes nuts, tough skins, and raw, crispy, or stringy foods
- Modified general: soft textures that do not require grinding or chopping

Fluid Consistencies and Thickening Agents
- Thin: regular fluids; no change in fluids
- Nectar-like: thin enough to be sipped through a straw or from a cup, but still spillable (eg, eggnog, buttermilk); 2–3 tsp of thickening powder to ½ cup (4 fl oz) of liquid
- Honey-like: thick enough to be eaten with a spoon, too thick for a straw, not able to independently hold its shape (eg, yogurt, tomato sauce, honey); 3–5 tsp of thickening powder to ½ cup (4 fl oz) of liquid
- Spoon-thick: pudding-like, must be eaten with a spoon (eg, thick milk pudding, thickened applesauce); 5–6 tsp of thickening powder to ½ cup (4 fl oz) of liquid

GASTROESOPHAGEAL REFLUX DISEASE (GERD)
Evaluation and Assessment
Empiric treatment is appropriate when hx is typical for uncomplicated GERD.
- Endoscopy (if symptoms are chronic or persist despite initial management, atypical presentation)
- Ambulatory pH testing

Symptoms Suggesting Complicated GERD and Need for Evaluation
- Dysphagia
- Bleeding
- Weight loss
- Anemia
- Choking, cough, shortness of breath, or hoarseness
- Chest pain
- Pain with swallowing

Management
- Antacids
- Avoid alcohol and fatty foods
- Avoid lying down for 3 h after eating
- Avoid tight-fitting clothes
- Change diet (avoid pepper, spearmint, chocolate, spicy or acidic foods)
- Drink 6–8 oz water with all medications
- Elevate head of the bed (6–8 in)
- Lose weight (if overweight)
- Stop drugs that may promote reflux
- Stop smoking
- Consider surgery

Table 38. Pharmacologic Management of GERD

Medication	Initial Oral Dosage	Formulations (Metabolism, Excretion)
Proton-pump Inhibitors		
✔ Esomeprazole (*Nexium*)	20 mg/d × 4 wk	C: ER 20, 40 (L)
✔ Lansoprazole (*Prevacid*)	15 mg/d × 8 wk	C: ER 15, 30; granules for susp: 15, 30/packet (L)
✔ Omeprazole (*Prilosec*)	20 mg/d × 4–8 wk	C: ER 10, 20,[a] 40; T: enteric-coated 20 (L)
✔ Pantoprazole (*Protonix*)	40 mg/d × 8 wk	T: enteric-coated 20, 40; inj (L)
✔ Rabeprazole (*AcipHex*)	20 mg/d × 4–8 wk; 20 mg/d maintenance, if needed	T: enteric-coated ER 20 (L)
H$_2$ Antagonists (for less severe GERD)		
Cimetidine (*Tagamet*)	400 or 800 mg q 12 h	S: 200 mg/20 mL, 300 mg/5 mL with alcohol 2.8%; T: 100, 200,[a] 300, 400, 800; inj (K, L)
✔ Famotidine (*Pepcid*)	20 mg q 12 h × 6 wk	S: oral sus 40 mg/5 mL; T: film-coated 10,[a] 20, 40, oral disintegrating 20, 40; C (gel): 10[a]; ChT: 10[a]; inj (K)
✔ Nizatidine (*Axid*)	150 mg q 12 h	C: 150, 300; T: 75 (K)
Ranitidine (*Zantac*)	150 mg q 12 h	Pk: gran, effervescent (EFFERdose) 150 mg; S: syr 15 mg/mL; T: 75,[a] 150, 300; T: effervescent (EFFERdose) 150; inj (K, F)
Mucosal Protective Agent		
Sucralfate (*Carafate*)	1 g q 6 h, 1 h ac, and hs	S: oral sus 1 g/10 mL; T: 1 g (F, K)
Prokinetic Agents		
Bethanechol (*Urecholine*)	25 mg q 6 h	T: 5, 10, 25, 50 (unknown)
Metoclopramide[b] (*Reglan*)	5 mg q 6 h, ac, and hs	S: syr, sugar-free 5 mg/5 mL, conc 10 mg/mL; T: 5, 10; inj (K, F)

✔ = preferred for treating older adults
[a] OTC strength
[b] Risk of EPS high in people >65 yr old.
Source: Data from DeVault KR, Castell DO. Updated guidelines for the diagnosis and treatment of gastroesophageal reflux disease. *Am J Gastroenterol* 2005;100(1):190–200.

PEPTIC ULCER DISEASE
Causes
Helicobacter pylori is the major cause. NSAIDs are the second most common cause.

Diagnosis of *H pylori*
• Endoscopic examination
• Serology
• Urea breath test

Initial Treatment Options

- Empiric anti-ulcer treatment for 6 wk
- Definitive diagnostic evaluation by endoscopy
- Noninvasive testing for *H pylori* and treatment with antibiotics for those that test positive (see **Table 39** for regimens)
- Review patient's chronic medications for drug interactions before selecting regimen; many potential drug interactions and adverse drug events.

Table 39. FDA-approved Treatments for *H pylori*–induced Ulcerations (all oral routes)

Lansoprazole 30 mg q 12 h + amoxicillin 1 g q 12 h + clarithromycin 500 mg q 8 h × 10 (or 14) d

or Omeprazole 20 mg q 12 h + clarithromycin 500 mg q 12 h + amoxicillin 1 g q 12 h × 10 d

or Lansoprazole 30 mg q 12 h + clarithromycin 500 mg q 12 h + amoxicillin 1 g q 12 h × 10 d (*Prevpac*)

or Omeprazole 40 mg/d + clarithromycin 500 mg q 8 h × 2 wk, then omeprazole 20 mg/d × 2 wk

or Lansoprazole 30 mg q 8 h + amoxicillin 1 g q 12 h × 2 wk (only for patients allergic to or who cannot tolerate clarithromycin)

or Ranitidine bismuth citrate (RBC) 400 mg q 12 h + clarithromycin 500 mg q 8 h × 2 wk, then RBC 400 mg q 12 h × 2 wk

or RBC 400 mg q 12 h + clarithromycin 500 mg q 12 h × 2 wk, then RBC 400 mg q 12 h × 2 wk

or Bismuth subsalicylate (*Pepto-Bismol*) 525 mg q 6 h (pc and hs) + metronidazole 250 mg q 6 h + tetracycline 500 mg q 6 h × 2 wk (*Helidac, Pylera*) + H₂ receptor antagonist or proton-pump inhibitor as directed × 4 wk

or Esomeprazole 20 mg q 12 h or 40 mg q 24 h + clarithromycin 500 mg q 12 h + amoxicillin 1 g q 12 h × 10 d

or Rabeprazole 20 mg q 12 h + clarithromycin 500 mg q 12 h + amoxicillin 1 g q 12 h × 7 d

---

Source: www.cdc.gov/ulcer/keytocure.htm#treatment.

Medications

Bismuth subsalicylate (*Pepto-Bismol*) [T: 324; ChT: 262; S: sus 262 mg/15 mL, 525 mg/15 mL]
Antibiotics: (for complete information, see **Table 53**)
Amoxicillin (*Amoxil*) [C: 250, 500; ChT: 125, 250; S: oral sus 125 mg/5 mL, 250 mg/5 mL]
Clarithromycin (*Biaxin*) [T: film-coated 250, 500; S: oral sus 125 mg/5 mL, 250 mg/5 mL]
Metronidazole (*Flagyl*) [T: 250, 500, 750; C: 375]
Tetracycline (*Achromycin, Sumycin*) [T: 250, 500; S: oral sus 125 mg/5 mL]
Proton-pump Inhibitors: See **Table 38**.

STRESS-ULCER PREVENTION IN HOSPITALIZED OLDER ADULTS
Risk Factors (in order of prevalence in older adults)

- Hx of GI ulceration or bleed in past year
- Sepsis
- Multiple organ failure
- Hypotension
- Mechanical ventilation for >48 h
- Kidney failure
- Major trauma, shock, or head injury
- Coagulopathy (platelets <50,000/μL, INR >1.5, or PTT >2 × control)
- Burns over >25% of body surface area
- Hepatic failure
- Intracranial hypertension
- Spinal cord injury
- Quadraplegia

Prophylaxis
- H$_2$ antagonists (see **Table 38**)
- Proton-pump inhibitors (see **Table 38**)
- Sucralfate (see **Table 38**)
- Antacids
- Enteral feedings

Discontinue H$_2$ antagonists, proton-pump inhibitors, and other treatments for stress-ulcer prevention before transfer or discharge from hospital.

Key Points
- Prophylaxis has not been shown to reduce mortality.
- No one regimen has shown superior efficacy.
- Choice of regimen depends on access to and function of GI tract and presence of nasogastric suction.

IRRITABLE BOWEL SYNDROME (IBS)
Signs and Symptoms
Symptoms should be present ≥12 wk.
Consistent with IBS:
- Abdominal pain
- Bloating
- Constipation
- Diarrhea

Not Consistent with IBS:
- Weight loss
- First onset after age 50
- Nocturnal diarrhea
- Family hx of cancer or inflammatory bowel disease
- Rectal bleeding or obstruction
- Laboratory abnormalities
- Presence of fecal parasites

Diagnosis (of exclusion)
Exclude ischemia, diverticulosis, colon cancer, inflammatory bowel disease by physical examination and testing (colonoscopy, CT scan, or small-bowel series)

Treatment
- Reassurance; not life threatening; focus on relief of physical and emotional symptoms
- Dietary modification
  - Avoid foods that trigger symptoms or produce excess gas or bloating
  - Consider a trial of a lactose-free diet
- Behavioral interventions: hypnosis, biofeedback, psychotherapy have been shown to be more effective than placebo
- Fiber supplements (see **Table 40**)
  - Synthetic: polycarbophil (*FiberCon* [caplet: 625], others), methylcellulose (*Citrucel, Fiber Ease* [C, sus, pwd])
  - Natural: psyllium (*Metamucil* [C, T, wafer, pwd], others)
- Antispasmodics (short-term use only)
  - Dicyclomine (*Bentyl* [C: 10; T: 20; syr: 10 mg/5 mL; inj]) 10–20 mg po q 6 h prn (L)
  - Hyoscyamine (*Anazpaz, Levsin, Levsin/SL,* others [T (sl): 0.125, 0.15; T ER, C: 0.375; inj: 125 sol]) 0.125–0.25 mg po/sl q 6–8 h prn (L, K)

- Antidiarrheals: may be helpful for diarrhea but not for global IBS symptoms, abdominal pain, or constipation
  - Loperamide (*Imodium A-D* [C, T: 2; sol 1 mg/5 mL]) 4 mg × 1, then 2 mg after each loose bowel movement; max 16 mg/24 h
- Antidepressants
  - TCAs and SSRIs may be beneficial for patients with diarrhea or pain. See Depression, p 61, for dosing.
- Serotonin agent
  - Alosetron (*Lotronex* [T: 0.5, 1]): serotonin 3 antagonist; treatment of women with severe diarrhea-predominant IBS who have not responded to conventional therapy; 0.5 mg po q 12 h × 4 wk, increase to 1 mg q 12 h × 4 wk, stop if no response (K, L)

CONSTIPATION

Medications That Constipate
- Analgesics—opiates
- Antacids with aluminum or calcium
- Anticholinergic drugs
- Antidepressants, lithium
- Antihypertensives
- Antipsychotics
- Barium sulfate
- Bismuth
- Calcium channel blockers
- Diuretics
- Iron

Conditions That Constipate
- Colon tumor or mechanical obstruction
- Dehydration
- Depression
- Diabetes mellitus
- Hypercalcemia
- Hypokalemia
- Hypothyroidism
- Immobility
- Low intake of fiber
- Panhypopituitarism
- Parkinson's disease
- Spinal cord injury
- Stroke
- Uremia

Management of Chronic Constipation
Step 1. Stop all constipating medications, when possible.

Step 2. Increase dietary fiber to 6–25 g/d, increase fluid intake to ≥1500 mL/d, and increase physical activity; or add bulk laxative (**Table 40**), provided fluid intake is ≥1500 mL/d. If fiber exacerbates symptoms or is not tolerated, go to Step 3.

Step 3. Add 70% sorbitol solution (15–30 mL q 12–24 h, max 150 mL/d).

Step 4. Add stimulant laxative (eg, senna, bisacodyl), 2–3 times/wk. (Alternative: saline laxative, but avoid if CrCl <30 mL/min.)

Step 5. Use tap water enema or saline enema 2 times/wk.

Step 6. Use oil-retention enema for refractory constipation.

Table 40. Medications That May Relieve Constipation

Medication	Onset of Action	Starting Dosage	Site and Mechanism of Action
Bulk laxatives—not useful in managing opiate-induced constipation			
Methylcellulose (*Citrucel**), Psyllium (*Metamucil**)	12–24 h (up to 72 h)	1–2 rounded tsp or packets q 8–24 h with water or juice	Small and large intestine; holds water in feces; mechanical distention
Polycarbophil (*FiberCon**, others)	12–24 h (up to 72 h)	1250 mg q 6–24 h	Small and large intestine; holds water in feces; mechanical distention
Chloride channel activator			
Lubiprostone (*Amitiza*)		24 mcg q 12 h with food	Enhances chloride-ion intestinal fluid secretion; does not affect serum Na^+ or K^+ concentrations. For idiopathic chronic constipation.
Osmotic laxatives			
Lactulose (*Chronulac*)	24–48 h	15–30 mL q 12–24 h	Colon; osmotic effect
Polyethylene glycol (*Miralax**)	48–96 h	17 g pwd q 24 h (~1 tbsp) dissolved in 8 oz water	GI tract; osmotic effect
Sorbitol 70%*	24–48 h	15–30 mL q 12–24 h	Colon; delivers osmotically active molecules to colon
Saline laxatives			Class effect: potential hyperphosphatemia in patients with renal insufficiency
Magnesium citrate (*Citroma**)	30 min–3 h	120–240 mL × 1; 10 oz q 24 h or 5 oz q 12 h followed by 8 oz water × ≤5 d	Small and large intestine; attracts, retains water in intestinal lumen
Magnesium hydroxide (*Milk of Magnesia**)	30 min–3 h	30 mL q 12–24 h	Osmotic effect and increased peristalsis in colon
Sodium phosphate/ biphosphate emollient enema (*Fleet**)	2–15 min	14.5-oz enema × 1, repeat prn	Colon, osmotic effect
Stimulant laxatives			
Bisacodyl tablet (*Dulcolax**)	6–10 h	5–15 mg × 1	Colon; increases peristalsis
Bisacodyl suppository (*Dulcolax**)	15 min–1 h	10 mg × 1	Colon; increases peristalsis
Senna (*Senokot**)	6–10 h	2 tabs or 1 tsp qhs	Colon; direct action on intestine; stimulates myenteric plexus; alters water and electrolyte secretion
Surfactant laxative (fecal softener)			
Docusate (*Colace**)	24–72 h	100 mg q 12–24 h	Small and large intestine; detergent activity; facilitates admixture of fat and water to soften feces (effectiveness questionable)

*Available OTC

NAUSEA AND VOMITING
Causes
- CNS disorders (eg, motion sickness, intracranial lesions)
- Drugs (eg, chemotherapy, NSAIDs, opioid analgesics, antibiotics, digoxin)
- GI disorders (eg, mechanical obstruction; inflammation of stomach, intestine, or gallbladder; pseudo-obstruction; motility disorders; dyspepsia; diabetic gastroparesis)
- Infections (eg, viral or bacterial gastroenteritis, hepatitis, otitis, meningitis)
- Metabolic conditions (eg, uremia, acidosis, hyperparathyroidism, adrenal insufficiency)
- Psychiatric disorders

Evaluation
- If patient is not seriously ill or dehydrated, can probably wait 24–48 h to see if symptoms resolve spontaneously.
- If patient is seriously ill, dehydrated, or has other signs of acute illness, hospitalize for further evaluation.
- If symptoms persist, evaluate on the basis of the most likely causes.

Pharmacologic Management
- If analgesic drug is suspected, decrease dosage, consider adding antiemetic until tolerance develops, or change to a different analgesic drug.
- Drugs that are useful in the management of nausea and vomiting are listed in **Table 41**.

Table 41. Antiemetic Therapy

Class/Site of Action	Dosage (Metabolism)	Formulation
Dopamine antagonists/CTZ[a] vomiting center		
Haloperidol	IV, IM, po: 0.5–1 mg q 6 h (L, K)	See page 199.
Droperidol	IV, IM: 2.5 mg, repeat with 1.25 mg prn (L)	Inj: 2.5 mg/mL
Metoclopramide (*Reglan*)	PONV[b]: 5–10 mg IM near the end of surgery Chemotherapy (IV): 1–2 mg/kg 30 min before and q 2–4 h or q 4–6 h (K)	T: 5, 10 S: 10 mg/mL; syr (sugar-free): 5 mg/mL Inj: 5 mg/mL
Prochlorperazine (*Compazine*)	IM, po: 5–10 mg q 6–8 h, usual max 40 mg/d IV: 2.5–10 mg, max 10 mg/dose or 40 mg/d; may repeat q 3–4 h prn (L)	T: 5, 10, 25 mg C: 10, 15, 30 mg Syr: 5 mg/5 mL Inj: 5 mg/mL
Serotonin (5-HT$_3$) antagonists/CTZ, gut		
Ondansetron (*Zofran*)	PONV: 16 mg po 1 h before anesthesia IM, IV: 4 mg immediately before anesthesia; repeat if needed (L)	T: 4, 8, 24 mg T: oral disintegrating; 4, 8 mg S: 4 mg/5 mL Inj: 2 mg/mL
Granisetron (*Kytril*)	PONV: 1 mg IV before anesthesia or anesthesia reversal Chemotherapy: 2 mg/d po (L, K)	T: 1 mg S: 2 mg/10 mL Inj: 1 mg/mL
Dolasetron (*Anzemet*)	PONV: 100 mg po 2 h before surgery; 12.5 mg IV 15 min before stopping anesthesia (L)	T: 50, 100 mg Inj: 20 mg/mL

(cont.)

Table 41. Antiemetic Therapy (cont.)		
Class/Site of Action	**Dosage (Metabolism)**	**Formulation**
Antimuscarinic/H₁ antagonist/vestibular apparatus		
Diphenhydrinate[c] (*Dramamine*)	IM, IV, po: 50–100 mg q 4–6 h; max 400 mg/d (L)	T, ChT: 50 mg S: 12.5 mg/4 mL, 16.62 mg/5 mL Inj: 10 mg/mL
Meclizine[c] (*Antivert*)	Motion sickness: 12.5–25 mg 1 h before travel, repeat dose q 12–24 h if needed Vertigo: 25–100 mg/d in divided doses (L)	T: 12.5, 25, 50 mg ChT: 25 mg C: 25, 30 mg
Scopolamine (*Transderm Scop*)	Motion sickness: apply 1 pch behind ear ≥4 h before travel/exposure; change q 3 d (L)	Pch: 1.5 mg

[a] Chemoreceptor trigger zone
[b] Postoperative nausea and vomiting
[c] Available OTC
Note: All have potential CNS toxicity.

DIARRHEA
Causes
• Drugs (eg, antibiotics [see **Table 53** and p 96], laxatives, colchicine)
• Fecal impaction
• GI disorders (eg, irritable bowel syndrome, malabsorption, inflammatory bowel disease)
• Infections (eg, viral, bacterial, parasitic)
• Lactose intolerance

Evaluation
• If patient is not seriously ill or dehydrated and there is no blood in the feces, can probably wait 48 h to see if symptoms resolve spontaneously.
• If patient is seriously ill, dehydrated, or has other signs of acute illness, hospitalize for further evaluation.
• If diarrhea persists, evaluate on the basis of the most likely causes.

Pharmacologic Management
Drugs that are useful in the management of diarrhea are listed in **Table 42**.

Table 42. Antidiarrheals

Drug	Dosage (Metabolism)	Formulations
✔ Attapulgite[a] (*Kaopectate*)	1200–1500 mg after each loose bowel movement or q 2 h; 15–30 mL up to 9 × /d, up to 9000 mg/24 h (not absorbed)	S: oral conc 600, 750 mg/15 mL; T: 750; ChT: 300, 600
✔ Bismuth subsalicylate[a] (*Pepto-Bismol*)	2 tabs or 30 mL q 30–60 min prn up to 8 doses/24 h (L, K)	S: 262 mg/15 mL, 525 mg/15 mL; T: 324; ChT: 262
Diphenoxylate with atropine (*Lomotil*)[b]	15–20 mg/d of diphenoxylate in 3–4 divided doses; maintenance 5–15 mg/d in 2–3 divided doses (L)	S: oral, diphenoxylate hydrochloride 2.5 mg + atropine sulfate 0.025 mg/5 mL; T: diphenoxylate hydrochloride 2.5 mg + atropine sulfate 0.025 mg
✔ Loperamide[a] (*Imodium A-D*)	Initial: 4 mg followed by 2 mg after each loose bowel movement, up to 16 mg/d (L)	Caplet: 2; C: 2; T: 2; S: oral, 1 mg/5 mL

✔ = preferred for treating older adults
[a] Available OTC
[b] Anticholinergic, potential CNS toxicity

ANTIBIOTIC-ASSOCIATED DIARRHEA
(Antibiotic-associated pseudomembranous colitis [AAPMC])

Definition
A specific form of *Clostridium difficile* pseudomembranous colitis

Risk Factors
Almost any oral or parenteral antibiotic and several antineoplastic agents, including cyclophosphamide, doxorubicin, fluorouracil, methotrexate

Prevention
Probiotic products (eg, *DanActive*) containing *Lactobacillus caseia, Streptococcus thermophilus*, and *L bulgaricus* have been shown to decrease the incidence of antibiotic-associated diarrhea and *C difficile* diarrhea.

Presentation

- Abdominal pain, cramping
- Dehydration
- Diarrhea (can be bloody)
- Fecal leukocytes
- Fever (100–105°F)
- Hypoalbuminemia
- Hypovolemia
- Leukocytosis

Symptoms appear a few days after starting to 10 wk after discontinuing the offending agent.

Evaluation and Empiric Management
- D/C unnecessary antibiotics, and agents that can slow gastric motility such as opioids and antidiarrheal agents.
- Perform *C difficile* toxin test on 2 separate bowel movements. If suspicion remains after 2 negative tests, a third toxin test can be performed.
- Place patient in contact isolation and observe infection control procedures. Hand washing is crucial and must be done with soap and water to remove spores. Hand sanitizers do not kill or remove spores.
- Provide adequate fluid and electrolyte replacement.
- Consider empiric metronidazole (see below for dosing).

Diagnosis
Isolation of *C difficile* or its toxin from symptomatic patient. At least two negative fecal examinations are needed to exclude diagnosis.

Treatment
C difficile toxin positive
- Begin or continue metronidazole (*Flagyl*) po 250 mg q 6 h or 500 mg po q 8 h × 10 d; alternative: vancomycin po 125–500 mg q 6 h × 10 d
- Continue contact isolation for 1 wk after symptoms resolve or treatment ends
- If no response after 5 d, D/C metronidazole and start vancomycin

C difficile toxin negative (2 or 3 tests)
- D/C contact isolation
- D/C metronidazole
- Begin antidiarrheal agent
- Evaluate other causes for diarrhea

Recurrence
- Experienced by up to 25% of patients 1–4 wk after treatment
- Re-treat with oral metronidazole or vancomycin

HEARING IMPAIRMENT

DEFINITION
The most common sensory impairment in old age. To quantify hearing ability, the necessary intensity (decibel = dB) and frequency (Hertz) of the perceived pure-tone signal must be described.

EVALUATION
Screening and Evaluation
- Note problems during conversation
- Ask about hearing dysfunction
- Use a standardized questionnaire (see p 244)
- Test with handheld audioscope
- Use whisper test—stand behind patient 2 ft from ear, cover untested ear, fully exhale, whisper an easily answered question
- Refer patients who screen positive for audiologic evaluation

Audiometry
- Documents the dB loss across frequencies
- Determines the pattern of loss (see Classification, below)
- Determines if loss is unilateral or bilateral (*Note:* If speech discrimination is <50%, results with hearing aids may be poor.)

Aggravating Factors
- Sensorineural loss—medication ototoxicity (eg, aminoglycosides, loop diuretics, quinine, cisplatin), cerumen impaction (see p 99)
- Conductive loss—cerumen impaction, external otitis

CLASSIFICATION
Sensorineural Hearing Loss
- Due to cochlear or retrocochlear pathology
- Thresholds for both air and bone conduction increased (Weber test lateralizes away from impaired ear, Rinne test normal in both ears)
- Causes: aging, cranial nerve VIII damage from syphilis, viral meningitis, trauma, vascular events to cranial nerve VIII or cortical tracts, acoustic neuroma, Ménière's disease

Conductive Hearing Loss
- Occurs when sound transmission to inner ear is impaired
- Bone conduction better than air conduction (Weber test lateralizes toward impaired ear, Rinne test abnormal in impaired ear)
- Causes: external or middle ear disorders, including otosclerosis; rheumatoid arthritis; Paget's disease

Central Auditory Processing Disorder
- Loss of speech discrimination in excess of that from loss in hearing sensitivity
- Involves the CNS
- Occurs in dementia and infrequently with presbycusis

Presbycusis (Old-age Hearing Loss, a Subtype of Sensorineural Loss)
- Mainly high-frequency loss
- Impaired speech discrimination
- Recruitment (an increase in sensation of loudness)

MANAGEMENT
Remove Ear Wax
Fill ear canal with 5–10 gtt water and cover with cotton q 12 h × ≥4 d. Liquid must stay in contact with ear for ≥15 min. Hearing may worsen as cerumen expands. Water is as effective as commercial preparations (eg, *Debrox, Cerumenex, Colace*). Use of any of the commercial preparations for >4 d may cause ear irritation.

Table 43. Effects and Rehabilitation of Hearing Loss, by Level of Loss

Level of Loss	Difficulty Understanding	Need for Hearing Aid
0–24 dB	None	None
25–40 dB (mild)	Normal speech	In specific situations
41–55 dB (moderate)	Loud speech	Frequent
56–80 dB (severe)	Anything but amplified speech	For all communication
≥81 dB (profound)	Even amplified speech	Plus speech reading, aural rehabilitation, sign language, or cochlear implants

Source: Data in part from *A Report on Hearing Aids: User Perspectives and Concerns*. Washington, DC: American Association of Retired Persons; 1993:2.

Hearing Devices
Hearing Aids: Appropriate for most hearing-impaired people; enhance select frequencies; should be individualized for each ear. Amplification in both ears (binaural) provides best speech understanding; unilateral aid may be appropriate if hearing loss is asymmetrical, if hearing-aid care is challenging, or if cost is a factor. New features that enhance sound and speech quality include directional microphones, open-fit hearing aids, and ear-to-ear wireless coordination.

Assistive Listening Devices: Microphone placed close to sound source transmits to headphones or earpiece. Transmission is by wire or wireless (FM or infrared); these systems increase signal-to-noise ratio, which is useful for people with central auditory processing disorder. Personal pocket devices (eg, *Pocket Talker*) are inexpensive; every care setting should have one.

Telephone Device for the Deaf (TDD): Receiver is a keyboard that allows the hearing-impaired person to respond.

Cochlear Implants: Bypass the middle ear, directly innervate auditory nerve. Reserved for severe and profound hearing loss (score ≤40% on the sentence recognition test in the ear to be implanted). Results after age 65 comparable to those in younger people. Failure rate <1%, but patient selection important. Hybrid devices that add an acoustic component to the electrical stimulation of traditional devices are being tested.

Tips for Communication with Hearing-impaired People
- Ask the person how best to communicate
- Stand 2–3 ft away
- Have the person's attention
- Have the person seated in front of a wall, which helps reflect sound
- Speak toward the better ear
- Use lower-pitched voice
- Speak slowly and distinctly; don't shout
- Rephrase rather than repeat
- Pause at the end of phrases or ideas
- Ask the person to repeat what was heard

TINNITUS
Definition
The perception of sound in the absence of external acoustic stimulation; may be ringing, crackling, or whistling; may be continuous or intermittent
Objective Tinnitus
Noise heard by both patient and examiner (rare); usually due to abnormal blood flow in or around ear (normal anatomic variants or a pathologic condition)
Subjective Tinnitus
- Cannot be heard externally by others (common)
- Normal tinnitus lasts <5 min, <once/week
- Pathologic tinnitus lasts >5 min, >weekly (usually in people with hearing loss)

Evaluation
- Auscultate the head and neck near ear orbits, mastoids for objective tinnitus.
  - If pulsatile, obtain CT/MRA for vascular cause.
  - If continuous, obtain MRI looking for patulous Eustachian tube; other causes include palatal myoclonus, stapedial muscle spasm.
  - Refer to otolaryngology
- Examine ear canals for cerumen, otitis externa or interna; treat and reassess.
- Assess hearing (as above); unilateral hearing loss and tinnitus suggest acoustic neuroma; obtain MRI.
- Audiometry (see p 98)
- Check medication list for drugs associated with tinnitus, eg, NSAIDs, ASA, antibiotics (especially erythromycin), loop diuretics (especially furosemide), chemotherapy, quinine.

Treatment
- Objective tinnitus: refer to otolaryngology.
- Subjective tinnitus without distress:
  - Normal tinnitus: reassure patient.
  - Pathologic tinnitus: educate patient, encourage amplification for those with hearing impairment.
- Subjective tinnitus with distress:
  - Severe complaints about tinnitus are often a sign of depression; treat if indicated (see p 61).
  - Refer to audiology for tinnitus control instruments and desensitization therapy.

ANEMIA
Evaluation

- Hematopoietic reserve capacity declines with age, eg, slower return of Hb to normal after phlebotomy.
- Evaluate people >65 yr old when Hb <13.
- Evaluate if Hb falls >1 g/dL in 1 yr.
- Physical examination and laboratory tests for kidney or liver disease.
- Evaluate GI and GU source if iron deficient.
- Check WBC and peripheral blood smear; pursue suspected causes as appropriate.
- Combined deficiencies are common in older adults; reasonable to check B_{12}, folate, and iron in all cases.
- Check reticulocyte count and reticulocyte index.
  - Reticulocyte count or index high: adequate response, suspect blood loss or RBC destruction
  - Reticulocyte count or index normal or low: check MCV
    - MCV >100 μm^3/cell: see **Figure 4**
    - MCV <100 μm^3/cell: see **Figure 5**

Common Anemias of Later Life: Diagnosis and Treatment

Iron deficiency anemia: Usual laboratory values (iron, TIBC, ferritin) less reliable in presence of inflammatory conditions (see **Figure 5**). Soluble transferrin receptors (sTfR) help differentiate anemia of chronic disease from that of iron deficiency; elevated receptors suggest iron deficiency. The ratio sTfR/log ferritin is the best test for identification of iron deficiency in the presence of chronic disease.

Chronic disease anemia:
- Most common causes in older adults:
  - Acute and chronic infection
  - Chronic inflammation
  - Malignancy
  - Protein calorie malnutrition
  - Unidentified chronic disease
- Laboratory tests: usually low iron, low or normal TIBC, high ferritin, low sTfR
- Type determines treatability:
  - "Rheumatoid arthritis type" responds to erythropoietin at usual dosages (see **Table 44**).
  - "Cancer type" may respond to erythropoietin at high dosages (see **Table 44**).
- Restoring Hb to 10–12 g/dL improves quality of life, function, and possibly survival.

Combined iron deficiency and anemia of chronic disease:
- Anemia often more severe than in chronic disease alone.
- Ferritin low to normal.
- Iron, transferrin, and saturation reduced.
- Elevated sTfR documents iron deficiency; if sTfR is normal, calculate ratio of sTfR/log ferritin (see **Figure 5**) or give iron trial and check reticulocyte count in 2 wk.

Figure 4. Evaluation of Hypoproliferative Anemia with High MCV

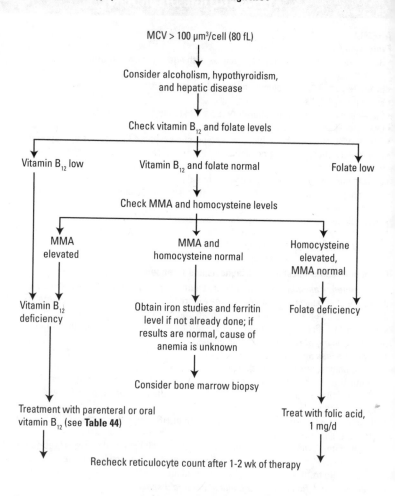

Source: Balducci L. Epidemiology of anemia in the elderly: Information on diagnostic evaluation. *J Amer Geriatr Soc* 2003; 51(3 Suppl):S2–9. Reprinted with permission.

Figure 5. Evaluation of Hypoproliferative Anemia with Normal or Low MCV

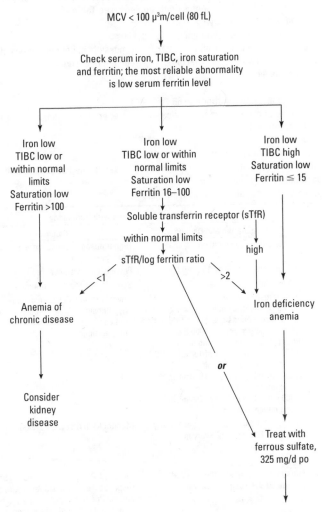

MCV < 100 μ³m/cell (80 fL)

Check serum iron, TIBC, iron saturation
and ferritin; the most reliable abnormality
is low serum ferritin level

Iron low
TIBC low or
within normal
limits
Saturation low
Ferritin >100

Iron low
TIBC low or within
normal limits
Saturation low
Ferritin 16–100

Iron low
TIBC high
Saturation low
Ferritin ≤ 15

Soluble transferrin receptor (sTfR)

within normal limits

high

sTfR/log ferritin ratio

<1

>2

Anemia of
chronic disease

Iron deficiency
anemia

or

Consider
kidney
disease

Treat with
ferrous sulfate,
325 mg/d po

Recheck reticulocyte count after 1–2 wk of therapy

Anemia of renal insufficiency:
- Caused by decreased erythropoietin production; check erythropoietin level.
- Restoring Hb levels increases survival, quality of life, and cognitive function, and decreases hospitalization, LVH, and HF. Treatment is erythropoietin (see **Table 44**).

Anemia of B_{12} and folate deficiency:
- Laboratory tests: anemia or pancytopenia, macrocytosis
- B_{12} deficiency definite at concentrations <100 pg/mL, possible at concentrations of 100–300 pg/mL; check MMA or give trial of B_{12} replacement (see **Figure 5**)
- Treatment: see **Table 44**

Anemia of unknown cause:
- Prevalence: 17% of all anemias after age 65
- May be age-related decline in hematopoietic reserve, low erythropoietin, or poor response to endogenous erythropoietin

Hemolytic anemia:
- Hallmark is high reticulocyte count.
- Causes if Coombs' test positive: chronic lymphocytic leukemia, medications, lymphoma, collagen vascular disease, idiopathic
- Causes if Coombs' test negative: vascular, intrinsic

Table 44. Treatment of Anemias Associated with Deficiency

Treatment	Formulation and Dosage	Comments
Iron	Ferrous sulfate 325 mg/d po	Higher dosages cause more GI adverse events
	Ferrous polysaccharide 150 mg/d po	Fewer GI adverse events
	Iron dextran	See full prescribing information.
	Iron sucrose (*Venofer*): 200 mg IV, injected undiluted over 2–5 min on 5 different occasions within 14-d period (total cumulative dose of 1000 mg) Other recommended dosing options: • 100 mg, dilute to max of 100 mL in NS and infuse over ≥15 min • 300 mg, dilute to max of 250 mL in NS and infuse over 1.5 h • 400 mg, dilute to max of 250 mL in NS and infuse over 2.5 h	Avoid fast infusion (can cause hypotension, cardiovascular collapse); do not administer concomitant iron preparations
B_{12}	1000 mcg IM daily × 5 days, then weekly × 4 wk, then 1000 mcg IM every mo or 1000 mcg/d po	Monitor K^+ in first wk of treatment
Folate	1 mg/d po	
Erythropoietin	Epoetin alfa (*Epogen, Procrit*) usual dosage 50–150 U/kg SC every wk	Monitor BP, adjust dosage based on response. For use in kidney failure and in anemia due to chemotherapy. Caution: target Hb 11–12 g/dL, not higher; use in anemic cancer patients not on chemotherapy increases risk of death.
	Darbepoetin alfa (*Aranesp*) 2.25–6.25 mcg/kg every wk	

PANCYTOPENIA
Unless due to B$_{12}$ deficiency, bone marrow aspirate is indicated; causes include cancer, fibrosis, myelodysplasia, sideroblastic anemia

Aplastic Anemia
- Increases in prevalence with age
- 50% respond to antithymocyte globulin and cyclosporine

Myelodysplasia
A group of stem cell disorders, refractory anemia with or without ringed sideroblasts
- Macrocytosis, mild leukopenia, normal or increased platelets
- Cytogenetic abnormalities common, most often 5q deletion
- Treatment supportive
- DiGugleilmo's syndrome related to myelodysplasia; red cell, white cell, and platelet dysplasia often evolves to erythroleukemia

PRIMARY MYELOPROLIFERATIVE DISORDERS
Polycythemia Vera
- Elevated RBC mass with normal arterial oxygen saturation and low plasma erythropoietin
- Splenomegaly, leukocytosis, and thrombocytosis may be seen
- Treatment: phlebotomy to achieve iron deficiency and hematocrit ≤45, and ASA 325 mg/d

Essential Thrombocytosis
- Platelet count >600,000/μL on two occasions ≥1 mo apart
- Normal RBC mass, iron marrow stores, and splenomegaly
- No Philadelphia or *bcr-abl* gene rearrangements or myelofibrosis in marrow
- Treatment: For patients at high risk of thrombohemorrhagic events, use ASA and anagrelide (*Agrylin*) or interferon-alpha or hydroxyurea.

Chronic Myelogenous Leukemia
- Leukocytosis with early myeloid forms evenly distributed in peripheral blood
- Philadelphia chromosome in >95% of cases
- Leukocyte alkaline phosphatase score low
- Treatment: chronic and acute phases—imatinib (*Gleevec*); acute-phase treatment for select patients is stem cell transplantation.

Myelofibrosis
- Pancytopenia, splenomegaly, and other extramedullary hematopoiesis
- Marrow fibrosis (dry tap) and peripheral blood: leukoerythroblastosis, tear-drop cells
- Acute leukemia develops in 5%–20%
- Treatment for patients with symptomatic anemia: androgens, steroids, erythropoietin

Monoclonal Gammopathy of Undetermined Significance (MGUS)
- Definition: monoclonal immunoglobulin concentration in serum ≤3 g/dL; no lytic bone lesions, anemia, hypercalcemia, or renal insufficiency; plasma cells in marrow ≤10%
- Prevalence increases with age: 3.2% at ≥50 yr; 6.6% at ≥80 yr.
- Evaluation: SPEP, urine and serum immunofixation, and serum κ:λ light-chain ratio. If serum monoclonal protein is ≥1.5 g/dL, obtain bone marrow aspirate and skeletal survey.
- 1%/yr progress to multiple myeloma.

- Risk of progression to myeloma increases with increasing number of these risk factors: monoclonal protein $\geq$1.5 g/dL, monoclonal immunoglobulin other than IgG, abnormal serum free light-chain ratio (κ:λ light chains) of <0.26 or >1.65.
- Monitor all patients indefinitely for progression to myeloma using quantitative serum immunoglobulins, calcium, creatinine.

URINARY INCONTINENCE (UI)

UI is not a normal part of aging. It is a loss of urine control due to a combination of:

- Genitourinary pathology
- Age-related changes
- Comorbid conditions and medications
- Environmental obstacles

Classification

Potentially Reversible Causes of Incontinence (DRIPP Mnemonic)

Delirium

Restricted mobility (illness, injury, gait disorder, restraint)

Infection (acute, symptomatic); **I**nflammation (atrophic vaginitis); **I**mpaction of feces

Polyuria (diabetes mellitus, caffeine intake, volume overload)

Pharmaceuticals (see **Table 45**)

Common Causes

- **Urge UI:** Detrusor muscle overactivity (uninhibited bladder contractions); small to large volume loss; may be idiopathic or associated with CNS lesions or bladder irritation from infection, stones, tumors. Detrusor hyperactivity with impaired contractility (DHIC) is urge incontinence with a weak detrusor muscle.
- **Stress UI:** Failure of sphincter mechanisms to remain closed during bladder filling (often due to insufficient pelvic support in women and to trauma from prostate surgery in men); loss occurs with increased intra-abdominal pressure.
- **Overflow UI:** Impaired detrusor contractility or bladder outlet obstruction. Impaired contractility—chronic outlet obstruction, diabetes mellitus, vitamin B_{12} deficiency, tabes dorsalis, alcoholism, or spinal disease. Outlet obstruction—in men, BPH, cancer, stricture; in women, prior incontinence surgery or large cystocele.
- **Mixed UI:** Combined urge and stress UI is common in older women; a similar syndrome may develop in men after prostatectomy.
- **Other (rare):** Bladder-sphincter dyssynergia, fistulas, reduced detrusor compliance

Table 45. Medications Commonly Associated with UI	
Medication/Class	**Effect on Continence**
Alcohol	Frequency, urgency, sedation, immobility
α-Adrenergic agonists	Outlet obstruction (men)
α-Adrenergic blockers	Stress leakage (women)
Anticholinergics	Impaired emptying, delirium, fecal impaction
Calcium channel blockers	Impaired detrusor contraction, edema with nocturnal diuresis
Loop diuretics	Polyuria, frequency, urgency
NSAIDs/thiazolidinediones	Edema, nocturnal diuresis
Sedative hypnotics	Sedation, delirium, immobility
Narcotic analgesics	Constipation, sedation, delirium
Antidepressants/antipsychotics	Anticholinergic effects, sedation, immobility

Risk Factors

- Age-related changes (eg, BPH, atrophic urethritis)
- Constipation
- Dementia, depression, stroke, Parkinson's disease
- HF, COPD, or chronic cough
- Impaired ADLs
- Obesity
- Parity

Evaluation

History

- Onset, frequency, volume, timing, precipitants (eg, caffeine, diuretics, alcohol, cough, medications)
- Sudden, compelling urgency suggests urge UI.
- Loss with cough, laugh, or bend suggests stress UI.
- Continuous leakage suggests intrinsic sphincter insufficiency or overflow.

Physical Examination

- Functional status (eg, mobility, dexterity)
- Mental status
- Findings:
  - Bladder distention
  - Cord compression (interosseus muscle wasting, Hoffmann's or Babinski's signs)
  - Rectal mass or impaction
  - Sacral root integrity (anal sphincter tone, anal wink, perineal sensation)
  - Volume overload, edema

Male GU

Prostate consistency; symmetry; in uncircumcised, check phimosis, paraphimosis, balanitis

Female GU

Atrophic vaginitis (see p 216); pelvic support (cystocele, rectocele, prolapse; see p 240)

Testing

- **Bladder Diary:** Record time and volume of incontinent and continent voids, activities and time of sleep; knowing oral intake is sometimes helpful.
- **Standing Full Bladder Stress Test (for patients with symptoms of stress UI):** Relax perineum and cough once—immediate loss suggests stress, several seconds delay suggests detrusor overactivity.
- **Postvoid Residual:** If available, bladder ultrasound after voiding is preferred to catheterization. If >100 mL, repeat; still >100 mL suggests detrusor weakness, neuropathy, medications, fecal impaction, outlet obstruction, or DHIC.
- **Laboratory:** UA and urine C&S; glucose and calcium if polyuric; renal function tests and B_{12} if urinary retention; urine cytology if hematuria or pain.
- **Urodynamic Testing:** Not routinely indicated; indicated before corrective surgery, when diagnosis is unclear, when empiric therapy is ineffective, or if postvoid residual volume >200–300 mL (possibly lower in men).

Management

In a stepped approach, treat all transient causes first (DRIPP); avoid caffeine, alcohol; if nocturia is a problem, minimize evening intake of fluids.

Nonpharmacologic Behavioral Therapy (First-line Therapy)

- **Urge and Stress UI:**
  - Bladder retraining, regular voiding (based on bladder diary, or every 2 hr), urgency control—when urgency occurs, sit or stand quietly, focus on letting urge pass, do pelvic muscle contraction, when no longer urgent walk slowly to the bathroom and void. When no incontinence for 2 d, increase voiding interval by 30–60 min until voiding every 3–4 h.
  - Pelvic muscle (Kegel's) exercises—isolate pelvic muscles (avoid thigh, rectal, buttocks contraction); perform slow velocity contraction, sustained for 6–8 sec in sets of 8–12 contractions, 3–4 times/wk for at least 15–20 wk (see www.healthinaging.org/public_education/tools/UItool10.pdf); follow up and encouragement necessary; consider biofeedback or electrical stimulation for training if initial instructions are not successful (refer to PT). Vaginal weights are an alternative for strengthening pelvic muscles; however, no data in postmenopausal women.
- **Cognitively Impaired Individuals:** Prompted toileting (ask if patient needs to void, take them to toilet) starting at 2- to 3-h intervals during day; encourage patients to report continence status; praise patient when continent and responds to toileting.
- **Pessaries:** May benefit women with vaginal (see p 240) or uterine prolapse who experience retention or stress UI (see p 107).
- **DHIC:** Treat urge first with behavioral methods; may add detrusor muscle-relaxing medications but follow postvoid residual; clean intermittent self-catheterization if needed.

Nocturnal Frequency in the Absence of HF

- Two voidings per night is probably normal for older adults.
- Exclude sleep difficulties (see Sleep Disorders, p 226), then consider if the condition is due to excessive output or urinary tract dysfunction.
- Bladder diary with measured voided volumes can be very helpful. If between bedtime and awakening, the patient voids more than one-third of his or her total 24-hr output, this is excessive fluid excretion.
  - All patients should restrict fluid intake 4 h before bedtime.
  - If stasis edema is present, have patient wear pressure-graded stockings.
  - If no stasis edema, a potent, short-acting loop diuretic can be used in the afternoon or early evening to induce a diuresis before bedtime, eg, bumetanide 0.5–1.5 mg titrated to achieve a brisk diuresis.
  - Evaluate for other factors contributing to volume overload or diuresis (eg, HF, poorly controlled diabetes).

Pharmacologic Therapy

Eliminate medications causing/exacerbating UI if possible (see **Table 45**). Data suggesting benefit of topical postmenopausal estrogen therapy in urge and possibly stress UI are limited. See **Table 93** for available preparations. See **Table 46** for other therapies.

Surgical Therapy

- Consider for the 50% of women whose stress UI does not respond adequately to behavioral treatment and exercise.
- Type of surgery depends on type of urethral function impairment, patient-related factors, and coexisting conditions (eg, prolapse).

Table 46. Medications to Treat Urge or Mixed Urinary Incontinence

Medication	Dosage	Formulations	Adverse Events (Metabolism)
Oxybutynin (*Ditropan, Ditropan XL, Oxytrol*)	2.5–5 mg q 8–12 h 5–20 mg/d 3.9 mg/d (apply pch 2 × /wk)	T: 5; S: 5 mg/5 mL SR: 5, 10, 15 Transdermal pch 39 cm²	Dry mouth, blurry vision, dry eyes, delirium/confusion, constipation Pch: side effects similar to those of placebo; may irritate skin (L)
Tolterodine (*Detrol, Detrol LA*)	2 mg q 12 h 4 mg/d	T: 1, 2 C: ER 2, 4	Dry mouth, blurry vision, dry eyes, constipation, delirium, hallucinations, P450 interactions (L, CYP3A4 and CYP2D6)
Trospium (*Sanctura, Sanctura XR*)	20 mg q 12–24 h (on empty stomach), dose once daily at hs in patients >75 yr or with CrCl <30 mL/min; 60 mg/d (XR)	T: 20 C: ER 60	Dry mouth, constipation, dyspepsia, headache; caution in liver dysfunction; XR formulation not recommended if CrCl <30 mL/min (L, K)
Darifenacin (*Enablex*)	7.5–15 mg/d	T: 7.5, 15	Dry mouth, constipation, urinary and gastric retention; not recommended in severe liver impairment (L, CYP3A4 and CYP2D6)
Solifenacin (*VESIcare*)	5–10 mg/d	T: 5, 10	Same as darifenacin; max dose 5 mg with CrCl <30 mL/min or moderate liver impairment (L, CYP3A4)

Note: For prostate obstruction UI, see benign prostatic hyperplasia, p 193.

Catheter Care

- Use catheter **only** for chronic urinary retention, to protect pressure ulcers, and when requested by patients or families to promote comfort (eg, at end of life).
- Leakage around catheter can be caused by large Foley balloon, too large catheter diameter, constipation, impaction.
- Bacteriuria is universal; treat only if symptoms (eg, fever, inanition, anorexia, delirium) or if bacteriuria persists after catheter removal.
- Suprapubic catheters reduce meatal and penile trauma but not infection. Condom catheters are less painful and have a somewhat lower complication rate.
- Replace catheter if symptomatic bacteriuria develops, then culture urine from new catheter.
- Nursing-facility patients with catheters should reside in separate rooms.
- For acute retention, catheterize for 7–10 d, then do voiding trial after catheter removal.

Replacing Catheter: Routine replacement not necessary. Changing q 4–6 wk is reasonable to prevent blockage. Patients with recurrent blockage need increased fluid intake, possibly acidification of urine, or change of catheter q 7–10 d.

FECAL INCONTINENCE (FI)
Definition
Involuntary or inappropriate passing of feces that impacts social functioning or hygiene

Prevalence
After age 65: 2% of community-dwelling, 14% of hospitalized, 54% of nursing-home residents

Risk Factors
Constipation, age >80 yr, female sex, UI, impaired mobility, dementia, neurologic disease

Age-related Factors
Decreased strength of external sphincter and weak anal squeeze; increased rectal compliance, decreased resting tone in internal sphincter, and impaired anal sensation

Causes: FI is commonly multifactorial.
- Overflow: from colonic distention by excessive feces, causing continuous soiling
- Loose feces: caused by medications, neoplasia, colitis, lactose intolerance
- Functional incontinence: associated with poor mobility
- Dementia related: uninhibited rectal contraction, often have UI
- Anorectal incontinence: weak external sphincter (surgery, multiparity, etc)
- Comorbidity: stroke, diabetes mellitus (autonomic neuropathy), sacral cord dysfunction

Evaluation
History
- Description of FI (eg, diarrhea, hard feces, etc), including usual bowel habit, change in habit, usual fecal consistency
- Frequency, urgency, ability to delay, difficulty wiping, post-defecation soiling, ability to distinguish feces and flatus
- Evacuation difficulties: straining, incomplete emptying, rectal prolapse or pain
- Functional: communication of needs, need for assistance, toilet access
- Other: bowel medications, other medications, UI, prior treatment (eg, pads)
Examination
- Examine/palpate abdomen for colonic distention, and visually inspect anus.
- Check for prolapse while patient seated on commode.
- Perform rectal examination for tone, volume, and consistency of feces; heme test.
- Observe gait, mobility, dressing, hygiene, mental status.
Laboratory
- TSH, electrolytes, calcium
Bowel investigations
- Abdominal radiograph: may identify colonic distention by excessive feces
- Colonoscopy: only when pathology suspected (unexplained loose feces, bleeding)
- Anorectal physiology tests: not generally needed for treatment

Treatment: Multiple interventions may be required.

Main approach
• Simulate the patient's usual bowel pattern.
• Use rectal evacuants to stimulate evacuation and to establish a bowel pattern.
• Use evacuants in the following order: glycerine suppository, bisacodyl suppository, microenemas (eg, *Enemeez*, docusate 5 mL), phosphate or tap water enemas; digital stimulation.
• Use antidiarrheals to slow an overactive bowel or to enable planned evacuation with rectal preparations.

Constipation (see p 92): often plays a role; evaluate (if needed) and treat

Modify fecal consistency to achieve soft, formed feces
• Loose feces: use fiber or loperamide titrated to effect, sometimes as little as q 48 h.
• Hard feces: modify diet; add osmotic agent (MgSO or MgOH are inexpensive). In poorly mobile people, bran and fiber may exacerbate constipation.

Patient education
• Respond promptly on urge to defecate, heed the gastrocolic reflex.
• Take loperimide 2–4 mg 45 min before meal or social event to prevent evacuation.
• Use coffee to stimulate the gut.
• Position on toilet with back support, foot stool to achieve squat position.
• Exercise to improve bowel motility.
• Those who are able may be taught rectal sphincter exercises (tighten rectal sphincter for 10 sec 50 times/d) or may use biofeedback.

Rectal evacuation and toilet training
• Following a regimen improves bowel control.
• When no spontaneous bowel action, stimulate with suppositories or enemas (see p 92); those with incompetent sphincters may not retain usual enemas.
• Bed pans should not be used; bedside commodes are not as good as toilets.

Nursing-home residents and very disabled older adults: FI is most often due to colonic loading and overflow. Treat as follows:
• Daily enemas until no more results.
• Add a daily osmotic laxative (see **Table 40**) and follow bowel training (above).
• Fecal transit can be stimulated with abdominal massage in direction of colonic transit.

Other therapies
• Manual evacuation may be appropriate in some patients.
• Skin care: Wet wipes better than dry; commercial preparations better than soap and water; toilet tongs and bottom wipers help those with shoulder disease.
• Surgery:
  ◦ Full-thickness rectal prolapse usually requires surgery using a transanal approach.
  ◦ Denervation of the sphincter can be repaired, but long-term results are often unsatisfactory.
  ◦ Division of the external anal sphincter or anal fissure can be repaired, but long-term results are less than satisfactory.
  ◦ Selected patients have improved quality of life through creation of a stoma.

PNEUMONIA
Presentation
Can range from subtle signs such as lethargy, anorexia, dizziness, falls, and delirium to septic shock or acute respiratory distress syndrome. Pleuritic chest pain, dyspnea, productive cough, fever, chills, or rigors are not consistently present in older adults.

Evaluation and Assessment
- Physical examination: Respiratory rate >20 breaths/min; low BP; chest sounds may be minimal, absent, or consistent with HF; 20% are afebrile.
- CXR: Infiltrate may not be present on initial film if the patient is dehydrated.
- Sputum: Gram's stain and culture (optional per ATS guidelines)
- CBC with differential: Up to 50% of patients have a normal WBC count, but 95% have a left shift.
- BUN, creatinine, electrolytes, glucose
- Blood culture × 2
- Oxygenation: arterial blood gas or oximetry
- Test for *Mycobacterium tuberculosis* with acid-fast bacilli stain and culture in selected patients.
- Test for *Legionella* spp in patients who are seriously ill without an alternative diagnosis, are immunocompromised, are nonresponsive to β-lactam antibiotics, have clinical features suggesting this diagnosis, or in outbreak setting. Urinary antigen testing is highly specific for serotype 1 but lacks specificity for other serotypes. Value and use vary by geographic region.
- Thoracentesis (if moderate to large effusion)

Aggravating Factors
- Age-related changes in pulmonary reserve
- Alcoholism
- Altered mental status
- Aspiration
- Comorbid conditions that alter gag reflexes or ciliary transport
- COPD or other lung disease
- Heart disease
- Heavy sedation or paralytic agents
- Hyperglycemia (maintain blood glucose between 80 and 110 mg/dL in patients in intensive care)
- Intubation, mechanical ventilation (orotracheal intubation and orogastric tubation preferred)
- Malnutrition
- Medications: immunosuppressants, sedatives, anticholinergic or other agents that dry secretions, agents that decrease gastric pH
- Nasogastric tubes
- Poor compliance with infection control (eg, hand disinfection)
- Supine positioning (semi-recumbent, 30–45 degrees preferred)

Expected Organisms (in order of frequency of occurrence)

Community-acquired:
- *Streptococcus pneumoniae*
- *Legionella* spp
- Respiratory viruses
- *Haemophilus influenzae*
- Gram-negative bacteria
- *Chlamydia pneumoniae*
- *Moraxella catarrhalis*
- *M tuberculosis*
- Endemic fungi

Nursing-home–acquired:
- Gram-negative bacteria
- *Staphylococcus aureus* (including methicillin-resistant *S aureus*)
- *Strep pneumoniae*
- Anaerobes
- *H influenzae*
- Group B streptococci
- *Chlamydia pneumoniae*

Hospital-acquired:
- Gram-negative bacteria
- Anaerobes
- Gram-positive bacteria
- Fungi

Supportive Management
- Chest percussion
- Inhaled β-adrenergic agonists
- Mechanical ventilation (if indicated)
- Oxygen as indicated
- Rehydration

Empiric Antibiotic Therapy (see Table 53)

Table 47. Treatment of Community-acquired Pneumonia for Immunocompetent Patients by Clinical Circumstances or Setting

Clinical Circumstances or Setting	Treatment Options
Outpatient, previously healthy and no antibiotic therapy in past 3 mo	Azithromycin, clarithromycin, or erythromycin Alternative: doxycycline
Outpatient, with comorbidities[a] or antibiotic therapy in past 3 mo[c]	A fluoroquinolone[b] alone **or** Azithromycin, clarithromycin, or erythromycin *plus* amoxicillin (high dose) or amoxicillin-clavulanate Alternative β-lactams: ceftriaxone, cefpodoxime, or cefuroxime Alternative to a macrolide: doxycycline
Hospitalized patient	A fluoroquinolone[b] alone **or** Azithromycin or clarithromycin *plus* cefotaxime, ceftriaxone, or ampicillin Alternative β-lactam: ertapenem Alternative to a macrolide: doxycycline
Hospitalized patient, intensive care unit	
No concern about *Pseudomonas*	Cefotaxime, ceftriaxone, or ampicillin-sulbactam *plus* azithromycin or a fluoroquinolone[b]
No concern about *Pseudomonas* but β-lactam allergy	A fluoroquinolone[b] plus aztreonam
Concern about *Pseudomonas*	Piperacillin-tazobactam, imipenem, meropenem, or cefepime *plus* ciprofloxacin or levofloxacin; **or** Piperacillin-tazobactam, imipenem, meropenem, or cefepime *plus* an aminoglycoside *and* azithromycin, ciprofloxacin, or levofloxacin

(cont.)

Clinical Circumstances or Setting	Treatment Options
Concern about *Pseudomonas* and β-lactam allergy	Aztreonam *plus* ciprofloxacin or levofloxacin *plus* an aminoglycoside
Nursing-home patient[d,e]	A fluoroquinolone[c] alone *or* Azithromycin, clarithromycin, or erythromycin *plus* amoxicillin (high dose) or amoxicillin-clavulanate

[a] Comorbidities: chronic heart, lung, liver, or kidney disease; diabetes mellitus; alcoholism; malignancies; asplenia; immunosuppressing conditions or drugs

[b] Fluoroquinolones (respiratory): moxifloxacin, levofloxacin, or gemifloxacin

[c] Choice of antibiotic should be from a different class

[d] Patients being treated in the nursing home; for treatment of nursing-home patients who are hospitalized, see hospitalized patient or intensive care unit.

[e] Because of the incidence of gram-negative and atypical bacterial pneumonia in nursing-home patients, experts in geriatric infectious disease often recommend expanded gram-negative antibiotic coverage.
Source: Mandell LA, Wunderink RG, Anzueto A, et al. Infectious Disease Society of America/American Thoracic Society consensus guidelines on the management of community-acquired pneumonia in adults. *Clin Infect Dis* 2007;44:S27–72.

Nursing-home or Hospital-acquired Pneumonia Requiring Parenteral Treatment: Alternative Recommendations

Antipseudomonal cephalosporin (cefepime or ceftazadime) *or*

Antipseudomonal carbepenem (imipenem or meropenem) *or*

β-Lactam/β-lactamase inhibitor (piperacillin-tazobactam)

plus

Antipseudomonal fluoroquinolone (ciprofloxacin or levofloxacin) *or*

Aminoglycoside (amikacin, gentamicin, or tobramycin)

plus

Linezolid or vancomycin (if risk factors for methicillin-resistant *S aureus* are present or if local incidence is high)

For both sets of empiric therapy guidelines, the choice of combination depends on local bacteriologic patterns.

Adapted from: ATS and IDSA Guidelines for the management of adults with hospital-acquired, ventilator-associated, and healthcare-associated pneumonia. *Am J Resp Crit Care Med* 2005;171:388–416.

Note: The empiric use of vancomycin should be reserved for patients with a serious allergy to β-lactam antibiotics or for patients from environments in which methicillin-resistant *S aureus* is known to be a problem pathogen. For all cases, antimicrobial therapy should be individualized once Gram's stain or culture results are known.

URINARY TRACT INFECTION OR UROSEPSIS
Definition
Bacteriuria is the presence of significant number of bacteria in the urine without reference to symptoms.

- **Symptomatic bacteriuria** usually has signs of dysuria and increased frequency of urination; fever, chills, nausea may be present; pyuria ($>10^5$ cfu/mL) supports the diagnosis of UTI.
- **Asymptomatic bacteriuria** is seen when the same organism(s) ($\geq 10^5$ cfu/mL) is found on 2 consecutive cultures in the absence of symptoms of a UTI; no treatment is necessary.

Risk Factors
- Abnormalities in function or anatomy of the urinary tract
- Catheterization or recent instrumentation
- Comorbid conditions (eg, diabetes mellitus, BPH)
- Female gender
- Limited functional status

Assessment and Evaluation
Choice is based on presenting symptoms and severity of illness.
- Urinalysis with culture (do not obtain sample from catheter bag)
- Blood culture × 2
- BUN, creatinine, electrolytes
- CBC with differential

Expected Organisms
Noncatheterized Patients: Most common: *Escherichia coli, Proteus* spp, *Klebsiella* spp, *Providencia* spp, *Citrobacter* spp, *Enterobacter* spp, and *Pseudomonas aeruginosa* if recent antibiotic exposure, known colonization, or known institutional flora
Nursing-Home–Catheterized Patients: *Enterobacter* spp and gram-negative bacteria

Empiric Antibiotic Management
Duration should be at least 7–10 d.
Community-Acquired or Nursing-Home–Acquired Cystitis or Uncomplicated UTI (oral route): TMP/SMZ DS, cephalexin, ampicillin, or amoxicillin. Amoxicillin-clavulanate should be reserved for patients with sulfa allergy and for settings with known β-lactam resistance. Fluoroquinolones should be reserved for patients with allergies to sulfa or β-lactams, or for settings with known resistance.
Suspected Urosepsis (IV route): Third-generation cephalosporin plus aminoglycoside, aztreonam, or fluoroquinolone ± aminoglycoside.

Vancomycin should be reserved for patients with a serious allergy to β-lactam antibiotics.

UTI Prophylaxis
Leads to antibiotic resistance; generally not recommended.

HERPES ZOSTER ("SHINGLES")
Definition
Cutaneous vesicular eruptions followed by radicular pain secondary to the recrudescence of varicella zoster virus.

Prevention

Zoster vaccine live (*Zostavax*) for individuals ≥60 yr who are immunocompetent and without prior zoster infection. (**See Table 75.**)

Clinical Manifestations

- Abrupt onset of pain along a specific dermatome (see **Figure 1**)
- Macular, erythematous rash that becomes vesicular and pustular (Tzanck cell test positive) after ~3 d, crusts over and clears in 10–14 d
- Complications: postherpetic neuralgia, visual loss or blindness if ophthalmic involvement

Pharmacologic Management

When started within 72 h of the rash's appearance, antiviral therapy (see **Table 48**) decreases the severity and duration of the acute illness and possibly shortens the duration and reduces the risk of postherpetic neuralgias. Corticosteroids may also decrease the risk and severity of postherpetic neuralgias. (See p 165 for treatment of postherpetic neuralgia.)

	Table 48. Antiviral Treatments for Herpes Zoster		
Medication, Route	**Dosage**	**Formulations**	**Comment**
Acyclovir (*Zovirax*)			
Oral	800 mg 5 ×/d for 7–10 d	T: 400, 800; C: 200; S: 200 mg/5 mL	Reduce dosage when CrCl[a] <25 mL/min
IV[b]	10 mg/kg q 8 h for 7–10 d	500 mg/10 mL	Reduce dosage when CrCl[a] <50 mL/min
Famciclovir (*Famvir*)			
Oral	500 mg q 8 h for 7 d	T: 125, 250, 500	Reduce dosage when CrCl[a] <60 mL/min
Valacyclovir[c] (*Valtrex*)			
Oral	1000 mg q 8 h for 7 d	C: 500, 1000	Reduce dosage when CrCl[a] <50 mL/min

[a] The CrCl listed is the threshold below which the dosage (amount or frequency) should be reduced. See package insert for detailed dosing guidelines.
[b] Use IV for serious illness, ophthalmic infection, or patients who cannot take oral medication.
[c] Preferred to po acyclovir; prodrug of acyclovir with serum concentrations equal to those achieved with IV administration.

INFLUENZA

Vaccine Prevention (ACIP Guidelines)

Yearly vaccination is recommended for all adults ≥65 yr old and all residents and staff of nursing homes, or residential or long-term–care facilities. Nursing-home residents admitted during the winter months after the vaccination program has been completed should be vaccinated at admission if they have not already been vaccinated. The influenza vaccine is contraindicated in people who have an anaphylactic hypersensitivity to eggs or any other component of the vaccine. Dose: 0.5 mL IM once in the fall for those living in the northern hemisphere.

Pharmacologic Prophylaxis and Treatment with Antiviral Agents
Indications:
- Prevention (during an influenza outbreak): people who are not vaccinated, are immunodeficient, or may spread the virus
- Prophylaxis: during 2 wk required to develop antibodies for people vaccinated after an outbreak of influenza A
- Reduction of symptoms, duration of illness when started within the first 48 h of symptoms
- During epidemic outbreaks in nursing homes

Duration: Treatment of symptoms: 3–5 d or for 24–48 h after symptoms resolve. Prophylaxis during outbreak: min 2 wk or until ~1 wk after outbreak ends.

Table 49. Antiviral Treatment of Influenza

Agent	Formulation	Dosage
Amantadine (*Symmetrel*)[a]	C: 100 mg S: 50 mg/5 mL	100 mg/d po[b]
✔ Oseltamivir (*Tamiflu*)[c]	C: 75 mg S: 12 mg/mL	Treatment: 75 mg po q 12 h × 5 d (75 mg/d po if CrCl 10–30 mL/min); not recommended if CrCl <10 mL/min
		Prophylaxis: 75 mg/d po × ≥7 d up to 6 wk (75 mg po q 48 h if CrCl 10–30 mL/min); not recommended if CrCl <10 mL/min
Rimantadine (*Flumadine*)[a]	T: 100 mg S: 50 mg/5 mL	100 mg/d po for frail older adults and nursing-home residents
		200 mg/d po for other adults, including those ≥65 yr old
		Decrease dose to 100 mg if adverse events appear
Zanamivir (*Relenza*)[c,d]	Inh: 5 mg/blister	2 × 5-mg inhalations q 12 h × 5 d
		Give doses on first day ≥2 h apart
		Prophylaxis: 2 × 5-mg inhalations q 24 h; household setting—start 36 h after onset of signs and symptoms of initial case, duration 10 d; community—begin within 5 d of outbreak, duration 30 d.

✔ = preferred for treating older adults
[a] No longer recommended for prophylaxis.
[b] Dosage adjustments for kidney function, CrCl (mL/min): ≥30 = 100 mg/d; 20–29 = 200 mg 2 ×/wk; 10–19 = 100 mg 3 ×/wk; <10 = 200 mg alternating with 100 mg q 7 d.
[c] Must be started within 2 d of symptom onset.
[d] Do not use in patients with COPD or asthma.

TUBERCULOSIS (TB)
TB in older adults may be the reactivation of old disease or a new infection due to exposure to an infected individual. Treatment recommendations differ; if a new infection is suspected or the patient has risk factors for resistant organisms, then bacterial sensitivities must be determined.

Risk or Reactivating Factors
- Chronic institutionalization
- Corticosteroid use
- Diabetes mellitus
- Malignancy
- Malnutrition
- Kidney failure

Risk Factors for Resistant Organisms

- HIV infection
- Homelessness, institutionalization (other than a nursing home)
- IV drug abuse
- Origin from geographic regions with a high prevalence of resistance (New York, Mexico, Southeast Asia)
- Exposure to INH-resistant TB or history of ineffective chemotherapy
- Previous treatment for TB
- AFB-positive sputum smears after 2 mo of treatment
- Positive cultures after 4 mo of treatment

Diagnosis

- Mantoux tuberculin skin test (TST): 0.1 mL of tuberculin purified protein derivative (PPD) intradermal injection into the inner surface of the forearm
- Read 48–72 h after injection (see **Table 50** for interpretation).
- Repeat ("booster") 1–2 wk after initial skin testing can be useful for nursing-home residents, healthcare workers, and others who are retested periodically to reduce the likelihood of misinterpreting a boosted reaction to subsequent TSTs.

Treatment

Latent Infection: See **Table 50** and **Table 51**.

Table 50. Identification of Patients at High Risk of Developing TB Who Would Benefit from Treatment of Latent Infection

Population	Minimum Induration Considered a Positive Test
Considered positive in any person, including those considered low risk	15 mm
Residents and employees of hospitals, nursing homes, and long-term facilities for older adults, residential facilities for AIDS patients, and homeless shelters	10 mm
Recent immigrants (<5 yr) from countries where TB prevalence is high	10 mm
Injectable-drug users	10 mm
People with silicosis; diabetes mellitus; chronic kidney failure; leukemia; lymphoma; carcinoma of the head, neck, or lung; weight loss of ≥10%; gastrectomy or jejunoileal bypass	10 mm
Recent contact with TB patients	5 mm
Fibrotic changes on CXR consistent with prior TB	5 mm
Immunosuppressed (receiving the equivalent of prednisone at ≥15 mg/d for ≥1 mo), organ transplant recipients, patients receiving TNF-α inhibitors	5 mm
HIV-positive patients	5 mm

Table 51. Treatment of Latent Tuberculosis

Drug	Dosage and Duration
INH*	5 mg/kg/d (max 300 mg/d) for 6 or 9 mo; or 15 mg/kg/d (max 900 mg/d) 2 × /wk with directly observed therapy for 6 or 9 mo
RIF	10 mg/kg/d (max 600 mg/d) for 4 mo

Note: INH = isoniazid; RIF = rifampin
*The preferred treatment for patients not infected with HIV.
Source: Data from: American Thoracic Society. Targeted tuberculin testing and treatment of latent tuberculosis. *Am J Respir Crit Care Med* 2000;161:S221–S247 (also available at www.atsjournal.org). *MMWR* 2003; 52:735–739.

Active Infection:

Initial treatment options for adults with active *Mycobacterium tuberculosis* infection in order of evidence-based preference are listed below. Daily observed therapy is preferred for all regimens and must be part of any 5 d/wk regimen.

• INH, RIF, PZA, EMB daily × 8 wk or 5 d/wk × 8 wk, then INH + RIF daily × 18 wk or 5 d/wk × 18 wk or 2 d/wk × 18 wk, or INH + RPT 1 d/wk × 18 wk
• INH, RIF, PZA, EMB daily × 2 wk, then INH + RIF 2 d/wk × 18 wk or INH + RPT 1 d/wk × 18 wk
• INH, RIF, PZA, EMB 3 d/wk × 8 wk, then INH + RIF 3 d/wk × 18 wk
• INH, RIF, EMB daily × 8 wk or 5 d/wk × 8 wk, then INH + RIF daily × 21 wk or 5 d/wk × 31 wk, or 2 d/wk × 31 wk

Note: EMB = ethambutol, INH = isoniazid, PZA = pyrazinamid, RIF = rifampin, RPT = rifapentine
Source: www.cdc.gov/mmwr/preview/mmwrhtml/rr5211a1.htm#tab2

Table 52. Dosing for Treatment Options for Active Tuberculosis

Agent	Route	Daily	2 × /Wk	3 × /Wk
INH	po, IM	5 mg/kg[a]	15 mg/kg[a]	15 mg/kg[a]
RIF	po, IM	600 mg[b]	600 mg[b]	600 mg[b]
RPT	po	10 mg/kg[c]	—	—
PZA	po	1.5 g (<50 kg)	2 g (<50 kg)	2 g (<50 kg)
		2 g (51–74 kg)	2.5 g (51–74 kg)	2.5 g (51–74 kg)
		2.5 g (≥75 kg)	3 g (≥75 kg)	3 g (≥75 kg)
Ethambutol	po	15–25 mg/kg[d]	50 mg/kg	30 mg/kg
Streptomycin	IM	10 mg/kg	—	—

[a] Max: daily = 300 mg; 2 × /wk = 900 mg; 3 × /wk = 900 mg
[b] Max: daily = 600 mg; 2 × /wk = 600 mg; 3 × /wk = 600 mg
[c] Max: daily = 600 mg
[d] Max: daily = 2.5 g

Table 53. Antibiotics

Antimicrobial Class, *Subclass*	Dosage	Adjust When CrCl[a] Is: (mL/min)	Formulations	Route of Elimination (%)
β-Lactams *Penicillins*				
Amoxicillin (*Amoxil*)	po: 250 mg–1 g q 8 h	<50	T: film coated 500, 875 C: 250, 500 ChT: 125, 200, 250, 400 S: 125, 200, 250, 400 mg/5 mL	K (80)
Ampicillin	po: 250–500 mg q 6 h IM/IV: 1–2 g q 4–6 h	<30	C: 250, 500 S: 125, 250 mg/5 mL Inj	K (90)
Penicillin G	IV: 3–5 × 10⁶ U q 4–6 h IM: 0.6–2.4 × 10⁶ U q 6–12 h	<30	Inj procaine for IM	K L (30)
Penicillin VK	po: 125–500 mg q 6 h	b	T: 250, 500 S: 125, 250 mg/5 mL	K, L
Antipseudomonal Penicillins				
Carbenicillin indanyl sodium (*Geocillin*)	po: 382–764 mg q 6 h	<50	T: 382	K (80–99)
Piperacillin (*Pipracil*)	IM: 1–2 g q 8–12 h IV: 2–4 g q 6–8 h	<40	Inj	K, F (10–20)
Ticarcillin (*Ticar*)	IM, IV: 1–4 g q 4–6 h	<60	Inj	K
Antistaphylococcal Penicillins				
Dicloxacillin (*Dycill, Pathocil*)	po: 125–500 mg q 6 h	NA	C: 125, 250, 500 S: 62.5 mg/5 mL	K (56–70)
Nafcillin	IM: 500 mg q 4–6 h IV: 500 mg–2 g q 4–6 h	NA	Inj	L
Oxacillin (*Bactocil*)	po: 500 mg–1 g q 4–6 h IM, IV: 250 mg–2 g q 6–12 h	<10	C: 250, 500 S: 250 mg/5 mL Inj	K
Monobactam (antipseudomonal)				
Aztreonam (*Azactam*)	IM: 500 mg–1 g q 8–12 h IV: 500 mg–2 g q 6–12 h	<30	Inj	K (70)

(cont.)

Table 53. Antibiotics (cont.)

Antimicrobial Class, *Subclass*	Dosage	Adjust When CrCl[a] Is: (mL/min)	Formulations	Route of Elimination (%)
Carbapenem (antipseudomonal)				
Ertapenem (*Invanz*)	IM, IV: 1 g q 24 h × 3–14 d IM × 7 d max IV × 14 d max	<30	Inj	K (80), F (10)
Imipenem-cilastatin (*Primaxin*)	IM: 500 mg–1 g q 8–12 h IV: 500 mg–2 g q 6–12 h	<70	Inj	K (70)
Meropenem (*Merrem IV*)	IV: 1 g q 8 h	≤50	Inj	K (75), L (25)
Penicillinase-resistant Penicillins				
Amoxicillin–clavulanate (*Augmentin*)	po: 250 mg q 8 h, 500 mg q 12 h, 875 mg q 12 h	<30	T: 250, 500, 875 ChT: 125, 200, 250, 400 S: 125, 200, 250, 400 mg/5 mL	K (30–40), L
Ampicillin–sulbactam (*Unasyn*)	IM, IV: 1–2 g q 6–8 h	<30	Inj	K (85)
Penicillinase-resistant and Antipseudomonal Penicillins				
Piperacillin–tazobactam (*Zosyn*)	IV: 3.375 g q 6 h	<40	Inj	K (70), F (10–20)
Ticarcillin–clavulanate (*Timentin*)	IV: 3 g q 4–6 h	<60	Inj	K, L
First-generation Cephalosporins				
Cefadroxil (*Duricef*)	po: 500 mg–1 g q 12 h	<50	C: 500 T: 1 g S: 125, 250, 500 mg/5 mL	K (90)
Cefazolin (*Ancef, Kefzol*)	IM, IV: 500 mg–2 g q 8 h	<55	Inj	K (80–100)
Cephalexin (*Keflex*)	po: 250 mg–1 g q 6 h	<40	C: 250, 500 T: 250, 500; 1 g S: 125, 250 mg/5 mL	K (80–100)
Cephalothin (*Keflin*)	IM, IV: 500 mg–2 g q 4–6 h	<50	Inj	K (50–75)

(cont.)

Table 53. Antibiotics (cont.)

Antimicrobial Class, *Subclass*	Dosage	Adjust When CrCl[a] Is: (mL/min)	Formulations	Route of Elimination (%)
Cephapirin (*Cefadyl*)	IM, IV: 1–3 g q 6 h	<10	Inj	K (60–85)
Cephradine (*Anspor*)	po, IM, IV: 500 mg–2 g q 6 h	<20	C: 250, 500 T: 1 g S: 125, 250 mg/5 mL Inj	K (80–90)
Second-generation Cephalosporins				
Cefaclor (*Ceclor*)	po: 250–500 mg q 8 h	<50	C: 250, 500 S: 125, 187, 250, 375 mg/5 mL T: ER 375, 500	K (80)
Cefotetan (*Cefotan*)	IM, IV: 1–3 g q 12 h or 1–2 g q 24 h (UTI)	<30	Inj	K (80)
Cefoxitin (*Mefoxin*)	IM, IV: 1–2 g q 6–8 h	<50	Inj	K (85)
Cefprozil (*Cefzil*)	po: 250–500 mg q 12–24 h	<30	T: 250, 500 S: 125, 250 mg/5 mL	K (60–70)
Cefuroxime axetil (*Ceftin*)	po: 125–500 mg q 12 h IM, IV: 750 mg–1.5 g q 6 h	<20	T: 125, 250, 500 S: 125, 150 mg/5 mL Inj	K (66–100)
Loracarbef (*Lorabid*)	po: 200–400 mg q 12–24 h	<50	C: 200, 400 S: 100, 200 mg/5 mL	K
Third-generation Cephalosporins				
Cefdinir (*Omnicef*)	po: 300 mg q 12 h or 600 mg/d × 10 d	<30	C: 300 S: 125 mg/5 mL	K
Cefditoren (*Spectracef*)	po: 400 mg q 12 h × 10 d (bronchitis) 400 mg q 12 h × 14 d (pneumonia) 200 mg q 12 h × 10 d (soft tissue or skin)	<50	T: 200	K
Cefixime (*Suprax*)	po: 400 mg/d	<60	T: 200, 400 S: 100 mg/5 mL	K (50)
Cefotaxime (*Claforan*)	IM, IV: 1–2 g q 6–12 h	<20	Inj	K, L
Cefpodoxime (*Vantin*)	po: 100–400 mg q 12 h	<30	T: 100, 250 S: 50, 100 mg/5 mL	K (80)

(cont.)

Table 53. Antibiotics (cont.)

Antimicrobial Class, *Subclass*	Dosage	Adjust When CrCl[a] Is: (mL/min)	Formulations	Route of Elimination (%)
Ceftazidime (*Ceptaz, Fortaz*)	IM, IV: 500 mg–2 g q 8–12 h UTI: 250–500 mg q 12 h	<50	Inj	K (80–90)
Ceftibuten (*Cedax*)	po: 400 mg/d	<50	C: 400 S: 100, 200 mg/5 mL	K (65–70)
Ceftizoxime (*Cefizox*)	IM, IV: 500 mg–2 g q 4–12 h	<80	Inj	K (100)
Ceftriaxone (*Rocephin*)	IM, IV: 1–2 g q 12–24 h	NA	Inj	K (33–65)
Fourth-generation Cephalosporins				
Cefepime (*Maxipime*)	IV: 500 mg–2 g q 12 h	<60	Inj	K (85)
Aminoglycosides				
Amikacin (*Amikin*)	IM, IV: 15–20 mg/kg/d divided q 12–24 h; 15–20 mg/kg q 24–48 h	<60, TDM	Inj	K (95)
Gentamicin (*Garamycin*)	IM, IV: 2–5 mg/kg/d divided q 12–24 h; 5–7 mg/kg q 24–48 h	<60, TDM	Inj ophth sus, oint	K (95)
Streptomycin	IM, IV: 10 mg/kg/d not to exceed 750 mg/d	<50	Inj	K (90)
Tobramycin (*Nebcin*)	IM, IV: 2–5 mg/kg/d divided q 12–24 h; 5–7 mg/kg q 24–48 h	<60, TDM	Inj ophth sus, oint	K (95)
Macrolides				
Azithromycin (*Zithromax*)	po: 500 mg day 1, then 250 mg/d IV: 500 mg/d	NA	C: 250 S: 100, 200 mg/5 mL, 1 g (single-dose pk) T: 600 Inj	L
Clarithromycin (*Biaxin, Biaxin XL*)	po: 250–500 mg q 12 h ER: 1000 mg/d	<30	S: 125, 250 mg/5 mL T: 250, 500 ER: 500	L, K (20–30)
Dirithromycin (*Dynabac*)	po: 500 mg/d with food	NA	T: 250	L, F

(cont.)

Antimicrobial Class, *Subclass*	Dosage	Adjust When CrCl[a] Is: (mL/min)	Formulations	Route of Elimination (%)
Erythromycin	po: Base: 333 mg q 8 h Estolate, stearate, or base: 250–500 mg q 6–12 h Ethylsuccinate: 400–800 mg q 6–12 h IV: 15–20 mg/kg/d divided q 6 h	NA	Base: C, T: 250, 333, 500 Estolate: 250 S: 125, 250 mg/5 mL T: 500 Ethylsuccinate: S: 100, 200, 400 mg/5 mL T: 400 ChT: 200 Stearate: T: 250, 500 Inj	L
Ketolide				
Telithromycin (*Ketek*)	po: 800 mg/d × 5–10 d	<30	T: 800	L, K
Quinolones				
Ciprofloxacin (*Cipro*)	po: 250–750 mg q 12 h\nophth: see **Table 99**\nIV: 200–400 mg q 12 h	po: <50\n\nIV: <30	T: 100, 250, 500, 750 S: 250 mg/5 mL, 500 mg/5 mL ophth sol: 3.5 mg/5 mL Inj	K (30–50), L, F (20–40)
Gemifloxacin (*Factive*)	po: 320 mg/d	≤40	T: 320 mg	K, L, F
Levofloxacin (*Levaquin*)	po, IV: 250–500 mg/d	<50	T: 250, 500	K
Lomefloxacin (*Maxaquin*)	po: 400 mg/d	<40	T: 400	K
Moxifloxacin (*Avelox*)	po: 400 mg/d	NA	T: 400	L (~55), F (25), K (20)
Norfloxacin (*Noroxin*)	po: 400 mg q 12 h ophth: see **Table 99**	<30	T: 400 ophth: 0.3%	K (30), F (30)
Ofloxacin (*Roxin*)	po, IV: 200–400 mg q 12–24 h ophth: see **Table 99**	<50	T: 200, 300, 400 ophth: 0.3% Inj	K
Sparfloxacin (*Zagam*)	po: 400 mg day 1, then 200 mg q 24 h	<50	T: 200	L
Trovafloxacin (*Trovan*)	po, IV: 200 mg/d × 10–14 d	NA	T: 100, 200 Inj	L

Table 53. Antibiotics (cont.)

(cont.)

Table 53. Antibiotics (cont.)

Antimicrobial Class, *Subclass*	Dosage	Adjust When CrCl[a] Is: (mL/min)	Formulations	Route of Elimination (%)
Tetracyclines				
Doxycycline (eg, *Vibramycin*)	po, IV: 100–200 mg/d given q 12–24 h	NA	C: 50, 100 T: 50, 100 S: 25 mg/5 mL, 50 mg/5 mL Inj	K (25), F (30)
Minocycline (*Minocin*)	po, IV: 200 mg once, then 100 mg q 12 h	NA	C: 50, 100 S: 50 mg/5 mL; inj	K
Tetracycline	po, IV: 250–500 mg q 6–12 h	NA	C: 100, 250, 500 T: 250, 500 S: 125 mg/5 mL; inj ophth: oint, sus topical: oint, sol	K (60)
Glycycline				
Tigecycline (*Tygacil*)	IV: 100 mg once, then 50 mg q 12 h × 5–14 d	NA	Inj	K (33), F (59), L
Other Antibiotics				
Chloramphenicol (*Chloromycetin*)	po, IV: 50 mg/kg/d given q 6 h; max: 4 g/d	NA	C: 250; topical; ophth; inj	L (90)
Clindamycin (*Cleocin*)	po: 150–450 mg q 6–8 h; max: 1.8 g/d IM, IV: 1.2–1.8 g/d given q 8–12 h; max: 3.6 g/d	NA	C: 75, 150, 300 S: 75 mg/5 mL crm, vaginal: 2% gel, topical: 1% Inj	L (90)
Co-trimoxazole (TMP/SMZ, *Bactrim*)	Doses based on the trimethoprim component: po: 1 double-strength tab q 12 h; IV: sepsis: 20 TMP/kg/d given q 6 h	≤50	T: SMZ 400, TMP 80 double-strength: SMZ 800, TMP 160 S: SMZ 200, TMP 40 mg/5 mL Inj	K, L
Daptomycin (*Cubicin*)	IV: 4 mg/kg/d × 7–14 d	<30	Inj	K (78), L (6)
Linezolid (*Zyvox*)	po: 400–600 mg q 12 h IV: 600 mg q 12 h	NA	T: 400, 600; S: 100 mg/5 mL; inj	L (65), K (30)

(cont.)

Table 53. Antibiotics (cont.)

Antimicrobial Class, *Subclass*	Dosage	Adjust When CrCl[a] Is: (mL/min)	Formulations	Route of Elimination (%)
Metronidazole (*Flagyl, MetraGel*)	po: 250–750 mg q 6–8 h Topical: apply q 12 h Vaginal: 1 applicator full (375 mg) qhs or q 12 h	≤10	T: 250, 500 ER: 750 C: 375 gel, topical: 0.75% (30 g) gel, vaginal: 0.75% (70 g) Inj	L (30–60), K (20–40), F (6–15)
Nitrofurantoin (*Macrodantin*)	po: 50–100 mg q 6 h	Do not use if <40	C: 25, 50, 100 S: 25 mg/5 mL	L (60), K (40)
Quinupristin-dalfopristin (*Synercid*)	Vancomycin-resistant *E faecium*: IV: 7.5 mg/kg q 8 h Complicated skin or skin structure infection: 7.5 mg/kg q 12 h	NA	Inj	L, B, F (75), K (15–19)
Vancomycin (*Vancocin*)	po: *C difficile:* 125–500 mg q 6–8 h IV: 500 mg–1 g q 8–24 h Peak: 20–40 mcg/mL Trough: 5–10 mcg/mL	<60	C: 125, 250 Inj	K (80–90)

Antifungals (see also **Table 32**)

Amphotericin

Amphotericin B (*Fungizone*)	IV: test dose: 1 mg infused over 20–30 min; if tolerated, initial therapeutic dosage is 0.25 mg/kg; the daily dosage can be increased by 0.25-mg/kg increments on each subsequent day until the desired daily dosage is reached Maintenance dosage: IV: 0.25–1 mg/kg/d or 1.5 mg/kg q 48 h; do not exceed 1.5 mg/kg/d	c	topical: crm, lot, oint 3% Inj	K

(cont.)

Table 53. Antibiotics (cont.)

Antimicrobial Class, *Subclass*	Dosage	Adjust When CrCl[a] Is: (mL/min)	Formulations	Route of Elimination (%)
Amphotericin B Lipid Complex (*Abelcet*)	2.5–5 mg/kg/d as a single infusion	c	Inj	K
Amphotericin B Liposomal (*AmBisome*)	3–6 mg/kg/d infused over 1–2 h	c	Inj	K
Amphotericin B Cholestreyl Sulfate Complex (*Amphotec*)	3–4 mg/kg/d infused at 1 mg/kg/h; max dosage 7.5 mg/kg/d	c	Inj	K
Azoles				
Fluconazole (*Diflucan*)	po, IV: first dose 200–800 mg, then 100–400 mg q 24 h for 14 d–12 wk, depending on indication Vaginal candidiasis: 150 mg as a single dose	<50	T: 50, 100, 150, 200 S: 10 and 40 mg/mL Inj	K (80)
Itraconazole (*Sporanox*)	po: 200–400 mg/d; dosages >200 mg/d should be divided. Life-threatening infections: loading dose: 200 mg q 8 h should be given for the first 3 d of therapy IV: 200 mg q 12 h × 4 d, then 200 mg/d	<30	C: 100 S: 100 mg/10 mL Inj	L
Ketoconazole (*Nizoral*)	po: 200–400 mg/d shp: 2/wk × 4 wk with ≥ 3 d between each shp Topical: apply q 12–24 h	NA	T: 200 shp: 2% crm: 2%	L, F
Miconazole (*Monistat IV*)	IT: 20 mg q 1–2 d IV: initial: 200 mg, then 1.2–3.6 g/d divided q 8 h for up to 2 wk	NA	Inj	L, F

(cont.)

Table 53. Antibiotics (cont.)				
Antimicrobial Class, *Subclass*	Dosage	Adjust When CrCl[a] Is: (mL/min)	Formulations	Route of Elimination (%)
Voriconazole (*VFEND*)	IV: loading dose 6 mg/kg q 12 h for 2 doses, then 4 mg/kg q 12 h po: >40 kg: 200 mg q 12 h; ≤40 kg: 100 mg q 12 h If on phenytoin, IV: 5 mg/kg q 12 h, and po: >40 kg: 400 mg q 12 h; ≤40 kg: 200 mg q 12 h	<50 (IV only)	Inj T: 50, 200 mg	L
Echinocandins				
Anidulafungin (*Eraxis*)	Esophageal candidiasis: 100 mg on day 1, then 50 mg/d × ≥13 d and 7 d after symptoms resolve	NA	Inj	L, F (30)
Caspofungin	Initial: 70 mg infused over 1 h; esophageal candidiasis: 50 mg/d; dosage with concurrent enzyme inducers: 70 mg/d	NA	Inj	L (50), F (35)
Micafungin (*Mycamine*)	Esophageal candidiasis: 150 mg/d; prophylaxis in stem cell transplant: 50 mg/d	NA	Inj	L, F (71), K (<15)
Other Antifungals				
Flucytosine (*Ancobon*)	po: 50–150 mg/kg/d divided q 6 h	<40	C: 250, 500	K (75–90)
Griseofulvin (*Fulvicin P/G, Grifulvin V*)	po: Microsize: 500–1000 mg/d in single or divided doses Ultramicrosize: 330–375 mg/d in single or divided doses Duration based on indication	NA	Microsize: S: 125 mg/5 mL T: 250, 500 Ultramicrosize: T: 125, 165, 250, 330	L

(cont.)

Table 53. Antibiotics (cont.)				
Antimicrobial Class, *Subclass*	Dosage	Adjust When CrCl[a] Is: (mL/min)	Formulations	Route of Elimination (%)
Terbinafine (*Lamisil*)	po: 250 mg/d × 6–12 wk for superficial mycoses; 250–500 mg/d for up to 16 mo Topical: apply q 12–24 h for max of 4 wk	<50	T: 250 mg crm: 1% topical S: 1%	L, K (70–75)

Note: NA = not applicable; TDM = adjust dose on basis of therapeutic drug monitoring principles and institutional protocols

[a] The CrCl listed is the threshold below which the dosage (amount or frequency) should be adjusted. See package insert for detailed dosing guidelines.

[b] Dosage should not exceed 250 mg q 6 h in kidney impairment.

[c] Adjust dosage if decreased kidney function is due to the medication, or give every other day.

ACUTE KIDNEY FAILURE
Definition
An acute deterioration in kidney function defined by decreased urine output or increased values of kidney function tests, or both

Precipitating and Aggravating Factors (Italicized type indicates most common.)
• *Acute tubular necrosis* due to hypoperfusion or nephrotoxins
• Medications (eg, aminoglycosides, radiocontrast materials, NSAIDs, ACEIs)
• Multiple myeloma
• Obstruction (eg, BPH)
• Vascular disease (thromboembolic, atheroembolic)
• *Volume depletion* or redistribution of extracellular fluid (eg, cirrhosis, burns)

Evaluation
• Review medication list
• Catheterize bladder, determine postvoid residual
• UA (see **Table 54** for likely diagnoses)
• Renal ultrasonography
• Renal biopsy in selected cases
• If patient is not on diuretics, determine fractional excretion of sodium (FENa):

$$FENa = \left[\frac{urine\ Na/plasma\ Na}{urine\ creatinine/plasma\ creatinine} \right] \times 100$$

FENa <1% indicates prerenal cause; FENa >3% indicates acute tubular necrosis; FENa 1%–3% is nondiagnostic. Note that some older adults who have prerenal cause may have FENa ≥1% because of age-related changes in sodium excretion.

• If patient is receiving diuretics, determine fractional excretion of urea (FEUrea):

$$FEUrea = \left[\frac{urine\ urea\ nitrogen/BUN}{urine\ creatinine/plasma\ creatinine} \right] \times 100$$

FEUrea ≤35% indicates prerenal azotemia; FEUrea >50% indicates acute tubular necrosis; FEUrea 36%–50% is nondiagnostic.

Table 54. Likely Diagnoses Based on UA Findings

Findings	Diagnoses
Hematuria, RBC casts, heavy proteinuria	Glomerular disease or vasculitis
Granular and epithelial cell casts, free epithelial cells	Acute tubular necrosis
Pyuria, WBC casts, granular or waxy casts, little or no proteinuria	Acute interstitial nephritis, glomerulitis, vasculitis, obstruction, renal infarction
Normal UA	Prerenal disease, obstruction, hypercalcemia, myeloma, acute tubular necrosis

Prevention of Radiocontrast-induced Acute Kidney Failure in High-risk Patients (Cr >1.5 mg/dL, GFR <60 mL/min/1.73 m² body surface area)

- Hold NSAIDs and diuretics for 24 h and metformin for 48 h before administration
- Use iso-osmolal contrast agents in low doses
- Avoid closely spaced repeat studies
- Avoid volume depletion (eg, give 0.9% saline IV 1 mL/kg/h for 24 h beginning 2–12 h before administration and continuing 6–12 h after procedure)
- Acetylcysteine *(Mucomyst)* (100, 200/mL) 600 mg po q 12 h the day before and the day of procedure (controversial)
- Sodium bicarbonate (154 mEq/L) 3 mL/kg/h for 1 h before procedure and 1 mL/kg/h for 6 h after procedure, especially if insufficient time for hydration before procedure
- Repeat serum creatinine 24–48 h after administration

Treatment

- D/C medications that are possible precipitants; avoid contrast dyes.
- If prerenal pattern, treat HF (see p 32) if present. Otherwise, volume repletion. Begin with fluid challenge 500–1000 mL over 30–60 min. If no response, give furosemide 100–400 mg IV.
- If obstructed, leave urinary catheter in place during evaluation and while specific treatment is implemented.
- If acute tubular necrosis, monitor weight daily, record intake and output, and monitor electrolytes frequently. Fluid replacement should be equal to urinary output plus other drainage plus 500 mL/d for insensible losses.
- Dialysis is indicated when severe hyperkalemia, acidosis, or volume overload cannot be managed with other therapies or when uremic symptoms (eg, pericarditis, coagulopathy, or encephalopathy) are present.

CHRONIC KIDNEY FAILURE
Evaluation

- Hx and physical examination: assess for diabetes mellitus, HTN, vascular disease, HF, NSAIDs, contrast dye exposure, angiographic procedures with possible cholesterol embolization, glomerulonephritis, myeloma, BPH or obstructive cancers, current or previous treatment with a nephrotoxic drug, hereditary kidney disease (eg, polycystic)
- Blood tests (CBC, comprehensive metabolic profile, cholesterol, ESR, SPEP, estimate CrCl or GFR (see p 1)
- If GFR <30 mL/min/1.73 m² body surface area, refer to a nephrologist for co-management.
- If CrCl 15–59 mL/min, then measure iPTH; if iPTH >100 pg/mL, then measure serum 25-hydroxy vitamin D
- UA and quantitative urine protein (protein:Cr ratio or 24-h urine for protein and Cr); urine immunoelectrophoresis, if indicated
- Renal ultrasound, consider Doppler to exclude renal artery stenosis
- Renal biopsy in selected cases

Treatment

- Attempt to slow progression of kidney failure
  - Control BP (target <125/75 if proteinuria or increased Cr); most important
  - ACEI or ARB (see **Table 17**), or both
  - Diabetes control, HbA_{1c} <7
  - Moderate dietary protein restriction, 0.8–1 g/kg/d, especially if diabetic nephropathy
  - Smoking cessation
  - Reduction of proteinuria to <1 g/d, if possible
- Prevent and treat symptoms and complications
  - Treat hyperkalemia if present; restrict orange juice, bananas, potatoes, cantaloupe, honeydew, tomatoes; diuretics and oral bicarbonate can also be helpful.
  - Normalize serum calcium with calcium carbonate (500 mg elemental calcium q 6–24 h) or calcium citrate if patient is on proton-pump inhibitor or has achlorhydria; if hypocalcemia is refractory, consider calcitriol (*Rocaltrol*) 0.25 mcg/d.
  - Normalize serum phosphate with target goal ≤6 mg/dL; restrict dairy products and cola. When hyperphosphatemia is refractory, begin:
    - If serum calcium is low, calcium carbonate (1250–1500 mg q 8 h with meals) or calcium acetate (*PhosLo*) (3 or 4 tabs q 8 h with meals).
    - If serum calcium is normal or calcium supplementation is ineffective:
      □ Sevelamer (*Renagel*) [T: 400, 800; C: 403]
        - If phosphate 6–7.5 mg/dL, 800 mg po q 8 h with each meal.
        - If phosphate 7.5–9.0 mg/dL, 1200–1600 po q 8 h with each meal.
        - If phosphate >9 mg/dL, 1600 mg po q 8 h with each meal.
      □ Lanthanum carbonate (*Fosrenol*) [ChT:250, 500] at initial dosage of 250–500 mg po q 8 h with each meal, then titrate in increments of 750 mg/d at intervals of 2–3 wk to max of 3750 mg/d.
  - Treat vitamin D insufficiency.
    - If GFR <30 mL/min, iPTH >100 pg/mL, and serum 25-hydroxy vitamin D is <30 ng/mL, then vitamin D (ergocalciferol) 50,000 U po every mo for 6 mo.
    - If iPTH remains >100 pg/mL, then oral vitamin D therapy with calcitriol at 0.25 mcg/d.
  - Correct metabolic acidosis if HCO_3 falls below 18–20 mEq/L (target is ≥22 mEq/L) with sodium bicarbonate 325–650 mg q 8 h.
  - Treat anemia with iron (if iron-deficient) or erythropoietin-darbopoetin (see **Table 44**).
  - Manage volume overload (see HF, p 33).
  - Prevent and treat cardiovascular disease (see p 28) with target LDL goal <100 mg/dL.
  - Treat secondary hyperparathyroidism; increased PTH can be treated with calcitriol as mentioned above.
  - Immunize with *Pneumovax* and, before dialysis, hepatitis B vaccines if hepatitis B surface antigen and antibody are negative.
  - Prepare for dialysis or transplant. Educate patients regarding options of hemodialysis, peritoneal dialysis, and kidney transplantation. If estimated GFR <25 mL/min, recommend referral for arteriovenous fistula access. If estimated GFR <20 mL/min, patients can be listed for cadaveric kidney transplant.

- Dialysis is indicated when severe hyperkalemia, acidosis, or volume overload cannot be managed with other therapies or when uremic symptoms (eg, pericarditis, coagulopathy, or encephalopathy) are present.

VOLUME DEPLETION (DEHYDRATION)
Definition
Losses of sodium and water that may be isotonic (eg, loss of blood) or hypotonic (eg, nasogastric suctioning)

Precipitating Factors
- Blood loss
- Diuretics
- GI losses
- Kidney or adrenal disease (eg, renal sodium wasting)
- Sequestration of fluid (eg, ileus, burns, peritonitis)
- Age-related changes (impaired thirst, sodium wasting due to hyporeninemic hypoaldosteronism, and free water wasting due to renal insensitivity to antidiuretic hormone)

Evaluation
Clinical Symptoms
- Anorexia
- Nausea and vomiting
- Orthostatic lightheadedness
- Delirium
- Weakness

Clinical Signs
- Dry tongue and axillae
- Oliguria
- Orthostatic hypotension
- Elevated heart rate
- Weight loss

Laboratory Tests
- Serum electrolytes
- Urine sodium (usually <10 mEq/L) and FENa (usually <1% but may be higher because of age-related sodium wasting)
- Serum BUN and creatinine (BUN:creatinine ratio often >20)

Management
- Weigh daily; monitor fluid losses and serum electrolytes, BUN, creatinine.
- If mild, oral rehydration of 2–4 L of water/d and 4–8 g Na diet; if poor oral intake, give IV D5W1/2 NS with potassium as needed.
- If hemodynamically unstable, give IV 0.9% saline 500 mL bolus and 200 mL/h until systolic BP ≥100 mm Hg and no longer orthostatic. Then switch to D5W1/2 NS. Monitor closely in patients with a hx of HF.

HYPERNATREMIA
Causes
- Pure water loss
  - Insensible losses due to sweating and respiration
  - Central (eg, post-traumatic, CNS tumors, meningitis) diabetes insipidus or nephrogenic (eg, hypercalcemia, lithium) diabetes insipidus

- Hypotonic sodium loss
  - Renal causes: osmotic diuresis (eg, due to hyperglycemia), postobstructive diuresis, polyuric phase of acute tubular necrosis
  - GI causes: vomiting and diarrhea, nasogastric drainage, osmotic cathartic agents (eg, lactulose)
- Hypertonic sodium gain (eg, treatment with hypertonic saline)
- Impaired thirst (eg, delirious or intubated) or access to water (eg, functionally dependent) may sustain hypernatremia

Evaluation
- Measure intake and output.
- Obtain urine osmolality:
  - >800 mOsm/kg suggests extrarenal (if urine Na <25 mEq/L) or remote renal water loss or administration of hypertonic Na^+ salt solutions (if urine Na >100 mEq/L).
  - <250 mOsm/kg and polyuria suggest diabetes insipidus.

Treatment
- Treat underlying causes.
- Correct slowly over at least 48–72 h using oral (can use pure water), nasogastric (can use pure water), or IV (D5W, 1/2 or 1/4 NS) fluids; correct at rate of no more than 1 mmol/L/h if acute (eg, developing over hours) and at no more than 10 mmol/L/d if of longer duration.
- Correct with NS only in cases of severe volume depletion with hemodynamic compromise; once stable, switch to hypotonic solution.
- When repleting fluids, use the following formula to estimate the effect of 1 L of any infusate on serum Na:

$$\text{Change in serum Na} = \frac{\text{infusate Na} - \text{serum Na}}{\text{total body water} + 1}$$

  - Infusate Na (mmol/L): D5W = 0; 1/4 NS = 34; 1/2 NS = 77; NS = 154
  - Calculate total body water as a fraction of body weight (0.5 kg in older men and 0.45 kg in older women).
- Divide treatment goal (usually 10 mmol/L/d) by change in serum Na/L (from formula) to determine amount of solution to be given over 24 h.
- Compensate for any ongoing obligatory fluid losses, which are usually 1–1.5 L/d.
- Divide amount of solution for repletion plus amount for obligatory fluid losses by 24 to determine rate per hour.

HYPONATREMIA
Causes
- With increased plasma osmolality: hyperglycemia (1.6 mEq/L decrement for each 100 mg/dL increase in plasma glucose)
- With normal plasma osmolality (pseudohyponatremia): severe hyperlipidemia, hyperproteinemia (eg, multiple myeloma)

- With decreased plasma osmolality:
  - With extracellular fluid (ECF) excess: kidney failure, HF, hepatic cirrhosis, nephrotic syndrome
  - With decreased ECF volume: renal loss from salt-losing nephropathies, diuretics, osmotic diuresis; extrarenal loss due to vomiting, diarrhea, skin losses, and third-spacing (usually urine Na <20 mEq/L, FENa <1%, and uric acid >4 mg/dL)
  - With normal ECF volume: primary polydipsia (urine osmolarity <100 mOsm/kg), hypothyroidism, adrenal insufficiency, SIADH (urine Na >40 mEq/L and uric acid <4 mg/dL)

Management

Treat underlying cause. Specific treatment only if symptomatic (eg, altered mental status, seizures) or severe acute hyponatremia (eg, <120 mEq/L):

- Goal is 0.5 mEq/L/h rise in Na (more rapid correction can result in central pontine myelinolysis); time (in hours) to correct = $(140 - Na)/0.5$ mEq/L/h.
- Calculate free water excess (liters) = $(0.5 \times$ current body weight in kg$) \times (1 - [Na/140])$.
- Target rate of free water removal (L/h) = free water excess/time to correct.
- Replace urine output with 3% saline or isotonic saline.
- Monitor Na closely and taper treatment when >120 mEq/L or symptoms resolve.
- Conivaptan (*Vaprisol*), an arginine vasopressin receptor antagonist, is effective in euvolemic hyponatremia in hospitalized patients; 20 mg IV over 30 min once, followed by continuous infusion of 20–40 mg over 24 h for 4 d max (L) (CYP3A4 interactions).

SYNDROME OF INAPPROPRIATE SECRETION OF ANTIDIURETIC HORMONE (SIADH)
Definition
Hypotonic hyponatremia (<280 mOsm/kg) with:

- Less than maximally dilute urine (usually >100 mOsm/kg)
- Elevated urine sodium (usually >40 mEq/L)
- Normal volume status
- Normal kidney, adrenal, and thyroid function

Precipitating Factors, Causes
- Medications (eg, SSRIs, venlafaxine, chlorpropamide, carbamazepine, oxcarbazepine, NSAIDs, barbiturates)
- Neuropsychiatric factors (eg, neoplasm, subarachnoid hemorrhage, psychosis, meningitis)
- Postoperative state, especially if pain or nausea
- Pulmonary disease (eg, pneumonia, tuberculosis, acute asthma)
- Tumors (eg, lung, pancreas, thymus)

Evaluation
- BUN, creatinine, serum cortisol, TSH
- CXR
- Review of medications
- Neurologic tests as indicated
- Urine sodium and osmolality

Management

Acute Treatment: See hyponatremia management (above).

Chronic Treatment:
- D/C offending medication or treat precipitating illness.
- Restrict water intake to 1000–1500 mL/d.
- Liberalize salt intake.
- Demeclocycline (*Declomycin*) 150–300 mg q 12 h [T: 150, 300] (may be nephrotoxic in patients with liver disease).

HYPERKALEMIA

Causes
- Kidney failure
- Addison's disease
- Hyporeninemic hypoaldosteronism
- Renal tubular acidosis
- Acidosis
- Diabetic hyperglycemia
- Hemolysis, tumor lysis, rhabdomyolysis
- Medications (potassium-sparing diuretics, ACEIs, trimethoprim-sulfamethoxazole, β-blockers, NSAIDs, cyclosporine, tacrolimus, pentamidine, heparin, digoxin toxicity)
- Pseudohyperkalemia from extreme thrombocytosis or leukocytosis
- Transfusions of stored blood
- Constipation

Evaluation
- ECG; peaked T waves typically occur when K^+ exceeds 6.5 mEq/L. ECG changes are more likely with acute increases of K^+ than with chronic increases.

Treatment

Minor elevations
- K^+ <6 mEq/L without ECG changes:
  - Low-potassium diet (restrict orange juice, bananas, potatoes, cantaloupe, honeydew, tomatoes)
  - Oral diuretics (eg, oral torsemide or bumetanide, combined oral loop and thiazide-like diuretics; metolazone is the most K^+ wasting); avoid hypovolemia
  - Oral $NaHCO_3$ (650–1300 mg q 12 h)
  - Reduce or D/C medications that increase K^+
- K^+ 6–6.5 mEq/L without ECG changes: above treatments plus sodium polystyrene sulfonate (*SPS, Kayexelate*) 15–30 g po q 6–24 h, or prn as enema 30–50 g in 100 mL of dextrose; full effect takes 4–24 h.
- K^+ 6.5 mEq/L with peaked T waves but no other ECG changes; hospitalization is decided case-by-case based on acuteness of onset, cause, and other patient factors.

Absolute indications for hospitalization
- K^+ >8 mEq/L
- ECG changes other than peaked T waves (eg, prolonged PR, loss of P waves, widened QRS)
- Acute deterioration of kidney function

Inpatient management of hyperkalemia
- Antagonism of cardiac effects of hyperkalemia (most rapid-acting acute therapy; use only for severe hyperkalemia with significant ECG changes when too dangerous to wait for redistribution therapies to take effect)
  - 10% calcium gluconate IV infused over 2–3 min (20–30 min if on digoxin) with ECG monitoring; effect lasts 30–60 min, may repeat if needed
- Reduction of serum K^+ by redistribution into cells (acute therapy; can be used in combination with calcium gluconate, and different redistribution therapies can be combined depending on severity of hyperkalemia)
  - Insulin (regular) 10 U in 500 mL of 10% dextrose over 30–60 min or bolus insulin (regular) 10 U IV followed by 50 mL of 50% dextrose
  - Albuterol 0.5 mg in 100 mL of 5% dextrose given over 10–15 min or nebulized 10–20 mg in 4 mL of NS over 10 min (should not be used as single agent)
  - Sodium bicarbonate use is controversial.
- Removal of potassium from body (definitive therapy; work more slowly)
  - Diuretics (eg, oral torsemide or bumetanide, IV furosemide, combined oral loop and thiazide-like diuretics; metolazone is the most K^+ wasting). Avoid hypovolemia.
  - Fludrocortisone (*Florinef*) 0.1–0.3 mg/d
  - Sodium polystyrene sulfonate (*SPS, Kayexalate*) 15–30 g po q 6–24 h or prn as enema 30–50 g in 100 mL of dextrose; full effect takes 4–24 h.
  - Dialysis

MALNUTRITION

DEFINITION
There is no uniformly accepted definition of malnutrition in older adults. Some commonly used definitions include the following:

Community-dwelling Older Adults
- Involuntary weight loss (eg, $\geq$10 lb over 6 mo, $\geq$4% over 1 yr)
- Abnormal body mass index (eg, BMI >27; BMI <22)
- Hypoalbuminemia (eg, $\leq$3.8 g/dL)
- Hypocholesterolemia (eg, <160 mg/dL)
- Specific vitamin or micronutrient deficiencies (eg, vitamin B_{12})

Hospitalized Patients
- Dietary intake (eg, <50% of estimated needed caloric intake)
- Hypoalbuminemia (eg, <3.5 g/dL)
- Hypocholesterolemia (eg, <160 mg/dL)

Nursing-home Patients (Triggered by the Minimum Data Set)
- Weight loss of $\geq$5% in past 30 d; $\geq$10% in 180 d
- Dietary intake <75% of most meals

EVALUATION
Multidimensional Assessment
In the absence of valid nutrition screening instruments, clinicians should focus on whether the following issues may be affecting nutritional status:
- Economic barriers to securing food
- Availability of sufficiently high-quality food
- Dental problems that preclude ingesting food
- Medical illnesses that:
  - interfere with digestion or absorption of food
  - increase nutritional requirements
  - require dietary restrictions (eg, low-sodium diet or npo)
- Functional disability that interferes with shopping, preparing meals, or feeding
- Food preferences or cultural beliefs that interfere with adequate food intake
- Poor appetite
- Depressive symptoms

Anthropometrics
Weight on each visit and yearly height (see p 1)

Biochemical Markers
Serum Proteins: All may drop precipitously because of trauma, sepsis, or major infection.
- Albumin (half-life 18–20 d) has prognostic value in all settings.
- Transferrin (half-life 7 d)
- Prealbumin (half-life 48 h) may be valuable in monitoring nutritional recovery.

Serum Cholesterol (Low or Falling Levels): Has prognostic value in all settings but may not be nutritionally mediated.

MANAGEMENT
Vitamin Supplementation
All older adults should receive a multivitamin supplement, calcium 1200 mg/d, and vitamin D 800 IU/d.

Calculating Basic Energy (Caloric) and Fluid Requirements
- WHO energy estimates for adults 60 yr old and older:
  - Women (10.5) (weight in kg) + 596
  - Men (13.5) (weight in kg) + 487
- Harris-Benedict energy requirement equations:
  - Women: 655 + (9.6) (weight in kg) + (1.7) (height in cm) − (4.7) (age in yr)
  - Men: 66 + (13.7) (weight in kg) + (5) (height in cm) − (6.8) (age in yr)
- Fluid requirements for older adults without heart or kidney disease are approximately 30 mL/kg/d.

Depending on activity and physiologic stress levels, these basic requirements may need to be increased (eg, 25% for sedentary or mild, 50% for moderate, and 100% for intense or severe activity or stress).

Appetite Stimulants
- No medications are FDA approved to promote weight gain in older adults.
- Dronabinol and megestrol acetate (not covered by Medicare Part D) have been effective in promoting weight gain in younger adults with specific conditions (eg, AIDS, cancer). Small clinical trials of megestrol in select groups (eg, after hospitalization, nursing home) have shown benefit for some nutritional markers (eg, prealbumin, weight) but not for clinical outcomes.
- A minority of patients receiving mirtazapine report appetite stimulation and weight gain.
- All medications used for appetite have substantial potential adverse events.

Nutritional Supplements
Protein and energy supplements in older adults at risk of malnutrition appear to have beneficial effects on weight gain and mortality, and shorten length of stay in hospitalized patients. Among those who are well nourished at baseline, the benefit is less clear. Supplements should be given between rather than with meals.

Many formulas are available (see **Table 55** and **Table 56**). Read the content labels and choose on the basis of calories/mL, protein, fiber, lactose, and fluid load.

- Oral: Many (eg, *Carnation Instant Breakfast, Health Shake*) are milk-based and provide approximately 1–1.5 calories/mL.
- Enteral: Commercial preparations have between 0.5 and 2 calories/mL; most contain no milk (lactose) products. For patients who need fluid restriction, the higher concentrated formulas may be valuable, but they may cause diarrhea. Because of reduced kidney function with aging, some recommend that protein should contribute no more than 20% of the formula's total calories. If formula is sole source of nutrition, consider one that contains fiber (25 g/d is optimal).

Table 55. Examples of Lactose-free Oral Products

Product	Kcal/mL	mOsm	Protein (g/L)	Water (mL/L)	Na (mEq/L)	K (mEq/L)	Fiber (g/L)
Low residue							
Boost Drink[a]	1.01	610–670	42.0	850	24.0	43.0	0
Boost Plus	1.52	670	59.0	780	31.0	41.0	<4
Ensure[b]	1.06	600	37.0	844	36.7	40.0	0
Ensure Plus	1.50	525	54.9	720	41.9	44.8	0
Carnation Instant Breakfast lactose-free	1.00	480	35.0	842	38.0	32.0	0
Carnation Instant Breakfast lactose-free Plus	1.50	620	52.4	776	50.8	48.0	0
Low volume (packaged as 45-mL supplements; nutrients are provided per serving)							
Resource Benecalorie	330	NA	7.0	0	0.7	0	0
Epulor	320	418	4.0	0	0.5	0	0
High fiber (can also be given enterally)							
Boost with Fiber	1.01	600–650	42.0	840	31.0	41.0	13.0
Ensure Fiber	1.06	500	37.0	823	36.7	40.0	12.0
Clear liquid							
CitriSource	0.76	700	37.0	876	10.0	1.6	0
Resource	1.06	430	33.0	842	24.0	1.3	0
Enlive	1.25	825	40.0	768	10.4	4.0	0
Diabetes formulation							
Glucerna shake[c]	0.83	660	40.0	800	38.8	43.0	20

NA = not available
[a] Also has "pudding" product that has 240 Kcal/5 oz and 0 fiber
[b] Also has "pudding" product that has 170 Kcal/4 oz and 1 g fiber/serving
[c] Institutional formulation has 530 mOsm and 38 mEq K/L.

Table 56. Examples of Lactose-free Enteral Products

Product	Kcal/mL	mOsm	Protein (g/L)	Water (mL/L)	Na (mEq/L)	K (mEq/L)	Fiber (g/L)
Diabetes formulations							
Diabetisource AC	1.20	450	60	818	46.0	44.0	15.0
Glucerna	1.00	355	41.8	853	40.4	40.2	14.4
Low residue							
Isosource	1.2	490	43.0	819	48.0	49.0	0
Osmolite[a]	1.06	300	37.1	841	27.8	26.1	0
Nutren 1.0[b]	1.00	315	40.0	848	38.1	32.0	0
Low volume							
Nutren 2.0	2.00	745	80.0	703	56.8	48.9	0
TwoCal HN	2.00	725	83.5	700	63.0	62.6	5.0
High fiber							
Jevity[a]	1.06	300	44.3	835	40.4	40.2	14.4
Fibersource HN	1.2	490	53.0	814	52.0	51.0	10
Nutren 1.0 with fiber[b]	1.00	330	40.0	840	38.1	32.0	14.0

[a] Also has 1.2 and 1.5 calorie formulations
[b] Also has 1.5 calorie formulation

Important Drug-enteral Interactions

- Soybean formulas increase fecal elimination of thyroxine; time administration of thyroxine and enteral nutrition as far apart as possible.
- Enteral feedings reduce absorption of phenytoin; administer phenytoin at least 2 h after a feeding and delay feeding at least 2 h after phenytoin is administered; monitor levels and adjust dosages, as necessary.
- Check with pharmacy about suitability and best way to administer sustained-release, enteric-coated, and micro-encapsulated products (eg, omeprazole, lansoprazole, diltiazem, fluoxetine, verapamil).

Gastrostomy/Jejunostomy Tube Feeding

- Chronic artificial nutrition and hydration is not a basic intervention and is associated with uncertain benefit and considerable risks and discomfort.
- Artificial nutrition and hydration should be used only for specific medical indications, not to increase patient comfort.
- Randomized trials have not shown benefit in stroke patients with dysphagia.

Tips for Successful Tube Feeding

- Gastrostomy tube feeding may be either intermittent or continuous.
- Jejunostomy tube feedings must be continuous.
- Continuous tube feeding is associated with less frequent diarrhea but with higher rates of tube clogging.
- To prevent clogging and to provide additional free water, flushing with at least 30–60 mL of water q 4–6 h is recommended. Sometimes sugar-free carbonated beverages, cranberry juice, or meat tenderizer can restore patency to clogged tubes.
- Diarrhea, which develops in 5%–30% of people receiving enteral feeding, may be related to the osmolality of the formula, the rate of delivery, high sorbitol content in liquid medications (eg, APAP, lithium, oxybutynin, furosemide), or other patient-related factors such as antibiotic use or impaired absorption.
- To help prevent aspiration, maintain ≥30-degree elevation of the head of the bed during continuous feeding and for at least 2 h after bolus feedings.
- Do not administer bulk-forming laxatives (eg, methylcellulose or psyllium) through feeding tubes.
- Check gastric residual volume before each bolus feeding and hold feeding for at least 1 h if residual is more than half of previous feeding volume. Metoclopramide (*Reglan*) 5–10 mg [5 mg/5 mL] q 6 h may be useful for problems with high gastric residual volume once mechanical obstruction has been excluded.

Parenteral Nutrition

Indicated in those with digestive dysfunction precluding enteral feeding. Delivers protein as amino acids, carbohydrate as dextrose (D5 = 170 kcal/L; D10 = 340 kcal/L), and fat as lipid emulsions (10% = 1100 kcal/L; 20% = 2200 kcal/L).

Peripheral Parenteral Nutrition: For short-term use; requires rotation of peripheral IV site q 72 h; solution osmolarity of <900 mOsm/L is recommended to reduce risk of phlebitis.

Total Parenteral Nutrition: Must be administered through a central catheter, which may be inserted peripherally.

SHOULDER PAIN: DIFFERENTIAL DIAGNOSIS AND TREATMENT

Rotator Cuff Tendinitis, Subacromial Bursitis, or Rotator Tendon Impingement on Clavicle

Dull ache radiating to upper arm. Painful arc (on abduction 60–120 degrees and external rotation) is characteristic. Also can be distinguished by applying resistance against active range of motion while immobilizing the neck with hand.

May cause shoulder impingement syndrome (insidious onset of anterolateral acromial pain frequently radiating to lateral mid-humerus). Pain is worse at night, exacerbated by lying on the involved shoulder or sleeping with the arm overhead. Active and passive range of motion are normal.

Treatment: Identify and eliminate provocative, repetitive injury (eg, avoid overhead reaching). A brief period of rest and immobilization with a sling may be helpful. Pain control with APAP or NSAIDs (**Table 57**), home exercises or PT (especially assisted range of motion and wall walking), and corticosteroid injections (see p 148) may be useful.

Rotator Cuff Tears

Mild to complete; characterized by diminished shoulder movement. If severe, patients do not have full range of active or passive motion. The "drop arm" sign (the inability to maintain the arm in an abducted 90-degree position) indicates supraspinatus and infraspinatus tear. Weakness of external rotation (elbows flexed, thumbs up with examiner's hands outside patient's elbows; patient is asked to resist inward pressure) is common. MRI establishes diagnosis.

Treatment: If due to injury, a brief period of rest and immobilization with a sling may be helpful. Pain control with APAP or NSAIDs (**Table 57**), home exercises or PT (especially assisted range of motion and wall walking) may be useful. If no improvement after 6–8 wk of conservative measures, consider surgical repair.

Bicipital Tendinitis

Pain felt on anterior lateral aspect of shoulder, tenderness in the groove between greater and lesser tuberosities of the humerus. Pain is elicited on resisted flexion of shoulder, flexion of the elbow, or supination (external rotation) of the hand and wrist with the elbow flexed at the side.

Treatment: Identify and eliminate provocative, repetitive activities (eg, avoid overhead reaching). A period of rest (at least 7 d with no lifting) and corticosteroid injections (see p 148) are major components of therapy. After rest period, PT should focus on stretching biceps tendon (eg, putting arm on doorframe and hyperextending shoulder, with some external rotation). Tendon sheath injection with corticosteroids may be helpful.

Frozen Shoulder (Adhesive Capsulitis)

Loss of passive external (lateral) rotation, abduction, and internal rotation of the shoulder to <90 degrees. Usually follows three phases: painful (freezing) phase lasting wks to a few mo; adhesive (stiffening) phase lasting 4–12 mo; resolution phase lasting 6–24 mo.

Treatment: Avoid rest and begin PT and home exercises for stretching the arm in flexion, horizontal adduction, and internal and external rotation. Corticosteroid injections (see p 148) may reduce pain and permit more aggressive PT. Consider surgical manipulation under anesthesia or arthroscopic dilation of capsule.

BACK PAIN: DIFFERENTIAL DIAGNOSIS AND TREATMENT
Acute Lumbar Strain (Low Back Pain Syndrome)
Acute pain frequently precipitated by heavy lifting or exercise. Pain may be central or more prominent on one side and may radiate to sacroiliac region and buttocks. Pain is aggravated by motion, standing, and prolonged sitting, and relieved by rest. Sciatic pain may be present even when neurologic examination is normal.

Treatment: Most can continue normal activities. If a patient obtains symptomatic relief from bed rest, generally 1–2 d lying in a semi-Fowler position or on side with the hips and knees flexed with pillow between legs will suffice. Treat muscle spasm with the application of ice, preferably in a massage over the muscles in spasm. APAP or NSAIDs (**Table 57**) can be used to control pain. Spinal manipulation is also effective for uncomplicated low back pain. As pain diminishes, encourage patient to begin isometric abdominal and lower-extremity exercises. Symptoms often recur. Education on back posture, lifting precautions, and abdominal muscle strengthening may help prevent recurrences.

Acute Disk Herniation
Over 90% of cases have herniation at L4–L5 or L5–S1 levels, resulting in unilateral impairment of ankle reflex, toe and ankle dorsiflexion, and pain (commonly sciatic) on straight leg raising (can be tested from sitting position by leg extension). Pain is acute in onset and varies considerably with changes in position.

Treatment: Initially same as acute lumbar strain (above). If unresponsive, administer epidural injection of a combination of a long-acting corticosteroid with an epidural anesthetic. Consider surgery if recurrence or neurologic signs persist beyond 6–8 wk after conservative treatment. The value of epidural injections and surgery for pain without neurologic signs is controversial. Surgery for severe sciatica provides faster pain relief and perceived recovery rates but no difference in perceived recovery and disability at 1 yr compared with conservative management. (See **Table 2** and **Table 3**.)

Osteoarthritis and Chronic Disk Degeneration
Characterized by aching pain aggravated by motion and relieved by rest. Occasionally, hypertrophic spurring in a facet joint may cause unilateral radiculopathy with sciatica.
Treatment: Identify and eliminate provocative activities. Education on back posture, lifting precautions, and abdominal muscle strengthening. APAP or NSAIDs (**Table 57**). Corticosteroid injections may be useful. Consider opioids and other pain treatment modalities for chronic refractory pain (see p 173).

Unstable Lumbar Spine
Severe, sudden, short-lasting, frequently recurrent pain often brought on by sudden, unguarded movements. Pain is reproduced when moving from the flexed to the erect position. Pain is usually relieved by lying supine or on side. Impingement on nerve roots by

spurs from facet joints or herniated disks can cause similar complaints, although symptoms in these conditions usually worsen over time. Symptoms can mimic disk herniation or degeneration, or osteoarthritis. Lumbar flexion radiographs can be diagnostic.

Treatment: Abdominal and paraspinal exercises, lumbrosacral corset. Surgery only in severe cases.

Lumbar Spinal Stenosis

Symptoms increase on spinal extension (eg, with prolonged standing, walking downhill, lying prone) and decrease with spinal flexion (eg, sitting, bending forward while walking, lying in the flexed position). Only symptom may be fatigue or pain in legs when walking (pseudo-claudication). May have immobility of lumbar spine, pain with straight leg raises, weakness of muscles innervated by L4 through S1 (see **Table 3**). Over 4 yr, 15% improve, 15% deteriorate, and 70% remain stable.

Treatment: APAP or NSAIDs (**Table 57**) and exercises to reduce lumbar lordosis are sometimes beneficial. Corticosteroid injections may be useful. Surgical intervention is more effective than conservative treatment in relieving moderate or severe symptoms; however, recurrence of pain several years after surgery is common.

Vertebral Compression Fracture

Immediate onset of severe pain; worse with sitting or standing; sometimes relieved by lying down.

Treatment: See Osteoporosis, p 166. Bed rest, analgesia, and mobilization as tolerated. Calcitonin may provide symptomatic improvement. May require hospitalization to control symptoms. Percutaneous vertebroplasty or kyphoplasty may be effective for pain relief in refractory cases.

Nonrheumatic Pain (eg, Tumors, Aneurysms)

Gradual onset, steadily expanding, often unrelated to position and not relieved by lying down. Night pain when lying down is characteristic. Upper motor neuron signs may be present. Involvement is usually in thoracic and upper lumbar spine.

HIP PAIN: DIFFERENTIAL DIAGNOSIS AND TREATMENT
Trochanteric Bursitis

Pain in lateral aspect of the hip that usually worsens when patient sits on a hard chair, lies on the affected side, or rises from a chair or bed; pain may improve with walking. Local tenderness over greater trochanter is often present, and pain is often reproduced on resisted abduction of the leg or internal rotation of the hip. However, trochanteric bursitis does not result in limited range of motion, pain on range of motion, pain in the groin, or radicular signs.

Treatment: Identify and eliminate provocative activities. Position pillow posterolaterally behind involved side to avoid lying on bursae while sleeping. Check for leg length discrepancy, prescribe orthotics if appropriate. Injection of a combination of a long-acting corticosteroid with an anesthetic is most effective treatment.

Osteoarthritis

"Boring" quality pain in the hip, often in the groin, and sometimes referred to the back or knee with stiffness after rest. Passive motion is restricted in all directions if disease is fairly advanced. In early disease, pain in the groin on internal rotation of the hip is characteristic.

Treatment: See also Osteoarthritis, p 148. Elective total hip replacement is indicated for patients who have radiographic evidence of joint damage and moderate to severe persistent pain or disability, or both, that is not substantially relieved by an extended course of nonsurgical management.

Guideline for the Management of Pain in Osteoarthritis, Rheumatoid Arthritis, and Juvenile Chronic Arthritis, 2nd ed., American Pain Society, 2002.

Hip Fracture

Sudden onset, usually after a fall, with inability to walk or bear weight, frequently radiating to groin or knee.

Treatment: Treatment is surgical with open reduction and internal fixation, hemiarthroplasty, or total hip replacement, depending on site of fracture and amount of displacement. For patients who were nonambulatory before the fracture, conservative management is an option.

Nonrheumatic Pain

Referred pain from viscera, radicular pain from the lower spine, avascular necrosis, Paget's disease, metastasis. Treatment based on identified etiology.

KNEE PAIN: DIFFERENTIAL DIAGNOSIS AND TREATMENT
Osteoarthritis

Pain usually related to activity (eg, climbing stairs, arising from chair, walking long distances). Morning stiffness lasts <30 min. Crepitation is common. Examination should attempt to exclude other causes of knee pain such as hip arthritis with referred knee pain (decreased hip range of motion), chondromalacia patellae (tenderness only over patellofemoral joint), iliotibial band syndrome (tenderness is lateral to the knee at site of insertion in fibular head or where courses over lateral femoral condyle), anserine bursitis (tenderness distal to knee over medial tibia), and determination of malalignment varus (bowlegged) or valgus (knock-kneed).

Treatment: See osteoarthritis treatment, p 148.

PLANTAR FASCIITIS
Definition

Strain or inflammation in plantar fascia causing foot pain that is worse when beginning to walk; 80% resolve spontaneously within 1 yr.

Causes/Risk Factors

- Jumping
- Running
- Rheumatic diseases
- Obesity
- Flat feet
- Plantar spurs

Evaluation
Examiner should dorsiflex toes and then palpate plantar fascia to elicit pain points; posterior heel pain is uncommon and suggests other diagnosis.

Treatment
Nonpharmacologic
- Rest and icing
- Exercises (calf plantar fascia stretch, foot/ankle circles, toe curls)
- Prefabricated silicone heel inserts
- Shoes (running, arch support, crepe sole)
- Short-leg walking cast
- Surgery (rarely needed)

Pharmacologic
- NSAIDs (short duration, 2–3 wk)
- Corticosteroid (eg, methylprednisolone 20–40 mg) and analgesic (eg, 1% lidocaine) injection of fascia; use only if conservative measures fail

CARPAL TUNNEL SYNDROME
Definition
Painful tingling or hypoesthesia, or both, in one or both hands in distribution innervated by median nerve

Causes
- Repetitive activities
- Diabetes mellitus
- Thyroid disease
- Amyloidosis
- Rheumatoid arthritis
- Space-occupying lesions (eg, lymphoma)
- Trauma (eg, Colles' fracture)

Evaluation and Assessment
Physical Examination
- Decreased sensation in palm, thumb, index finger, middle finger, and thumb side of ring finger
- Weak handgrip
- Tapping over median nerve at wrist causes pain to shoot from wrist to hand (Tinel's sign)
- Acute flexion of wrist for 60 sec (Phalen's test) should also cause pain

Laboratory Studies
- Fasting glucose
- TSH
- Nerve conduction velocity testing confirms diagnosis

Treatment
Nonpharmacologic
- Modify work or leisure activities to avoid repetitive movements
- Splinting in neutral position, especially at night
- Surgery (more effective than splinting)

Pharmacologic
- Injectable corticosteroids, eg, methylprednisolone 15 mg (more effective than oral)
- Oral corticosteroids, eg, prednisone 20 mg/d for 1 wk followed by 10 mg/d for a second wk

OSTEOARTHRITIS
Nonpharmacologic Approaches
- Superficial heat: hot packs, heating pads, paraffin, or hot water bottles (moist heat is better)
- Deep heat: microwave, shortwave diathermy, or ultrasound
- Biofeedback and transcutaneous electrical nerve stimulation
- Exercise (especially water-based), PT, OT: strengthening, stretching, range of motion, functional activities
- Weight loss: especially for low back, hip, and knee arthritis
- Splinting: Avoid splinting for long periods of time (eg, >6 wk) because periarticular muscle weakness and wasting may occur. Bracing (eg, neoprene sleeves over the knee, valgus brace) to correct malalignment is often helpful.
- Assistive devices: Cane should be used in the hand contralateral to the affected knee or hip. Cane length should be to the level of the wrist crease. Use walker if moderate or severe balance impairment, bilateral weakness, or unilateral weakness requiring support of >15%–20% of body weight.
- Surgical intervention (eg, debridement, meniscal repair, prosthetic joint replacement).
- Acupuncture as an adjunct to NSAIDs or analgesics for knee osteoarthritis or chronic low back pain.

Pharmacologic Intervention (see **Figure 6**)
Topical Analgesics: Liniments containing methylsalicylates (see **Table 73**), capsaicin cream, lidocaine 5% pch *(Lidoderm)*.

Intra-articular Bursal and Trigger-point Injections:
- Corticosteroids: May be particularly effective if monoarticular symptoms (eg, methylprednisolone acetate, triamcinolone acetonide, and triamcinolone hexacetonide [longest acting]); 20–40 mg for large joints (eg, knee, ankle, shoulder), 10–20 mg for wrists and elbows, and 5–15 mg for small joints of hands and feet; often mixed with lidocaine 1% or its equivalent (in equal volume with corticosteroids) for immediate relief. Effect typically lasts 1–2 mo. Usually given ≥ q 3 mo.
- Hyaluronic acid preparations (*Euflexxa, Hyalgan, Orthovisc, Synvisc, Supartz*) 3–5 injections 1 wk apart for knee osteoarthritis. Benefit is usually modest but may last ≥6 mo.

Nutriceuticals: Glucosamine sulfate (500 mg q 8 h) or chondroitin (400 mg q 8 h), or both, have been effective for some patients. Combination tabs and timed-release formulations (1500 mg and 1200 mg, respectively) are available. Results of clinical trials have been variable. Combination may be more effective in moderate to severe knee pain.

NSAIDs: Often provide pain relief but have higher rates of adverse events compared with APAP (see **Table 57**). Misoprostol (*Cytotec*) 100–200 mg q 6 h with food [T: 100, 200], or a proton-pump inhibitor (see **Table 38**) may be valuable prophylaxis against NSAID-induced ulcers in high-risk patients. Selective COX-2 inhibitors have lower likelihood of causing gastroduodenal ulcers than nonselective NSAIDs but increase risk of MI. All may increase INR in patients receiving warfarin.

Oral Opioids: Use requires careful risk-benefit analysis (see **Table 71**).

Figure 6. Pharmacologic Management of Osteoarthritis*

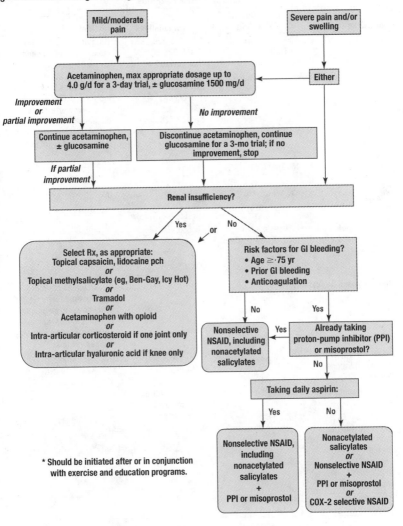

Source: Adapted from original material courtesy of Catherine MacLean, MD, PhD. Reprinted with permission.

Table 57. APAP and NSAIDs

Class, Drug	Usual Dosage for Arthritis	Formulations	Comments (Metabolism, Excretion)
✔APAP (*Tylenol***)	650 mg q 4–6 h (q 8 h if CrCl <10 mg/mL)	T: 80, 325, 500, 650; C: 160, 325, 500; S: elixir 120/5 mL, 160/5 mL, 167/5 mL, 325/5 mL; S: 160/5 mL, 500/15 mL; Sp: 120, 325, 600	Drug of choice for chronic musculoskeletal conditions; no anti-inflammatory properties; hepatotoxic above 4 g/d; at high dosages (≥2 g/d) may increase INR in patients receiving warfarin; reduce dosage 50%–75% if liver or kidney disease or if harmful or hazardous alcohol intake (L, K)
Extended release (*Tylenol ER***)	1300 mg q 8 h	ER: 650	
ASA	650 mg q 4–6 h	T: 81, 325, 500, 650, 975; Sp: 120, 200, 300, 600	(K)
Extended release (*ZORprin***)	1300 mg q 8 h or 1600–3200 mg q 12 h	CR: 650, 800	
Enteric-coated*	1000 mg q 6 h	T: 81, 162, 325, 500, 650, 975	
Nonacetylated Salicylates			Do not inhibit platelet aggregation; fewer GI and renal adverse events; no reaction in ASA-sensitive patients; monitor salicylate concentrations
✔Choline magnesium salicylate (*Tricosal, Trilisate, CMT*)	3 g/d in 1, 2, or 3 doses	T: 500, 750, 1000; S: 500 mg/5mL	(K)
✔Choline salicylate (*Arthropan*)	4.8–7.2 g/d divided	T: 325, 545, 600, 650 S: 870 mg/5 mL	(L, K)
✔Magnesium salicylate* (eg, *Doan's Extra Strength***, *Keyigesic***, *Momentum***, *Novasal*)	2 tabs q 6–8 h, max 4800 mg q 24 h	T: 467, 600, 650	Avoid in kidney failure
✔Salsalate (eg, *Amigesic*)	1500 mg to 4 g/d in 2 or 3 doses	T: 500, 750	(K)

(cont.)

Table 57. APAP and NSAIDs (cont.)

Class, Drug	Usual Dosage for Arthritis	Formulations	Comments (Metabolism, Excretion)
Nonselective NSAIDs			
Diclofenac (*Cataflam, Voltaren*)	50–150 mg/d in 2 or 3 doses	T: 50, 75; 50, enteric coated	(L)
(*Voltaren-XR*)	100 mg/d	T: ER 100	(L)
↵Enteric coated (*Arthrotec 50*)	1 tab q 8–12 h	50 mg with 200 mcg misoprostol	(L)
(*Arthrotec 75*)	1 tab q 12 h	75 mg with 200 mcg misoprostol	(L)
Diflunisal (*Dolobid*)	500–1000 mg/d in 2 doses	T: 500	(K)
↵Etodolac (*Lodine*)	200–400 mg q 6–8 h	T: 400, 500; ER 400, 500, 600	Fewer GI adverse events (L)
(*Lodine XL*)	400–1000 mg/d	C: 200, 300	
Fenoprofen (*Nalfon*)	200–600 mg q 6–8 h	C: 200, 300; T: 600	Higher risk of GI adverse events (L)
Flurbiprofen (*Ansaid*)	200–300 mg/d in 2, 3, or 4 doses	T: 50, 100	(L)
↵Ibuprofen (eg, *Advil, Motrin, Nuprin*)**	1200–3200 mg/d in 3 or 4 doses	T: 100, 200, 300, 400, 600, 800; ChT: 50, 100; S: 100 mg/5 mL	Fewer GI adverse events (L)
↵Ketoprofen (*Orudis*)	50–75 mg q 8 h	T: 12.5; C: 50, 75	(L)
Sustained release (*Oruvail* [Canadian brand])	200 mg/d	C: 200	(L)
Ketorolac (*Toradol*)	10 mg q 4–6 h, 15 mg IM or IV q 6 h	T: 10 Inj	Duration of use should be limited to 5 d (K)
Meclofenamate sodium	200–400 mg/d in 3 or 4 doses	C: 50, 100	High incidence of diarrhea (L)
Mefenamic acid (*Ponstel*)	250 mg q 6 h	C: 250	(L)
↵Meloxicam (*Mobic*)	7.5–15 mg/d	T: 7.5, 15 S: 7.5 mg/5mL	Has some COX-2 selectivity; fewer GI adverse events (L)
↵Nabumetone (*Relafen*)	500–1000 mg q 12 h	T: 500, 750	Fewer GI adverse events (L)
↵Naproxen (*Aleve,*** *Naprosyn*)	220–500 mg q 12 h	T: 220**, 375, 500, 750; S: 125 mg/5 mL	(L)
Delayed release (*EC-Naprosyn*)	375–500 mg q 12 h	T: 375, 500	(L)
Extended release (*Naprelan*)	750–1000 mg/d	T: 250, 375, 500	(L)

(cont.)

Table 57. APAP and NSAIDs (cont.)

Class, Drug	Usual Dosage for Arthritis	Formulations	Comments (Metabolism, Excretion)
Naproxen sodium (*Anaprox*)	275 mg or 550 mg q 12 h	T: 275, 550	(L)
✔Oxaprozin (*Daypro*)	1200 mg/d	C: 600	(L)
Piroxicam (*Feldene*)	10 mg/d	C: 10, 20	Can cause delirium (L)
Sulindac (*Clinoril*)	150–200 mg q 12 h	T: 150, 200 C: 200	May have higher rate of renal impairment (L)
Tolmetin (*Tolectin*)	600–1800 mg/d in 3 or 4 doses	T: 200, 600; C: 400	(L)
Selective COX-2 Inhibitor			
✔Celecoxib (*Celebrex*)	100–200 mg q 12 h	C: 50, 100, 200, 400	Increased risk of MI; less GI ulceration; do not inhibit platelets; may increase INR if taking warfarin; avoid if moderate or severe hepatic insufficiency; may induce renal impairment; contra-indicated if allergic to sulfonamides (L)

✔ = preferred for treating older adults
 * Also OTC in a lower tab strength.
** OTC

RHEUMATOID ARTHRITIS
Diagnosis
Diagnosis established if ≥4 of the following 7 criteria are met (ACR):

1. Morning stiffness in and around the joints, lasting ≥1 hr before max improvement and present for ≥6 wk.
2. Arthritis of 3 or more joint areas simultaneously with soft-tissue swelling or fluid (not bony overgrowth alone), observed by a physician and present for ≥6 wk; the 14 possible joint areas are right or left proximal interphalangeal (PIP) joints, metacarpophalangeal (MCP) joints, wrist, elbow, knee, ankle, and metatarsophalangeal (MTP) joints.
3. Arthritis of hand joints (as defined above) in a wrist, MCP, or PIP joint and present for ≥6 wk.
4. Symmetric arthritis defined as simultaneous involvement of the same joint areas (see #2 above) on both sides of the body (bilateral involvement of PIPs, MCPs, or MTPs is acceptable without absolute symmetry) and present for ≥6 wk.
5. Rheumatoid nodules (which are subcutaneous) over bony prominences or extensor surfaces, or in juxta-articular regions, observed by a physician.
6. Serum rheumatoid factor present (anti-cyclic citrullinated peptide [anti-CCP] may be positive before rheumatoid factor but is not currently a criterion for diagnosis of RA).
7. Radiographic changes typical of RA on posteroanterior hand and wrist radiographs, which must include erosions or unequivocal bony decalcification localized to or most marked adjacent to the involved joints (osteoarthritis changes alone do not qualify).

Management
Nonpharmacologic
- Patient education
- Exercise
- Physical and occupational therapy
- Splints and orthotics
- Surgery for severe functional abnormalities due to synovitis or joint destruction

Pharmacologic
All patients with established disease should be offered disease-modifying anti-rheumatoid drugs (DMARDs) as soon as possible; goal is to induce remission and then lower dosages to maintain remission.

- Analgesics (see **Table 57** and Pain, p 170)
- NSAIDs (see **Table 57**)
- Glucocorticoids (eg, prednisone ≤15 mg/d or equivalent) with osteoporosis prevention measures (see Osteoporosis, p 166)
- DMARDs (may use ≥1 class; no clear guidelines on which combinations are best and which patients need combination therapy)
  - Hydroxychloroquine [T: 200], begin 200–400 mg/d; dose at <6.5 mg/kg/d to reduce risk of retinal toxicity; annual eye examination to screen for retinal toxicity; contraindicated in G6PD deficiency.
  - Sulfasalazine (*Azulfidine, Azulfidine* EN-tabs) [T: 500], to avoid GI upset, begin at 500 mg/d, increasing dose by 500 mg every 3–4 d until taking 2–3 g/d split between 2 doses; check CBC, LFTs q 8 wk.
  - Methotrexate (*Rheumatrex* [T: 2.5], *Trexall* [T: 2.5, 5, 7.5, 10, 15]), 10–25 mg/wk, adjust dosage for renal impairment; may cause oral ulcers, hepatotoxicity, pulmonary toxicity, cytopenias, thrombocytopenia (rare), and anemia (rare); avoid in patients with liver disease; check CBC, LFTs q 8 wk; folic acid 1 mg/d should be given with methotrexate to reduce adverse events.
  - Leflunomide *(Arava)* [T: 10, 20], begin 100 mg/d × 3 d, then 20 mg/d; may cause hepatotoxicity, cytopenias, thrombocytopenia (rare), and anemia (rare); avoid in patients with liver disease; check CBC, LFTs q 8 wk.
  - Anticytokine therapies: increased risk of serious infections and reactivation of latent infections; check PPD and make sure patient is up to date on all vaccinations before starting; hold therapy for any infection.
    - Anti-TNF-α agents:
      - Etanercept *(Enbrel)* 50 mg SC once/wk or 25 mg SC twice/wk
      - Infliximab *(Remicade)* 3 mg/kg IV in conjunction with methotrexate; repeat in 2–6 wk, then q 8 wk
      - Adalimumab *(Humira)* 40 mg SC every other week, or 40 mg SC every wk if not taking methotrexate
    - Interleukin-1 receptor antagonist: anakinra *(Kineret)* 100 mg SC daily
- Medications used when response to DMARD has been inadequate:
  - T-cell activation inhibitor: abatacept (*Orencia*)—<60 kg: 500 mg; 60–100 kg: 750 mg; >100 kg: 1 g IV at 0, 2, and 4 wk, then q 4 wk (do not use with anti-TNF-α agents or with anakinra)
  - Anti-CD20 monoclonal antibody: rituximab (*Rituxam*) 1000 mg IV in conjunction with methotrexate; repeat in 2 wk

GOUT
Definition
Urate crystal disease that may be expressed as acute gouty arthritis, usually in a single joint of foot, ankle, knee, or olecranon bursa; or chronic arthritis.

Precipitating Factors
- Alcohol, heavy ingestion
- Allopurinol, stopping or starting
- Binge eating
- Dehydration
- Diuretics
- Fasting
- Infection
- Serum uric acid concentration, any change up or down
- Surgery

Evaluation of Acute Gouty Arthritis
Joint aspiration to remove crystals and microscopic examination to establish diagnosis; serum urate (can be normal during flare).

Management
Treatment of Acute Gouty Flare: Experts differ regarding order of choices:
- Intra-articular injections (see p 148)
- NSAIDs (see **Table 57**)
- Colchicine (more toxic in older adults; more effective if given within 24 hr of symptom onset)
  - Oral 0.5–0.6 mg (1 tab) q 1–2 h until symptoms abate, GI toxicity develops, or max dose of 6 mg/24-h period has been given.
  - IV 1–2 mg in 10–20 mL NS given over 3–5 min
    - may repeat the following day but patients should receive no more colchicine by any route for 7 days
    - contraindicated in patients who have had recent oral colchicine
    - avoid in patients with kidney or liver disease
    - potential for severe bone marrow toxicity, disseminated intravascular coagulation
- Prednisone 20–40 mg/d po until response, then rapid taper
- ACTH 75 IU SC or cosyntropin (*Cortrosyn*) 75 mcg SC; may repeat daily for 3 d

Treatment of Hyperuricemia After Acute Flare: Colchicine 0.5–0.6 mg/d for 2–4 wk before beginning any treatment in **Table 58** and continued until serum urate has returned to normal.

	Table 58. Medications Useful in Managing Chronic Gout		
Medication	**Usual Dosage**	**Formulations**	**Comments (Metabolism, Excretion)**
✔Allopurinol (*Zyloprim, Lopurin*)	100–800 mg/d in divided doses if >300 mg/d	T: 100, 300	Do not initiate during flare; reduce dosage in renal or hepatic impairment; increase dose by 100 mg every 2–4 wk to normalize serum urate level; monitor CBC; rash is common (K)
Colchicine*	0.5–0.6 mg/d	T: 0.5, 0.6; Inj	May also be effective in prevention of recurrent pseudogout; monitor CBC (L)

(cont.)

Table 58. Medications Useful in Managing Chronic Gout (cont.)

Medication	Usual Dosage	Formulations	Comments (Metabolism, Excretion)
Losartan (Cozaar)	12.5–100 mg q 12–24 h	T: 25, 50, 100	Modest uricosuric effect that plateaus at 50 mg/d; may be useful in patients with HTN or HF
Probenecid* (Benemid)	500–1500 mg in 2–3 divided doses	T: 500	Adjust dose to normalize serum urate level or increase urine urate excretion; inhibits platelet function; may not be effective if renal impairment (K, L)
Sulfinpyrazone (Anturane)	50 mg po q 12 h to 100 mg q 6 h	T: 100; C: 200	Inhibits platelet function; may not be effective if renal impairment (K)

✔ = preferred for treating older adults
* Probenecid (500 mg) and colchicine (0.5 mg) combinations (*ColBenemid, Col-Probenecid, Proben-C*) are available.

PSEUDOGOUT
Definition
Crystal-induced arthritis (especially affecting wrists and knees) associated with calcium pyrophosphate

Risk Factors
- Advanced osteoarthritis
- Diabetes mellitus
- Gout
- Hemochromatosis
- Hypercalcemia
- Hyperparathyroidism
- Hypomagnesemia
- Hypophosphatemia
- Hypothyroidism
- Neuropathic joints
- Older age

Precipitating Factors
- Acute illness
- Dehydration
- Minor trauma
- Surgery

Evaluation of Acute Arthritis
Joint aspiration and microscopic examination to establish diagnosis; radiograph indicating chondrocalcinosis (best seen in wrists, knees, shoulder, symphysis pubis)

Management of Acute Flare
If single joint, aspiration and intra-articular glucocorticoid may be effective. If multiple joints, see Gout, management (p 154). Colchicine is less effective in pseudogout.

POLYMYALGIA RHEUMATICA, GIANT CELL (TEMPORAL) ARTERITIS
Definitions and Evaluation
Polymyalgia Rheumatica: Proximal limb and girdle stiffness usually lasting ≥30 min without tenderness but with constitutional symptoms (eg, fatigue, malaise, weight loss) for ≥1 mo and sedimentation rate elevated to >50 mm/hr (7%–22% will have normal sedimentation rate), and C-reactive protein; consider ultrasound to demonstrate effusions within shoulder bursae if diagnosis is uncertain.

Giant Cell (Temporal) Arteritis: Medium to large vessel vasculitis that presents with symptoms of polymyalgia rheumatica, headache, scalp tenderness, jaw or tongue claudication, visual disturbances, TIA or stroke, and elevated sedimentation rate and C-reactive protein. The presence of synovitis suggests an alternative diagnosis. Giant cell arteritis is confirmed by temporal artery biopsy.

Management
- Polymyalgia rheumatica management is low-dosage (eg, 5–20 mg/d) prednisone or its equivalent. Increase dosage if symptoms are not controlled within 1 wk. Methylprednisolone 120 mg IM q 3–4 wk is also effective. After 2–4 wk, begin gradual taper to lowest dose that will control symptoms and C-reactive protein or sedimentation rate. Once-daily dose is 10 mg, taper in 1-mg decrements. Maintain therapy for ≥1 yr to prevent relapse. Some patients with milder symptoms may respond to NSAIDs alone. Monitor symptoms and C-reactive protein or sedimentation rate. Maintain therapy for ≥1 yr to prevent relapse. Relapse occurs in 25%–50%, and resuming or increasing steroid dosage is necessary. Consider osteoporosis prevention medication (see p 167).
- Giant cell arteritis treatment should not be delayed while waiting for pathologic diagnosis from temporal artery biopsy. Begin prednisone (40–60 mg/d) or its equivalent while biopsy and pathology are pending. Consider adding methotrexate po 10 mg/wk and folate 5–7.5 mg/d, which may have a steroid-sparing effect. After 2–4 wk, begin taper with target of moderate dosage (eg, 20 mg prednisone/d) at 2 mo and gradual taper over 9–12 mo. Once-daily dose is 10 mg, taper in 1-mg decrements. High-dose parenteral steroids (eg, 1000 mg methylprednisolone IV daily for 3 days) for visual loss is controversial. Use low-dosage aspirin (81–100 mg/d) to reduce risk of visual loss, TIA, or stroke. Combine with PPI or misoprostol. Maintain therapy for ≥1 yr to prevent relapse. Consider osteoporosis prevention medication (see p 167). Monitor for development of thoracic aortic aneurysm with CXR yearly for up to 10 yr.

TREMORS

Table 59. Classification of Tremors

Tremor Type	Hz	Associated Conditions	Features	Treatment
Cerebellar	3–5	Cerebellar disease	Present only during movement; ↑ with intention; ↑ amplitude as target is approached	Symptomatic management
Essential	4–12	Familial in 50% of cases	Varying amplitude; common in upper extremities, head, neck; ↑ with antigravity movements, intention, stress, medications	Long-acting propranolol or atenolol (see **Table 20**); or primidone (*Mysoline*) 100 mg qhs start, titrate to 0.5–1.0 g/d in 3–4 divided doses [T: 50, 250; S: 250 mg/5 mL]; or gabapentin (see **Table 64**)
Parkinson's	3–7	Parkinson's disease, parkinsonism	"Pill rolling;" present at rest; ↑ with emotional stress or when examiner calls attention to it; commonly asymmetric	See Parkinson's disease (p 160)
Physiologic	8–12	Normal	Low amplitude; ↑ with stress, anxiety, emotional upset, lack of sleep, fatigue, toxins, medications	Treatment of exacerbating factor

DIZZINESS

Table 60. Classification of Dizziness

Primary Symptom	Features	Duration	Diagnosis	Management
Dizziness	Lightheadedness 1–30 min after standing	Seconds to minutes (E)	Orthostatic hypotension	See **Table 37**
	Impairment in >1 of the following: vision, vestibular function, spinal proprioception, cerebellum, lower-extremity peripheral nerves	Occurs with ambulation (C)	Multiple sensory impairments	Correct or maximize sensory deficits; PT for balance and strength training
	Unsteady gait with short steps; ↑ reflexes and/or tone	Occurs with ambulation (C)	Ischemic cerebral disease	Aspirin; modification of vascular risk factors; PT
	Provoked by head or neck movement; reduced neck range of motion	Seconds to minutes (E)	Cervical spondylosis	Behavior modification; reduce cervical spasm and inflammation

(cont.)

Table 60. Classification of Dizziness (cont.)

Primary Symptom	Features	Duration	Diagnosis	Management
Drop attacks	Provoked by head or neck movement, reduced vertebral artery flow seen on Doppler or angiography	Seconds to minutes (E)	Postural impingement of vertebral artery	Behavior modification
Vertigo	Brought on by position change, positive Dix-Hallpike test	Seconds to minutes (E)	Benign paroxysmal positional vertigo	Epley maneuver to reposition crystalline debris (see www.audiometrics.com/bppv.htm); exercises provoking symptoms may be of help
	Acute onset, nonpositional	Days	Labyrinthitis (vestibular neuronitis)	Methylprednisolone, 100 mg/d po × 3 d with subsequent gradual taper over 3 wk to improve vestibular function recovery; meclizine (see **Table 41**) for acute symptom relief
	Low-frequency sensorineural hearing loss and tinnitus	Minutes to hours (E)	Ménière's disease	Meclizine (see **Table 41**) for acute symptom relief; diuretics and/or salt restriction for prophylaxis
	Vascular disease risk factors, cranial nerve abnormalities	10 min to several hours (E)	TIAs	Aspirin; modification of vascular risk factors

Note: C = chronic; E = episodic

MANAGEMENT OF ACUTE STROKE
Attempt to Diagnose Cause
Examination
- Cardiac (murmurs, arrhythmias, enlargement)
- Neurologic (serial examinations)
- Optic fundi
- Vascular (carotids and other peripheral pulses)

Tests
- ABG
- Brain imaging
- BUN
- CBC
- LFTs
- Creatinine
- ECG
- Glucose
- Electrolytes
- ESR
- PT, PTT, INR

Transesophageal echocardiography is preferred over transthoracic echocardiography for detection of cardiogenic emboli. Carotid duplex and transcranial Doppler studies can detect carotid and vertebrobasilar embolic sources, respectively. Magnetic resonance angiography is indicated if emergent thrombolytic therapy is being considered to reverse stroke progression within 3 h of onset of symptoms (thrombolytic therapy is of unproven benefit in older adults).

Provide Supportive Care
- Do not lower BP if SBP ≤220 or if DBP <120; higher BP should be lowered *gently*, with the goal of a 10%–15% reduction in BP.
  ○ For SBP >220 or DBP 121–140, use labetolol (*Normodyne, Trandate*) 10–20 mg IV over 1–2 min, repeating q 10 min prn (max dose 300 mg); alternative is nicardipine (*Cardene*) 5 mg/h IV infusion initially, increasing by 2.5 mg/h q 5 min to max of 15 mg/h.
  ○ For DBP >140, use nitroprusside (*Nitropress*) IV infusion at starting dosage of 0.5 mg/kg/min with continuous BP monitoring.
- Correct metabolic and hydration imbalances.
- Detect and treat coronary ischemia, HF, arrhythmias.
- Monitor and treat for hypoxia and hyperthermia.
- Monitor for depression.
- Refer to rehabilitation when medically stable.
- Discharge on statin drug (**Table 19**) if not contraindicated with goal of LDL <70 mg/dL.

Stop or Reverse Progression
Acute Cardioembolic or Noncardioembolic Stroke, Progressing Stroke, Crescendo TIAs, or TIA: Use ASA, 325 mg/d, begun within 24–48 h of onset. Anticoagulants are not recommended.
Hemorrhagic Stroke: supportive care

STROKE PREVENTION
Risk Factor Modification
- Stop smoking.
- Reduce BP to at least 140/90; <120/80 is desirable.
- Treat dyslipidemia (see **Table 18** and **Table 19**).
- Start anticoagulation (see p 21) or antiplatelet therapy for atrial fibrillation.
- Low-sodium (≤2–3 g/d), high-potassium (≥4.7 g/d) diet
- Exercise (≥30 min of moderate intensity activity daily)
- Weight reduction (BMI <25 kg/m²)

Antiplatelet Therapy for Patients With Prior TIA or Stroke
- First-line therapy is ASA 81–325 mg/d.
- Clopidogrel (*Plavix*) 75 mg/d [T: 75] if intolerant to ASA or ASA ineffective.
- Ticlopidine (*Ticlid*) 250 mg q 12 h [T: 250]; monitor CBC and differential.
- Addition of a combination form of ASA and long-acting dipyridamole (*Aggrenox*) 1 tab q 12 h [T: 25/200] may provide additional benefit.
- In the absence of atrial fibrillation, warfarin therapy is no more effective and is associated with more bleeding than ASA in preventing strokes.

Table 61. Treatment Options for Carotid Stenosis

Presentation	% Stenosis	Preferred Treatment	Comments
Prior TIA or stroke	≥70	CA	CE superior to medical therapy only if patient is reasonable surgical risk and facility has track record of low complication rate for CE (<6%)
Prior TIA or stroke	50–69	CE or MM	Serial carotid Doppler testing may identify rapidly developing plaques
Prior TIA or stroke	<50	MM	CE of no proven benefit in this situation
Asymptomatic	≥80	CE or MM	CE should be considered only for the most healthy
Asymptomatic	<80	MM	CE of no proven benefit in this situation

Note: CA = carotid angioplasty with stent placement in patients with multiple comorbidities and/or at high surgical risk; CE = carotid endarterectomy; MM = medical management

PARKINSON'S DISEASE
Diagnosis Requires:
- Bradykinesia, eg,
  - Slowness of initiation of voluntary movements (eg, glue-footedness when starting to walk)
  - Reduced speed and amplitude of repetitive movements (eg, tapping index finger and thumb together)
  - Difficulty switching from one motor program to another (eg, multiple steps to turn during gait testing)
- **and** one or more of the following:
  - Muscular rigidity (eg, cogwheeling)
  - 4–6 Hz resting tremor
  - Impaired righting reflex (eg, retropulsed during sternal nudge)

Table 62. Distinguishing Early Parkinson's Disease From Other Parkinsonian Syndromes

Condition	Tremor	Asymmetric Involvement	Early Falls	Early Dementia	Postural Hypotension
Parkinson's disease	+	+	−	−	−
Drug-induced parkinsonism	+/−	−	−	−	−
Vascular parkinsonism	−	+/−	+/−	+/−	−
Dementia with Lewy bodies	+/−	+/−	+/−	+	+/−
Progressive supranuclear palsy	−	−	+	+/−	−
Multiple system atrophy	−	+/−	+/−	−	+

Note: + = usually or always present, +/− = sometimes present, − = absent
Adapted from Christine CW, Aminoff MJ. *Am J Med* 2004;117:412–419.

Nonpharmacologic Management

- Patient education is essential, and support groups are often helpful; see p 259 for telephone numbers, Web sites.
- Monitor for orthostatic hypotension (see p 50).
- Exercise program
- Surgical therapies can be considered for disabling symptoms refractory to medical therapy. Tremor can be improved by thalamotomy or thalamic stimulation (fewer adverse events). Dyskinesias can be treated by pallidotomy or pallidal and subthalamic stimulation.

Pharmacologic Treatment (see Table 63)

- Begin treatment when symptoms interfere with function.
- Start at low dose and titrate upward gradually.
- Monitor orthostatic BP during titration of medications.

Class, Medication	Initial Dosage	Formulations	Comments (Metabolism, Excretion)
Table 63. Medications for Parkinson's Disease			
Dopamine			
✔ Carbidopa-levodopa* (*Sinemet*)	1/2 tab of 25/100 q 12–24 h	T: 10/100, 25/100, 25/250	Mainstay of Parkinson's disease therapy; increase dose by 1/2-1 tab q 1-2 wk to achieve minimal target dose of 1 tab q 8 h; then titrate upward gradually as needed; watch for GI adverse events, orthostatic hypotension, confusion (L)
✔ Sustained-release carbidopa-levodopa* (*Sinemet CR*)	1 tab/d	T: 25/100, 50/200	Useful at daily dopamine requirement ≥300 mg; slower absorption than carbidopa-levodopa; can improve motor fluctuations (L)
Dopamine Agonists			More CNS adverse events than dopamine
Apomorphine (*Apokyn*)	2 mg SC	Inj: 10 mg/mL	Use with extreme caution; can cause severe orthostasis; indicated only for "off" episodes associated with levodopa therapy
Bromocriptine (*Parlodel*)	1.25 mg q 12–24 h	T: 2.5 C: 5	Increase by 1.25-mg increments every 2–5 d, titrating to effective dosage (10–30 mg/d) (L)
✔ Pramipexole* (*Mirapex*)	0.125 mg/d	T: 0.125, 0.25, 0.5, 1, 1.5	Increase gradually to effective dosage (0.5–1.5 mg q 8 h) (K)
✔ Ropinirole* (*Requip*)	0.25 mg/d	T: 0.25, 0.5, 1, 2, 3, 4, 5	Increase gradually to effective dosage (up to 1–8 mg q 8 h) (L)
Rotigotine (*Neupro*)	2 mg/d	Pch: 2, 4, 6	Watch for orthostatic hypotension, syncope, dizziness, nausea, local site reaction (K)
Catechol O-Methyl-transferase (COMT) Inhibitors			Adjunctive therapy with L-dopa
✔ Tolcapone (*Tasmar*)	100 mg q 8 h	T: 100, 200	Monitor LFTs q 6 mo (L, K)
✔ Entacapone (*Comtan*)	200 mg with each L-dopa dose	T: 200	Watch for nausea, orthostatic hypotension (K)

(cont.)

Table 63. Medications for Parkinson's Disease (cont.)

Class, Medication	Initial Dosage	Formulations	Comments (Metabolism, Excretion)
Anticholinergics			
Benztropine (*Cogentin*)	0.5 mg/d	T: 0.5, 1, 2	Can cause confusion and delirium; helpful for drooling (L, K)
Trihexyphenidyl (*Artane, Trihexy*)	1 mg/d	T: 2, 5 S: 2 mg/5 mL	Same as above (L, K)
Dopamine Reuptake Inhibitor			
Amantadine (*Symmetrel*)	100 mg q 12–24 h	T: 100 C: 100 S: 50 mg/5 mL	Useful in early and late Parkinson's disease; watch closely for CNS adverse events; do not D/C abruptly (K)
MAO B Inhibitors			
Rasagilene (*Azilect*)	0.5 mg/d	T: 0.5, 1	Interactions with numerous drugs and tyramine-rich foods; expensive (L, K)
Selegiline (*Carbex, Eldepryl, Zelapar*)	5 mg q am; 1.25 mg/d for orally disintegrating tab	T: 5; orally disintegrating tab: 1.25	Use as adjunctive therapy with dopamine; do not exceed a total dosage of 10 mg/d (L, K)
Combination Medication			
Carbidopa-levodopa + entacapone (*Stalevo*)	1 tab/d	T: 12.5/50/200; 25/100/200; 37.5/150/200	Should be used only after individual dosages of carbidopa, levodopa, and entacapone have been established (L, K)

✔ = preferred for treating older adults
* = first-line therapy

SEIZURES
Classification
- Generalized: All areas of brain affected with alteration in consciousness.
- Partial: Focal brain area affected, not necessarily with alteration in consciousness; can progress to generalized type.

Initial Evaluation, Assessment
- History: neurologic disorders, trauma, drug and alcohol use
- Physical examination: general, with careful neurologic
- Routine tests: BUN, calcium, CBC, creatinine, ECG, EEG, electrolytes, glucose, head CT, LFTs, magnesium
- Tests as indicated: head MRI, lumbar puncture, oxygen saturation, urine toxic or drug screen

Common Causes
- Advanced dementia
- CNS infection
- Drug or alcohol withdrawal
- Idiopathic causes
- Metabolic disorders
- Prior stroke (most common)
- Toxins
- Trauma
- Tumor

Management

- Treat underlying causes.
- Institute anticonvulsant therapy (see **Table 64**). Virtually all anticonvulsant medications can cause sedation and ataxia.

		Target Blood		
Medication	Dosage (mg)	Concentration (mcg/mL)	Formulations	Comments (Metabolism, Excretion)
◆Carbamazepine (Tegretol) (Tegretol XR)	200–600 q 12 h	4–12	T: 200 ChT: 100 S: 100/5 mL T: 100, 200, 400 C: CR 200, 300	Many drug interactions; mood stabilizer; may cause SIADH, thrombocytopenia, leukopenia (L, K)
◆Gabapentin (Neurontin)	300–600 q 8 h	NA	C: 100, 300, 400 T: 600, 800 S: 250/5 mL	Used as adjunct to other agents; adjust dosage on basis of CrCl (K)
Lamotrigine (Lamictal)	100–300 q 12 h	2–4	T: 25, 100, 150, 200 ChT: 2, 5, 25	Prolongs PR interval; risk of severe rash; when used with valproic acid, begin at 25 mg q 48 h, titrate to 25–100 mg q 12 h (L, K)
Levetiracetam (Keppra)	500–1500 q 12 h	NA	T: 250, 500, 750	Reduce dosage in renal impairment: CrCl 30–50: 250–750 q 12 h CrCl 10–29: 250–500 q 12 h CrCl <10: 500–1000 q 24 h
Oxcarbazepine (Trileptal)	300–1200 q 12 h	NA	T: 150, 300, 600 ChT: 2, 5, 25 S: 300/5 mL	Can cause hyponatremia, leukopenia (L)
Phenobarbital (Luminal)	30–60 q 8–12 h	20–40	T: 15, 16, 30, 32, 60, 100 S: 20/5 mL	Many drug interactions; not recommended for use in older adults (L)
Phenytoin (Dilantin)	200–300/d	5–20*	C: 30, 100 ChT: 50 S: 125/5 mL	Many drug interactions; exhibits nonlinear pharmacokinetics (L)
◆Pregabalin (Lyrica)	50–200 q 8–12 h		C: 25, 50, 75, 100, 150, 200, 225, 300	Indicated as adjunct therapy for partial-onset seizures only; not well studied in older adults (K)
Tiagabine (Gabitril Filmtabs)	2–12 q 8–12 h	NA	T: 2, 4, 12, 16, 20	Adverse-event profile in older adults less well described (L)
Topiramate (Topamax)	25–100 q 12–24 h	NA	T: 25, 100, 200 C, sprinkle: 15, 25	May affect cognitive functioning at high dosages (L, K)
Valproic acid (Depacon, Depakene, Depakote) (Depakote ER)	250–750 q 8–12 h	50–100	T: 125, 250, 500 C: 125, 250 S: 250/5 mL T: 500	Can cause weight gain, tremor, hair loss; several drug interactions; mood stabilizer; monitor LFTs and platelets (L)

Table 64. Anticonvulsant Therapy in Older Adults

(cont.)

Table 64. Anticonvulsant Therapy in Older Adults (cont.)

Medication	Dosage (mg)	Target Blood Concentration (mcg/mL)	Formulations	Comments (Metabolism, Excretion)
Zonisamide (*Zonegran*)	100–400/d	NA	C: 25, 100	Anorexia; contraindicated in patients with sulfonamide allergy (K)

Note: NA = not available ◆ = also has primary indication for neuropathic pain.
*Phenytoin is extensively bound to plasma albumin. In cases of hypoalbuminemia or marked renal insufficiency, calculate adjusted phenytoin concentration (*C*):

$$C_{adjusted} = \frac{C_{observed}(mcg/mL)}{0.2 \times albumin\ (g/dL) + 0.1}$$

If creatinine clearance <10 mL/min, use:

$$C_{adjusted} = \frac{C_{observed}(mcg/mL)}{0.1 \times albumin\ (g/dL) + 0.1}$$

Obtaining a free phenytoin level is an alternative method of monitoring phenytoin in cases of hypoalbuminemia or marked renal insufficiency.

APHASIA

Table 65. Aphasias in Which Repetition Is Impaired

Type	Fluency	Auditory Comprehension	Associated Neurologic Deficits	Comments
Broca's	−	+	Right hemiparesis	Patient aware of deficit; high rate of associated depression; message board helpful for communication
Wernicke's	+	−	Often none	Patient frequently unaware of deficit; speech content usually unintelligible; therapy often focuses on visually based communication
Conduction	+	+	Occasional right facial weakness	Patient usually aware of deficit; speech content usually intelligible
Global	−	−	Right hemiplegia with right field cut	Most commonly due to left middle cerebral artery thrombosis, which has a poor prognosis for meaningful speech recovery

Note: + = present; − = absent

PERIPHERAL NEUROPATHY
Diagnosis
• Establish pattern of involvement:
  ○ Focal (entrapment syndromes, compression neuropathies, vasculitis)
  ○ Multifocal (vasculitis, diabetes)
  ○ Symmetric
• If symmetric, determine location:
  ○ Proximal—many causes, including Guillain-Barré syndrome, porphyria, chronic inflammatory demyelinating polyneuropathy, Lyme disease

- Distal—nerve conduction studies can help distinguish the more common axonal pathologies (diabetes, medication effects, alcohol abuse, kidney failure, malignancy) from demyelinating ones (including Guillain-Barré syndrome and chronic inflammatory demyelinating polyneuropathy)

Treatment
Prevention of Complications:
- Protect distal extremities from trauma—appropriate shoe size, daily foot inspections, good skin care, avoidance of barefoot walking.
- Maintain tight glycemic control in diabetic neuropathy.

Treatment of Painful Neuropathy: Start at low dosage, increase as needed and tolerated:
- Nortriptyline (*Aventyl, Pamelor*) 10–100 mg qhs [T: 10, 25, 50, 75]; desipramine (*Norpramin*) 10–75 mg qam [T: 10, 25, 50, 75]
- Gabapentin (*Neurontin*) can begin 100–200 mg qhs but may need up to 100–600 mg q 8 h [C: 100, 300, 400; T: 600, 800; S: 250/5 mL]
- Pregabalin *(Lyrica)* 75–300 mg po q 12 h [C: 25, 50, 75, 100, 150, 200, 225, 300]: primary indication is for management of postherpetic neuralgia and for diabetic peripheral neuropathy
- Other oral agents that may be effective include:
  - Carbamazepine (*Tegretol*) 200–400 mg q 8 h [T: 200; ChT: 100; S: 100 mg/5 mL]; (*Tegretol XR*) 200 mg q 12 h [T: 100, 200, 400; C: CR 200, 300]
  - Duloxetine (*Cymbalta*) 60 mg/d [C: 20, 30, 60]
  - SSRIs have not been shown to be as effective as tricyclics (**Table 29**)
  - Lamotrigine (*Lamictal*, see **Table 64**) 400–600 mg/d
  - Opioids (**Table 71**); watch for adverse events of itching, mood changes, weakness, confusion
  - Tramadol (*Ultram*, see **Table 71**) 200–400 mg/d
- Topical agents that may be effective include:
  - Capsaicin cream (eg, *Zostrix*) 0.075% applied q 6–8 h [0.025%, 0.075%]
  - Transcutaneous electrical nerve stimulation
  - Lidocaine 5% pch (*Lidoderm*) 1–3 patches covering the affected area up to 24 h/d [700-mg pch]

OSTEOPOROSIS

COMMONLY USED DEFINITIONS
- Established osteoporosis: occurrence of a minimal trauma fracture of any bone (WHO).
- Osteoporosis: a skeletal disorder characterized by compromised bone strength (bone density and bone quality) predisposing to an increased risk of fracture (NIH Consensus Development Panel. Osteoporosis prevention, diagnosis, and therapy. *JAMA* 2001; 285 (6):785–795.)
- Osteoporosis: BMD 2.5 SD or more below that of younger normal individuals (T score) (WHO). Scores between 1 and 2.5 SD below are termed osteopenia. Some experts prefer to use Z score, which compares an individual with a population adjusted for age, sex, and race. For each SD decrement in BMD, hip fracture risk increases about 2-fold; for each SD increment in BMD, hip fracture risk is about halved.

RISK FACTORS FOR OSTEOPOROTIC FRACTURE
- Previous fracture as adult
- Dementia
- Depression
- Low calcium intake
- Impaired vision
- Low physical activity
- Fracture in 1st-degree relative
- Frailty
- Alcoholism
- Female sex
- Weight <127 lb if female
- Cigarette smoking
- Early menopause (<45 yr)
- Recurrent falls

TOXINS AND MEDICATIONS THAT CAN CAUSE OR AGGRAVATE OSTEOPOROSIS
- Alcohol (>2 drinks/d)
- Anticonvulsants
- Corticosteroids
- Heparin
- Lithium
- Nicotine (ie, smoking)
- Phenytoin
- PPIs (if ≥1 yr)
- SSRIs
- Thyroxine (if overreplaced or in suppressive dosage)

EVALUATION
BMD at least once after age 65 (see **Table 75**). Uncertain how often to repeat. Some suggest in 3 yr for patients with osteopenia and in 5 yr for those with normal bone density. The value of monitoring BMD in patients already receiving treatment is unproved. Some experts recommend excluding secondary causes (serum 25-hydroxy vitamin D, serum PTH, TSH, calcium, phosphorus, albumin, alkaline phosphatase, bioavailable testosterone in men, kidney and liver function tests, CBC, UA, electrolytes, protein electrophoresis). Less consensus on 24-h urinary calcium excretion, cortisol, antibodies associated with gluten enteropathy.

MANAGEMENT
Universal Recommendations
- Calcium (elemental) 1200 mg/d. For most patients, calcium carbonate is sufficient and least expensive. For patients on proton-pump inhibitors (see **Table 38**) or who have achlorhydria, calcium citrate should be used. For patients who have difficulty swallowing calcium citrate tabs, smaller tabs of 125 mg (*Freeda Mini Cal-citrate*) and granules, 1 tsp = 760 mg (*Freeda Calcium Citrate Fine Granular*), are available.

- Vitamin D 800 IU
- Most calcium plus vitamin D preparations contain 500–600 mg of calcium and 100–200 IU of vitamin D.
- Avoid tobacco
- Weight-bearing exercise
- Falls prevention (see **Table 37**)
- No more than moderate alcohol use

Pharmacologic Prevention

- Most organizations have recommended initiating pharmacologic management (**Table 66**) in women with BMD T scores below −2 in the absence of risk factors and in women with T scores below −1.5 if other risk factors are present.

Table 66. Pharmacologic Prevention and Treatment of Osteoporosis*

Medication	Dosage	Formulations	Comments
Bisphosphonates			Consider discontinuing after 5 yr
Alendronate (*Fosamax*)	Prevention: 5 mg/d or 35 mg/wk Treatment: 10 mg/d or 70 mg/wk	T: 5, 10, 35, 40, 70; 70 sol	Must be taken fasting with water; patient must remain upright and npo for ≥30 min after taking; do not use if CrCl <35 mL/min; relatively contraindicated in GERD
Ibandronate (*Boniva*)	po: 150 mg/mo or 2.5 mg/d IV: 3 mg q 3 mo	T: 2.5, 150 IV: 1 mg/mL (available in 3-mL prefilled syringes)	Must be taken fasting with water; patient must remain upright and npo for ≥60 min after taking; do not use if CrCl <30 mL/min
Risedronate (*Actonel*)	35 mg/wk, 75 mg on 2 consecutive days/mo, or 5 mg/d	T: 5, 30, 35, 75	Must be taken fasting or ≥2 h after evening meal; patient must remain upright and npo for 30 min after taking; do not use if CrCl <30 mL/min
Zoledronic acid (*Reclast*)	5 mg IV given over >15 min every yr	5 mg/100 mL	Not recommended if CrCl <35 mL/min
Others			
Raloxifene (*Evista*)	60 mg/d	T: 60	
Calcitonin (*Calcimar, Cibacalcin, Miacalcin, Osteocalcin, Salmonine*)	Treatment: 100 IU/d SC (human) or 200 IU intranasally (salmon) in alternate nostrils q 48 h	Inj: human (*Cibacalcin*) 0.5 mg/vial Intranasal: salmon 200 units/mL (*Miacalcin*)	May also be helpful for analgesic effect in patients with acute vertebral fracture (see also p 145)
Estrogen	See **Table 102**		For use in select patients
Teriparatide (*Forteo*)	Treatment: 20 mcg/d for up to 24 mo	Inj 3 mL, 28-dose disposable pen device	For high-risk patients; contraindicated in patients with Paget's disease or prior skeletal radiation therapy (L, K); treatment for 1 yr followed by 1 yr of bisphosphonates can maintain 1-yr gains in BMD

* Unless specified, medication can be used for prevention or treatment.

Nonpharmacologic Treatment of Vertebral Fracture

Vertebroplasty (injection of bone cement into a collapsed vertebra) or kyphoplasty (inflation of a balloon tamp before cement injection) has short-term improvements in pain and function but this treatment is expensive and may have adverse effects. Short-term complications are usually due to extravasation of cement. Long-term complications include local acceleration of bone resorption and increased fracture risk in treated or adjacent vertebrae.

Pharmacologic Treatment Regimens for Those with Prior Osteoporotic Fractures

- BMD measurement is unnecessary. See **Table 66** for treatment regimens.
- Combination therapy (eg, estrogen plus bisphosphonate or calcitonin) is slightly more effective in improving BMD but has not been proved to affect fracture rates.

Table 67. Bone Outcomes of Medications for Osteoporosis Based on Randomized Clinical Trials*

Medication	Spine BMD and Fracture	Hip BMD	Hip Fracture	All Nonspinal Fractures
Estrogen	improved	improved	reduced	no effect
Raloxifene	improved	improved	no data	no effect
Alendronate	improved	improved	reduced	reduced
Ibandronate	improved	improved	no data	no effect
Risedronate	improved	improved	reduced	reduced
Calcitonin (nasal)	improved	no effect	no effect	no effect
Zolendronic acid	improved	improved	reduced	reduced
Teriparatide	improved	improved	no data	reduced

* The populations studied, sample sizes of individual studies, and duration of follow-up vary considerably; hence, this summary must be interpreted cautiously. Moreover, several randomized clinical trials are currently in progress and new findings may appear. Although different classes of drugs vary in effectiveness on BMD, effectiveness on fracture rates are similar.

Table 68. Effects on Other Outcomes, Level of Evidence,[a] and Risks of Medications for Osteoporosis

Medication	CHD Risk Factors	CHD Prevention	CHD Treatment	Breast Cancer	Deep-vein Thrombosis	Other
Estrogen[b]	improved–R	↑ risk–R	no effect–R	↑ risk–R	↑ risk–R	↑ vaginal bleeding, stroke, PE; ↓ colorectal cancer–R
Raloxifene	improved–R	↓ risk–R[c]	↓ risk–R	↓ risk–R	↑ risk–R	↑ hot flushes–R
Bisphos-phonates[d]	no data	no data	no data	no data	no data	Esophagitis; bone, joint, or muscle pain; osteonecrosis of jaw; occipital inflammation
Calcitonin (nasal)	no data	no data	no data	no data	no data	Rhinitis in 10%–12%

Note: CHD = coronary heart disease; R = randomized clinical trial

[a] The populations studied, sample sizes of individual studies, and duration of follow-up vary considerably; hence, this summary must be interpreted cautiously. Moreover, several randomized clinical trials are currently in progress and new findings may appear.

[b] In the Women's Health Initiative estrogen-alone trial, only stroke and pulmonary embolism risk were increased.

[c] Reduced risk demonstrated for high-risk women only.

[d] Alendronate, ibandronate, risedronate

PAIN

DEFINITION

An unpleasant sensory and emotional experience associated with actual or potential tissue damage (International Association for Study of Pain taxonomy)

Acute Pain

Distinct onset, usually evident pathology, short duration; common causes: trauma, postsurgical pain

Persistent Pain

Pain due to ongoing nociceptive, neuropathic, or mixed pathophysiologic processes, often associated with functional and psychologic impairment; can fluctuate in character and intensity over time (see **Table 69**)

Table 69. Types of Pain, Examples, and Treatment			
Type of Pain and Examples	**Source of Pain**	**Typical Description**	**Effective Drug Classes and Treatment**
Nociceptive: somatic			
Arthritis, acute postoperative, fracture, bone metastases	Tissue injury, eg, bones, soft tissue, joints, muscles	Well localized, constant; aching, stabbing, gnawing, throbbing	Nonopioids, NSAIDs, opioids Physical and cognitive-behavioral therapies
Nociceptive: visceral			
Renal colic, bowel obstruction	Viscera	Diffuse, poorly localized, referred to other sites, intermittent, paroxysmal; dull, colicky, squeezing, deep, cramping; often accompanied by nausea, vomiting, diaphoresis	Nonopioids, NSAIDs, opioids Physical and cognitive-behavioral therapies
Neuropathic			
Cervical or lumbar radiculopathy, post-herpetic neuralgia, trigeminal neuralgia, diabetic neuropathy, post-stroke syndrome, herniated intervertebral disc	Peripheral or central nervous system	Prolonged, usually constant, but can be paroxysmal; sharp, burning, pricking, tingling, squeezing; associated with other sensory disturbances, eg, paresthesias and dysesthesias; allodynia, hyperalgesia, impaired motor function, atrophy, or abnormal deep tendon reflexes	Tricyclic antidepressants, anticonvulsants, opioids, topical anesthetics Physical and cognitive-behavioral therapies
Undetermined			
Myofascial pain syndrome, somatoform pain disorders	Poorly understood	No identifiable pathologic processes or symptoms out of proportion to identifiable organic pathology; widespread musculoskeletal pain, stiffness, and weakness	Antidepressants, antianxiety agents Physical, cognitive-behavioral, and psychological therapies

EVALUATION
Key Points, Approach
- Perform comprehensive evaluation for cause of pain, pain characteristics, and impact of physical and psychosocial function.
- Consider patient's report as the most reliable evidence of pain intensity.
- Assess for pain on each presentation (older adults may be reluctant to report pain).
- Use synonyms for pain (eg, burning, aching, soreness, discomfort).
- Use a standard pain scale (eg, Numeric Rating Scale, Verbal Descriptor Scale, or Faces Pain Scale; see www.geriatricsatyourfingertips.org); adapt for sensory impairments (eg, large print, written versus spoken).
- Assess cognitively impaired patients by:
  - Using simple tools or questions with yes/no answers.
  - Using a structured approach to assessment and management (see **Figure 7**).
  - Asking caregiver about recent changes in function, gait, behavior patterns, mood.
- Reassess regularly for improvement, deterioration, and complications/adverse events, and document.

History and Physical Examination
- Focus on a complete examination of pain source and on musculoskeletal and neurologic systems.
- Distinguish new illness from chronic condition.
- Analgesic history: effectiveness and adverse events, current and previous prescription drugs, OTC drugs, "natural" remedies.
- Assess effectiveness of prior nondrug treatments.
- Laboratory and diagnostic tests to establish etiologic diagnosis.

Characteristics of Pain Complaint
Provocative (aggravating) and **P**alliative (relieving) factors
Quality (eg, burning, stabbing, dull, throbbing)
Region (eg, pain map)
Severity (eg, scale of 0 for no pain to 10 for worst pain possible)
Timing (eg, when pain occurs, frequency and duration)

Psychosocial Assessment
Depression (see p 247 for screen), anxiety, mental status (see p 244 for screen). Impact on family or significant other. Enabling behaviors by others (eg, oversolicitousness, codependency, reinforcing debility).

Assess for Risk of Addiction with Opioid Use
- Addiction is rare in those without prior hx of substance abuse.
- Risk factors include men who exceed 4 drinks/d or 16 drinks/wk; women who exceed 3 drinks/d or 12 drinks/wk; admission to marijuana or hashish use in the past year; hx of alcohol abuse, drug abuse, or significant psychiatric illness.
- Observe for behavior that may suggest nonadherence to prescribed medication schedule (eg, early refill requests, frequent lost prescriptions).
- Record any suspicious drug-seeking or other aberrant behaviors observed or reported by others, along with action(s) taken.
- Document evaluation process, rationale for long-term opioid therapy, and periodic review of patient status.

Figure 7. Pain Assessment in Older Adults with Severe Cognitive Impairment

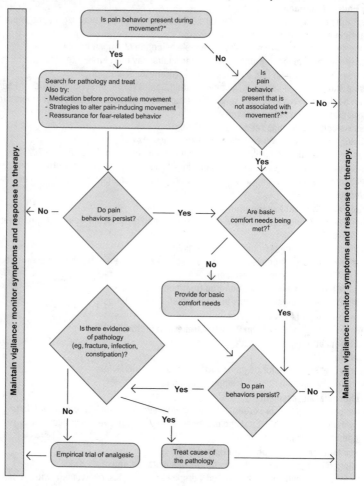

* Examples: grimacing, guarding, combativeness, groaning with movement; resisting care
** Examples: agitation, fidgeting, sleep disturbance, diminished appetite, irritability, reclusiveness, disruptive behavior, rigidity, rapid blinking
† Examples: toileting, thirst, hunger, visual or hearing impairment

Sources: American Geriatrics Society. The management of persistent pain in older persons. *J Amer Geriatr Soc* 2002; 50(6, Suppl): S205–S240; and Weiner D, Herr K, Rudy T, eds. Persistent Pain in Older Adults: An Interdisciplinary Guide for Treatment, 2002, Copyright Springer Publishing Company, Inc., New York 10036.

Functional Assessment
ADLs, impact on activities (see pp 245-247, for screens), and quality of life

Brief Pain Inventory
Use for comprehensive assessment of pain and its impact (see www.geriatricsatyourfingertips.org).

MANAGEMENT
Goal: To find optimal balance in pain relief, functional improvement, and adverse events.

Acute Pain and Short-term Management
- Use fixed schedule of APAP, NSAIDs (consider nonselective versus COX-2 inhibitors depending on risk factors and comorbidities, see **Figure 6**), or opioids.
- Include nonpharmacologic strategies (eg, relaxation, heat or cold).
- Patient-controlled analgesia (PCA): Requires patient comprehension of PCA instructions
  - Indications
    - Acute pain (eg, postoperative pain, trauma)
    - Persistent pain in patients who are npo
  - Dosing strategies (see **Table 70**)
    - Titrate up PCA dose 25%–50% if pain still not well controlled after 12 h.
    - Unless patient is awakened by pain during sleep, continuous opioid infusion not recommended because of increased risk of opioid accumulation and toxicity.
    - If basal rate used, hourly monitoring of sedation and respiratory status is warranted.
    - D/C PCA when patient able to take oral analgesics or unable to self medicate due to altered mental status or physical limitations.

Table 70. Typical Initial Dosing of PCA for Older Adults with Severe Pain

Medication (usual concentration)	Usual Dose Range*	Usual Lockout (min)
Morphine (1 mg/mL)	0.5–2.5 mg	5–10
Hydromorphone (0.2 mg/mL)	0.05–0.3 mg	5–10

* For opioid-naive patients, consider lower end of dosage range.

Persistent Pain
- Use multidisciplinary assessment and treatment (eg, pharmacists, physical therapists, psychologists) when possible.
- Educate patient for self-management and coping.
- Combine pharmacologic and nonpharmacologic strategies.
- Anticipate and attend to depression and anxiety.

Nonpharmacologic Treatment
- Educate patient and caregiver.
  - www.healthinaging.org/public_education/pef/persistent_pain.php
  - Explain difference between addiction, physical dependence, and tolerance.
  - www.ampainsoc.org/advocacy/opioids2.htm
- Emphasize self-administered therapies (eg, heat, cold, massage, liniments and topical agents, distraction, relaxation, music).

- Prescribe exercise, especially for persistent pain (see p 191).
- Add therapy taught and/or conducted by professionals (eg, coping skills, biofeedback, imagery, hypnosis) as needed.
- When appropriate, obtain:
  ○ Rehabilitation medicine consult (OT, PT) for mechanical devices to minimize pain and facilitate activity (eg, splints), transcutaneous electrical nerve stimulation, range-of-motion and ADL programs.
  ○ Psychiatric pain management consult for somatization or severe mood or personality disorder.
  ○ Anesthesia pain management consult for possible interventional therapy (eg, neuroaxial analgesia, injection therapy, neuromodulation) when more conservative approaches are ineffective.
  ○ Pain or chemical dependency specialist referral for management of at-risk patients and ongoing chemical dependency, "chemical coping," aberrant drug-related behaviors, and drug withdrawal.

Pharmacologic Treatment
Selection of Agent(s)
- Base initial choice of analgesic on the severity and type of pain; consider cost, availability, patient preference, comorbidity, and impairments (see **Figure 6**):
  ○ Consider nonopioids for mild pain (rating 1–3) (see **Table 57**).
  ○ Consider low-dose combination agents (see **Table 71**) for mild to moderate pain (rating 4–6).
  ○ Consider potent and titratable opioid agonists (see **Table 71**) for more severe pain (rating 7–10).
  ○ Consider adjuvant drugs (see **Table 73**) alone or in conjunction with opioids or nonopioids for neuropathic pain and other selected chronic conditions.
  ○ Select agents with lowest adverse-event profiles.
- Select least invasive route (usually oral) and fast-onset, short-acting analgesics for episodic or breakthrough pain.
- Use long-acting or sustained-release analgesics for continuous pain after stabilizing dose with short-acting opioid.
- Avoid long-term use of nonselective NSAIDs for chronic conditions (see **Figure 6**).
- Consider COX-2 inhibitor for patients who would benefit from anti-inflammatory medication on a continuous, long-term basis based on risk/benefit assessment (see Musculoskeletal Disorders, p 143).
- Consider fixed-dose combinations (eg, APAP and hydrocodone or tramadol) for mild to moderate pain; do not exceed max dose for APAP.
- Avoid using multiple opioids or nonopioids.
- Medications with long half-life or depot effects (eg, methadone, levorphanol, transdermal fentanyl) should be used and titrated cautiously, with close supervision of effects; duration of effect may exceed usual dose intervals because of reduced metabolism and clearance.
- Methadone is an option if other long-acting agents are not affordable but should be used with extreme caution and only with expertise and monitoring ability because of highly variable half-life and risk of dose accumulation.

Adjustment of Dosage
- Begin with lowest dose possible, usually 25%–50% adult dose, increasing slowly.

- Titrate dose on basis of persistent need for and use of medications for breakthrough pain. If using ≥3 doses/d of breakthrough pain medication, consider increased dosage of sustained-release medication.
- Dose to therapeutic ceiling of nonopioid or NSAID as limited by drug adverse events or risk factors.
- Increase opioid dosage until pain relief achieved or adverse events unmanageable before changing medications (there is no max dose or analgesic ceiling with opioids).
- Use morphine equivalents as a common denominator for all dose conversions to avoid errors, and titrate to effectiveness. See www.hopkinsopioidprogram.org.
- When changing opioids, decrease equivalent analgesic dose by 25%–50% because of incomplete cross-tolerance.
- Administer around-the-clock for continuous pain.
- Reassess, re-examine, and readjust therapy until pain is relieved.
- Opioid analgesics should not be discontinued abruptly. Gradual tapering is necessary to avoid withdrawal symptoms (eg, nausea, abdominal cramps, irritability, anxiety, diaphoresis, tachycardia, hypertension). Decreasing the daily dosage by 10%–20% each day for 10 d can wean most patients without adverse responses. Tapering may require conversion to short-acting opioids. For patients at cardiovascular risk, a slower taper with close monitoring for sympathetic hyperactivity is recommended, and low-dose clonidine may be useful in preventing some of the physiological (and symptomatic) stress related to opioid withdrawal.

Management of Adverse Events
- Anticipate, prevent, and vigorously treat adverse events; expect older adults to be more sensitive to adverse events.
- Warn patient about risk of sedation with opioids and that gradual resolution occurs within a week.
- Warn about risk of APAP toxicity and importance of including all OTC products with APAP in daily total (not to exceed 4 g/d in healthy older adults, 2 g/d in frail older adults or those with reduced CrCl).
- Begin prophylactic, osmotic, or stimulant laxative when initiating opioid therapy (see **Table 40**); if patient has sufficient fluid intake, cautiously increase fiber or psyllium; titrate laxative dose up with opiate dose. Instances of severe opioid-induced constipation may respond to oral naloxone 0.8–2 mg q 12 h, titrated to a max of 12 mg/d given in water or juice, along with routine bowel regimen. Careful titration and observation are necessary because some patients may experience partial analgesia reversal. (See also p 92.)
- Monitor for dry mouth, constipation, sedation, nausea, delirium, urinary retention, and respiratory depression; tolerance develops to mild sedation, nausea, and impaired cognitive function. Reduce dosage and/or consider adding medication to counter adverse medication events if troublesome until tolerance develops.
- On long-term NSAID use, monitor periodically for GI blood loss, renal insufficiency, and other drug-drug and drug-disease interactions.
- Avoid the following medications: carisoprodol, chlorzoxazone, cyclobenzaprine, indomethacin, meperidine, metaxalone, methocarbamol, nalbuphine, pentazocine, propoxyphene (see also p 252 for CMS guidance on unnecessary drugs in the nursing home).

Table 71. Short-acting Opioid Analgesic Drugs

Class, Medication	MS Equiv[a] (Route)	Starting Oral Dosage in Opioid-naive Patients	Formulations	Indication for Pain[b]
Codeine	200 mg (po)	15 mg q 4–6 h	T: 15, 30, 60; S: 15/5 mL; inj	A
Codeine + APAP[c]	200 mg (po)	1–2 15/325 tabs q 4–6 h; if 1 tab used, add 325 mg APAP	T: 15/325, 30/325, 60/325, 30/500, 30/650, 7.5/300, 15/300, 30/300, 60/300; S: 12/120/5 mL	A
Hydrocodone + APAP[c] (eg, *Lorcet, Lortab, Norco, Vicodin*)	30 mg (po)	5–10 mg q 4–6 h	T: 10/325, 5/400, 7.5/400, 10/400, 2.5/500, 5/500, 7.5/500, 10/500, 7.5/650, 7.5/750, 10/650, 10/660; C: 5/500; S: 2.5/167/5 mL (contains 7% alcohol)	A
Oxycodone (*Oxy IR, Roxicodone*)	20–30 mg (po)	2.5–5 mg q 3–4 h	T: 5, 15, 30; C: 5; S: 5 mg/mL, 20 mg/mL	A
Oxycodone + APAP[c] (*Percocet, Tylox*)	20 mg (po)	2.5–5 mg oxycodone q 6 h	T: 2.5/325, 5/325, 5/500, 7.5/325, 7.5/500, 10/325, 10/650; C: 5/500; S: 5/325/5 mL	A
Oxycodone + ASA (*Percodan*)	20 mg (po)	2.25–4.5 mg oxycodone q 6 h	T: 2.25/325, 4.5/325	A
Oxycodone + ibuprofen (*Combunox*)	20 mg (po)	1 tab po q 24 h	T: 5/400	B
Morphine (*MSIR, Astramorph PF, Duramorph, Infumorph, Roxanol, OMS Concentrate, MS/L, RMS, MS/S*)	30 mg (po), 10 mg (IV, IM, SC)	5 mg (po), 1–2 mg (IV) q 4–6 h	C: 15, 30; soluble T: 15, 30; S: 10 mg/5 mL, 20 mg/5 mL, 100 mg/5 mL, 4 mg/mL, 20 mg/mL; Sp: 5, 10, 20, 30; inj	B
Hydromorphone (*Dilaudid, Hydrostat*)	7.5 mg (po), 1.5 mg (IV, IM, SC), 6 mg (rectal)	0.5–1 mg q 3–4 h	T: 2, 4, 8; S: 5 mg/5 mL; Sp: 3; inj	B
Oxymorphone (*Opana, Opana* injectable)	10 mg (po), 1 mg (IV, IM, SC)	5–10 mg q 4–6 h 0.5 mg IM, IV, SC q 4–6 h	T: 5, 10; Sp: 5; inj	B
Tramadol (*Ultram*)	150–300 mg (po)	25–50 mg q 4–6 h; not >300 mg for age 75+	T: 50	B
Tramadol + APAP[c] (*Ultracet*)	37.5/325 mg (po)	2 tabs po q 4–6 h; max 8 tabs/d[d]	T: 37.5/325	B

[a] MS Equiv = morphine sulphate (MS) equivalent dose: morphine equivalency = dose of opioid equivalent to 10 mg of parenteral morphine or 30 mg of oral morphine with chronic dosing. The parenteral:oral ratio is greater (1:6) during acute dosing, ie, 10 mg IM MS = 60 mg po MS.

[b] A = mild to moderate pain; B = moderate to severe pain

[c] Caution: total APAP dose should not exceed 4 g/d.

[d] Treatment not to exceed 5 d; if CrCl <30 mL/min, max is 2 tab q 12 h, not to exceed 5 d.

Table 72. Opioids for Opioid-tolerant Patients

Class, Medication	MS Equiv[a] (Route)	Starting Oral Dose	Formulations	Indication for Pain[b]
Short-acting				
Hydrocodone + ibuprofen (eg, *Vicoprofen*)	30 mg	7.5/200	T: 7.5/200	A
Fentanyl (*Actiq, Fentora*)	NA	Suck on 200 mcg loz over 15 min, effect begins within 10 min	Loz on a stick: 200, 400, 600, 800, 1200, 1600 mcg	B
Fentanyl HCl iontophoric transdermal system (ITS)	NA	40 mcg dose with 10-min lockout through electrical stimulus	System pch with battery contains 80 doses of 40 mcg ea	B
Long-acting				
ER Morphine (*MS Contin, Kadian, Oramorph SR, Avinza*)	30 mg (po) *MS Contin, Kadian, Oramorph SR;* 60 mg (po) *Avinza*	20–30 mg q 24 h, 15 mg q 12 h (*MS Contin* CR and XR tabs), 20 mg q 24 h (*Kadian* SR caps), 15 mg q 24 h (*Oramorph SR*), 30 mg q 24 h (*Avinza* caps)	T: CR 15, 30, 60, 100, 200, XR 15, 30, 60; C: SR 5, 20, 30, 60, 100; C: 30, 60, 90, 120; T: SR 15, 30, 60, 100 (tab must be swallowed whole)	B
ER Oxycodone (*OxyContin*)	20–30 mg (po)	20 mg q 24 h, 10 mg q 12 h	T: CR 10, 20, 40, 80, 160	B
Oxymorphone ER (*Opana* ER)	10 mg	5 mg q 12 h; titrate dosage by 5-mg increments q 12 h	T: 5, 10, 20, 40	B
Transdermal fentanyl[c] (*Duragesic*)	NA (see package insert)	25 mcg/h or higher (if able to tolerate 50 mg oral morphine equiv/24 h)	12 mcg/h, 25 mcg/h, 50 mcg/h, 75 mcg/h, 100 mcg/h	B

[a] MS Equiv = morphine sulphate (MS) equivalent dose: morphine equivalency = dose of opioid equivalent to 10 mg of parenteral morphine or 30 mg of oral morphine with chronic dosing. The parenteral:oral ratio is greater (1:6) during acute dosing, ie, 10 mg IM MS = 60 mg po MS. NA = not applicable.
[b] A = mild to moderate pain; B = moderate to severe pain
[c] Caution: Active ingredient accumulates in subcutaneous fat; thus, duration of action may be >17 hr. Do not use in opioid-naive patients. Not recommended for treatment of acute pain.

Table 73. Adjuvant Medications for Pain Relief in Older Adults

Class, Medication	Formulations and Dosage	Comments
Anticonvulsants (see **Table 64** and pp 164–165)		If one does not work, try another.
Antidepressants (see **Table 29**)		Use low-dose desipramine or nortryptyline; data on SSRIs lacking.

(cont.)

Table 73. Adjuvant Medications for Pain Relief in Older Adults (cont.)

Class, Medication	Formulations and Dosage	Comments
Duloxetine (*Cymbalta*)	C: 20, 30, 60 30 mg/d	For management of pain associated with diabetic peripheral neuropathy; most common adverse events: nausea, dry mouth, constipation, diarrhea, urinary hesitancy; significant drug-drug interactions.
Corticosteroids (see **Table 33**)		Low-dose medical management may be helpful in inflammatory conditions.
Counterirritants		
✔Camphor-menthol-phenol (*Sarna*)*	lot: camphor 5%, menthol 5%, phenol 5% prn; max q 6 h	May be effective for arthritic pain, but effect limited when pain affects multiple joints; can cause skin injury, especially if used with heat or occlusive dressing.
✔Camphor and phenol (*Campho-Phenique*)*	S: camphor 5%, phenol 4.7% prn; max q 8 h	
✔Methylsalicylate and menthol		
(*Ben-Gay* oint*, *Icy Hot* crm*)	methylsalicylate 18.3%, menthol 16% q 6–8 h	Apply to affected area.
(*Ben-Gay* extra strength crm*)	methylsalicylate 30%, menthol 10% q 6–8 h	Apply to affected area.
✔Trolamine salicylate (*Aspercreme* rub*)	trolamine salicylate 10% q 6 h or more frequently	Apply to affected area.
Other		
Baclofen (*Lioresal*)	T: 10, 20; inj 2.5–5 mg q 8–12 h	Probably increased sensitivity and decreased clearance; monitor for weakness, urinary dysfunction; avoid abrupt discontinuation because of CNS irritability.
✔Capsaicin (eg, *Capsin, Capzasin, No Pain-HP, R-Gel, Zostrix*)	crm, lot, gel, roll-on: 0.025%, 0.075% q 6–8 h	Renders skin and joints insensitive by depleting and preventing reaccumulation of substance P in peripheral sensory neurons; may cause burning sensation up to 2 wk; instruct patient to wash hands after application to prevent eye contact; do not apply to open or broken skin.
✔Lidocaine (*Lidoderm*)	transdermal pch 5% 12 h on, 12 h off; up to 24 h on	Apply over affected area; used for neuropathic pain, may be helpful for low back pain, osteoarthritis.

✔ = preferred for treating older adults
* Available OTC
Note: Various adjuvant classes are useful for treatment of neuropathic pain. TCAs are often helpful for migraine or tension headaches and arthritic conditions. Baclofen is particularly useful for muscle-related problems, such as spasms.

PALLIATIVE AND END-OF-LIFE CARE

DEFINITION

"Palliative care means patient and family-centered care that optimizes quality of life by anticipating, preventing and treating suffering. Palliative care throughout the continuum of illness involves addressing physical, intellectual, emotional, social and spiritual needs to facilitate patient autonomy, access to information and choice." (From National Quality Forum's *National Framework and Preferred Practices for Palliative and Hospice Care*, 2006.)

PRINCIPLES

- Support, educate, and treat both patient and family.
- Address physical, psychologic, social, and spiritual needs.
- Use multidisciplinary team (physicians, nurses, social workers, chaplain, pharmacist, physical and occupational therapists, dietitian, family and caregivers, volunteers).
- Focus on symptom management, comfort, meeting goals, completion of "life business," healing relationships, and bereavement.
- Make care available 24 h/d, 7 d/wk.
- Educate, plan, and document advance directives; health care proxy; family awareness of decisions.
- Coordinate care among various providers. Help integrate potentially curative, disease-modifying, and palliative therapies.
- Offer bereavement support.
- Provide therapeutic environment (palliation can be given in any location).
- Advocate comprehensive palliative care for all dying patients.

QUALITY OF LIFE

Ways to help patient and family enhance quality of life at the end of life:

- Communicate, listen
- Teach stress management, coping
- Use all available resources
- Support decision making
- Encourage conflict resolution
- Help complete unfinished business
- Urge focus on nonillness-related affairs
- Urge a focus on one day at a time
- Help anticipate grief, losses
- Help focus on attainable goals
- Encourage spiritual practices
- Promote physical, psychologic comfort

END-OF-LIFE DECISIONS

Follow principles involved in informed decision making (see **Figure 2**).

Communicating Bad News

1. Prepare for discussion by ensuring all information/facts/data are available. Deliver in person in private area without interruptions. Determine individuals that patient may want involved.
2. Establish patient knowledge and understanding of illness.
3. Establish what/how much patient wants to know.

4. Deliver information in sensitive, straightforward manner, avoiding technical language and euphemisms. Check for understanding and clarify concepts and terms.
5. Respond by using active listening, encouraging expression of emotions, acknowledging patient's feelings.
6. Organize an immediate therapeutic plan addressing patient's concerns and agenda.
7. Reassess understanding of condition and treatment plan and determine need for further education and follow-up with patient and family.

Hospice Referral

- Patients, families, or other health care providers can refer, but a physician's certification of limited life expectancy (prognosis of ≤6 mo for most hospice programs; a requirement for the Medicare Hospice Benefit and Medicaid programs) is required for admission to a hospice program (see **Table 74**).
- Encourage nursing home staff to interview residents to determine goals, preferences, and palliative care needs suggestive of appropriateness for hospice. Fax request for hospice referral to primary health care provider.
- Referral is appropriate when curative treatment is no longer indicated (ie, ineffective, adverse events too burdensome) and life is limited to months.
- Hospice must be accepted by the patient or family, or both, and can be rescinded at any time.
- Hospice provides palliative medications, durable medical supplies and equipment, team member visits as needed and desired by patient and family (physician, nurses, home health aide, social worker, chaplain), and volunteer services.
- Optimal hospice care requires adequate time in the program; referral when death is imminent does not take full advantage of hospice care.
- Hospice care is usually delivered in patient's home, but it can be delivered in a nursing home or residential care facility (long-term care, assisted living) or in an inpatient setting (hospice-specific or contracted facility) if acuity or social circumstances warrant.

Table 74. Typical Trajectory and Hospice Eligibility for Selected Diseases	
Disease	**Typical Determinants for Hospice Eligibility***
Cancer	Clinical findings of malignancy with widespread, aggressive, or progressive disease evidenced by increasing symptoms, worsening laboratory values, and/or evidence of metastatic disease
	Impaired performance status with a Palliative Performance Scale (PPS; see p 248) value of ≤70%
	Refuses further curative therapy or continues to decline in spite of definitive therapy
Dementia	FAST Scale Stage 7 (loss of speech, locomotion, and consciousness; see p 249) **and**
	Comorbid or secondary conditions that contribute to structural or functional impairments suggesting a prognosis of ≤6 mo
Failure to thrive	BMI (kg/m²) <22
	Karnofsky score < 40 or PPS value < 40% (see p 248)

(cont.)

Table 74. Typical Trajectory and Hospice Eligibility for Selected Diseases (cont.)

Disease	Typical Determinants for Hospice Eligibility*
End-stage heart disease	Optimally treated with diuretics and vasodilators, which may include ACEIs or combination of hydralazine and nitrates *or* has angina pectoris at rest, resistant to standard nitrate treatment and is either not candidate for or declines invasive procedures *and* Significant symptoms of recurrent HF at rest and classified as NYHA Class IV (ie, unable to carry on any physical activity without symptoms, symptoms present at rest, symptoms increase if any physical activity is undertaken) Additional support needed for treatment-resistant symptomatic supraventricular or ventricular arrhythmia, history of cardiac arrest or resuscitation or unexplained syncope, brain embolism of cardiac origin, concomitant HIV disease, documented ejection fraction of $\leq 20\%$
End-stage pulmonary disease	Disabling dyspnea at rest, poorly or unresponsive to bronchodilators, resulting in decreased functional capacity, eg, bed to chair existence, fatigue, and cough (documentation of FEV_1, after bronchodilator, $<30\%$ of predicted is objective evidence for disabling dyspnea, but is not necessary to obtain) Progression of end-stage pulmonary disease, as evidenced by *prior* increased visits to emergency department or *prior* hospitalization for pulmonary infections and/or respiratory failure (documentation of serial decrease of FEV_1 >40 mL/yr is objective evidence for disease progression, but is not necessary to obtain) *and* Hypoxemia at rest on room air, as evidenced by $pO_2 \leq 55$ mm Hg or O_2 sat $\leq 88\%$ or hypercapnia, as evidenced by $pCO_2 \geq 50$ mm Hg Additional support needed for cor pulmonale and right heart failure secondary to pulmonary disease, unintentional progressive weight loss of $>10\%$ of body weight over preceding 6 mo, resting tachycardia >100 beats/min
Acute renal failure	Not seeking dialysis or renal transplant CrCl <10 mL/min (<15 mL/min for diabetes) Serum creatinine >8 mg/dL (>6 mg/dL for diabetes) Additional support needed for comorbid conditions such as malignancy, chronic lung disease (eg, mechanical ventilation), advanced cardiac disease, advanced liver disease
Chronic renal failure	Not seeking dialysis or renal transplant CrCl <10 mL/min (<15 mL/min for diabetes) Serum creatinine >8 mg/dL (>6 mg/dL for diabetes) Additional support needed for following signs and symptoms of renal failure: uremia, oliguria (<400 mL/day), intractable hyperkalemia (>7) not responsive to treatment, uremic pericarditis, hepatorenal syndrome

* May vary depending on fiscal intermediary; additional supportive indications available for most diagnoses. Adapted from Palmetto GBA (www.palmettogba.com).

Advance Directives

Designed to respect patient's autonomy and determine his/her wishes about future life-sustaining medical treatment if unable to indicate wishes.

Oral Statements

• Conversations with relatives, friends, clinicians are most common form; should be thoroughly documented in medical record for later reference.

• Properly verified oral statements carry same ethical and legal weight as those recorded in writing.

Instructional Advance Directives (DNR Orders, Living Wills)
- Written instructions regarding the initiation, continuation, withholding, or withdrawal of particular forms of life-sustaining medical treatment.
- May be revoked or altered at any time by the patient.
- Clinicians who comply with such directives are provided legal immunity for such actions.

Durable Power of Attorney for Health Care or Health Care Proxy
A written document that enables a capable person to appoint someone else to make future medical treatment choices for him or her in the event of decisional incapacity (see **Figure 2**).

Key Interventions, Treatment Decisions to Include in Advance Directives
- Resuscitation procedures
- Mechanical respiration
- Chemotherapy, radiation therapy
- Dialysis
- Simple diagnostic tests
- Pain control
- Blood products, transfusions
- Intentional deep sedation

Withholding or Withdrawing Therapy
- There is no ethical or legal difference between withholding an intervention (not starting it) and withdrawing life-sustaining medical treatment (stopping it after it has been started).
- Beginning a treatment does not preclude stopping it later; a time-limited trial may be appropriate.
- Palliative care should not be limited, even if life-sustaining treatments are withdrawn or withheld.
- Decisions on artificial feeding should be based on the same criteria applied to use of ventilators and other medical treatment.

Euthanasia
- Active euthanasia: direct intervention, such as lethal injection, intended to hasten a patient's death; a criminal act of homicide.
- Passive euthanasia: withdrawal or withholding of unwanted or unduly burdensome life-sustaining treatment; appropriate in certain circumstances.
- Assisted suicide: the patient's intentional, willful ending of his or her own life with the assistance of another; a criminal offense in most states.

MANAGEMENT OF COMMON END-OF-LIFE SYMPTOMS
Pain
- Primary goal: to alleviate suffering at end of life. See Pain (p 170) for assessment and interventions.
- The most distressing symptom for patients and caregivers.
- If intent is to relieve suffering, the risk that sufficient medication appropriately titrated will produce an unintended effect (hastening death) is morally acceptable (double effect).
- Alternate routes may be needed, eg, transdermal, transmucosal, rectal, vaginal, topical, epidural, and intrathecal.
- Recommend expert pain management consult if pain not adequately relieved with standard analgesic guidelines and interventions.
- Additional treatment may include:
  - radionuclides and bisphosphonates (for metastatic bone pain)
  - treatments (eg, radiotherapy, chemotherapy) directed at source of pain

- Pain crisis: Sedation at end of life for intractable pain and suffering is an important option to discuss with patients. Ketamine (*Ketalar*) 0.1 mg/kg IV bolus. Repeat as needed q 5 min. Follow with infusion of 0.015 mg/kg/min IV (if IV access not available, SC at 0.3–0.5 mg/kg). Decrease opioid dosage by 50%. A benzodiazepine may be useful. Observe for problems with increased secretions and treat (see p 184).

Weakness, Fatigue
Nonpharmacologic
- Modify environment to decrease energy expenditure (eg, placement of phone, bedside commode, drinks).
- Adjust room temperature to patient's comfort.
- Teach reordering tasks to conserve energy (eg, eating first, resting, then bathing).
- Modify daily procedures (eg, sitting while showering rather than standing).
Pharmacologic
- Treat remediable causes such as pain, medication toxicity, insomnia, anemia, and depression.
- Consider psychostimulants (eg, dextroamphetamine [*Dexedrine*] 2.5 mg po qam or q 12 h, methylphenidate [*Ritalin*] 5–10 mg po qam or q 12 h, or modafinil [*Provigil*] 200 mg qam); monitor for signs of psychosis, agitation, or sleep disturbance.

Dysphagia (see also p 87)
Nonpharmacologic
- Feed small, frequent amounts of pureed or soft foods.
- Avoid spicy, salty, acidic, sticky, and extremely hot or cold foods.
- Keep head of bed elevated for 30 min after eating.
- Instruct patient to wear dentures and to chew thoroughly.
- Use suction machine when necessary.
Pharmacologic
- For painful mucositis: 1:2:8 mixture of diphenhydramine elixir: lidocaine [2%–4%]: magnesium-aluminum hydroxide (eg, *Maalox*) as a swish-and-swallow suspension before meals.
- For candidiasis: clotrimazole 10-mg troches, 5 doses/d, *or* fluconazole 150 mg po followed by 100 mg/d po × 5 d.
- For severe halitosis: antimicrobial mouthwash; fastidious oral and dental care; treat putative respiratory tract infection with broad-spectrum antibiotics.

Dyspnea (see p 202)
Nonpharmacologic
- Teach positions to facilitate breathing, elevate head of bed.
- Teach relaxation techniques.
- Eliminate smoke and allergens.
- Assure brisk air circulation (facial breeze) with a room fan; oxygen is indicated only for symptomatic hypoxemia (ie, SaO_2 <90% by pulse oximetry).

Pharmacologic
- Opioids: oral morphine concentration (20 mg/mL: 1/4 to 1/2 mL sl, po; repeat in 10–15 min prn); if oral route not tolerated, nebulized morphine 2.5 mg in 2–4 mL NS *or* fentanyl 25–50 mcg in 2–4 mL NS; *or* IV morphine 1 mg or equivalent opioid q 5–10 min.
- Bronchodilators (see **Table 89**).
- Diuretics, if evidence of volume overload (see **Table 20**).
- Anxiolytics (eg, lorazepam po, sl, SC 0.5–2 mg q 2–4 h or prn); titrate slowly to effect.

Constipation (see p 92)
Most common cause: adverse effects of opioids, medications with anticholinergic adverse effects. Use stimulant or osmotic laxative (see **Table 40**). Consider enema if no bowel movement for 4 d. Evaluate for bowel obstruction or fecal impaction.

Bowel Obstruction
Indications for Radiographic Evaluation
- To differentiate between constipation and mechanical obstruction
- To confirm the obstruction, determine site and nature if surgery is being considered
Nonpharmacologic Management
- Nasogastric intubation: only if surgery is being considered, for high-level obstructions, and poor response to pharmacotherapy
- Percutaneous venting gastrostomy: for high-level obstructions and profuse vomiting not responsive to antiemetics
- Palliative surgery
- Hydration: IV or hypodermoclysis
Pharmacologic Management (aimed at specific symptoms)
- Nausea and vomiting: haloperidol (*Haldol*) po, IM 0.5–5 mg (≤10 mg) q 4–8 h prn; ondansetron (*Zofran*) IV (over 2–5 min) 4 mg q 12 h, po 8 mg q 12 h [inj; T: 4, 8, 24; S: 4 mg/5 mL], but costly; see also **Table 41**.
- Spasm, pain, and vomiting: scopolamine IM, IV, SC 0.3–0.65 mg q 4–6 h prn; oral 0.4–0.8 mg q 4–8 h prn; transdermal 2.5 cm^2 pch applied behind the ear q 3 d [inj; T: 0.4; pch 1.5 mg] *or* hyoscyamine (*Levsin/SL*) sl [T: 0.125; S: 0.125 mg/mL] 0.125–0.25 q 6–8 h.
- Diarrhea and excessive secretions: loperamide (*Imodium A-D*), see **Table 42**; octreotide (*Sandostatin*) SC 0.15–0.3 mg q 12 h [inj], very expensive.
- Pain: see **Table 71**.
- Inflammation due to malignant obstruction: dexamethasone (*Decadron*) po: 4 mg q 6 h × 5–7 d.

Excessive Secretions
Nonpharmacologic: Positioning and suctioning, as needed
Pharmacologic: Glycopyrrolate 0.1–0.4 mg IV, SC q 4 h prn *or* scopolamine 0.3–0.6 mg SC prn *or* transdermal scopolamine pch q 72 h *or* atropine 0.3–0.5 mg SC, sl, nebulized q 4 h prn

Cough (see p 201)

Nausea, Vomiting (see p 94)
Determine cause to select appropriate antiemetic based on pathway-mediating symptoms and neurotransmitter involved (see **Table 41**).

Anorexia, Cachexia, Dehydration
See also Malnutrition (p 139) and volume depletion (p 134). Universal symptom of patients with serious and life-threatening illness.
Nonpharmacologic
• Educate patient and family on effects of disease progression resulting in lack of appetite and weight loss.
• Promote interest, enjoyment in meals (eg, alcoholic beverage if desired, involve patient in meal planning, small frequent feedings, cold or semi-frozen nutritional drinks).
• Good oral care is important.
• Alleviate dry mouth with ice chips, popsicles, moist compresses, or artificial saliva.
Pharmacologic
• Corticosteroids: dexamethasone 1–2 mg po q 8 h; methylprednisolone 1–2 mg po q 12 h; prednisone 5 mg po q 8 h
• Hormone therapy: megestrol acetate 200–800 mg/d

Altered Mental Status, Delirium (see Delirium, p 52)

Anxiety, Depression
• Provide opportunity to discuss feelings, fears, existential concerns
• Referral to appropriate team members (spiritual, nursing)
• Medicate (see Anxiety, p 25, and Depression, p 61)

Source: Fine P. *Hospice Companion—Processes to Optimize Care During the Last Phase of Life*. 2nd ed. Scottsdale, AZ: VistaCare, Inc.; 2000.

PREOPERATIVE CARE
Cardiac Risk Assessment

Figure 8. Reducing Cardiac Risk in Noncardiac Surgery

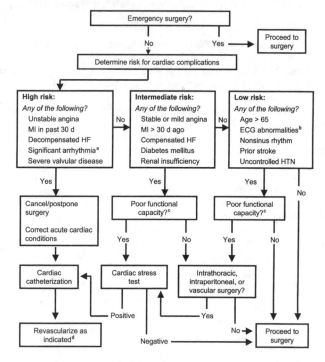

[a] High-grade AV block, symptomatic ventricular arrhythmias in the presence of underlying heart disease, or supraventricular arrhythmias with uncontrolled rate

[b] LVH, left bundle branch block, or ST-T abnormalities

[c] Unable to climb 1 flight of stairs or do light housework

[d] Left main or severe 3-vessel disease, or confirmed CAD accompanied by aortic stenosis, or severe left ventricular dysfunction; CABG preferred over PTCA

Adapted from: Eagle KA, Berger PB, Calkins H et al. ACC/AHA guideline update for perioperative cardiovascular evaluation for noncardiac surgery—executive summary. *Circulation* 2002;105:1257–1267.

Pulmonary Risk Assessment

Risk factors for postoperative pulmonary complications:

- Smoking
- COPD
- ASA Class II-V (I – healthy; II – mild systemic disease; III – moderate/severe systemic disease; IV – life-threatening systemic disease; V – moribund)
- ADL dependence
- HF
- Prolonged (>3 h) surgery; abdominal, thoracic, neurologic, head and neck, or vascular surgery; AAA repair; emergency surgery
- General anesthesia
- Serum albumin <3.5 mg/dL

Reducing risk of postoperative pulmonary complications:

- Smoking cessation 6–8 wk before surgery
- Preoperative training in incentive spirometry, active-cycle breathing techniques, and forced-expiration techniques has been shown to reduce complications in high-risk patients undergoing CABG.
- Postoperative incentive spirometry, chest physical therapy, coughing, postural drainage, percussion and vibration, suctioning and ambulation, intermittent positive-pressure breathing, and/or continuous positive-airway pressure
- Nasogastric tube use for patients with postoperative nausea or vomiting, inability to tolerate oral intake, or symptomatic abdominal distention

Other Assessments

Anticoagulation Status: See pp 21–24.

Cognitive Status: Unrecognized dementia is a risk factor for postoperative delirium. Measure preoperative cognitive status with Mini-Cog (see p 244) or MMSE.

Nutritional Status: Poor nutritional status can impair wound healing. Measure height, weight, serum albumin.

Routine Laboratory Tests: Recommended—Hb, hematocrit, electrolytes, creatinine, BUN, ECG, CXR, albumin. Optional—CBC, platelets, ABG, PT, PTT.

Cataract Surgery: Routine laboratory testing or cardiopulmonary risk assessment is unneccessary for cataract surgery performed under local anesthesia.

Advance Directives: Establish or update.

PERIOPERATIVE MANAGEMENT

β-Blocker Use

- Perioperative β-blockade is appropriate for patients at high or intermediate risk of cardiac complications (see **Figure 8**) who are undergoing emergent, vascular, head and neck, intrathoracic, intraperitoneal, orthopedic, or prostate surgery.
- Consider perioperative β-blockade for patients at low risk of cardiac complications (see **Figure 8**) who are undergoing vascular surgery.

- Begin β-blocker (eg, atenolol or bisoprolol) po 1–2 wk before surgery to achieve heart rate <70 beats/min. Continue therapy until 2 wk after surgery, with a goal of <80 beats/min in the postoperative period. Withhold β-blockers if heart rate is <55 beats/min; SPB <100; or the patient has asthma, decompensated HF, or third-degree heart block.
- Perioperative β-blockade is not indicated in patients undergoing endoscopic procedures, superficial procedures, cataract surgery, or breast surgery.

Statin Use
Statins have been associated with lower perioperative mortality in patients with known or suspected CAD undergoing noncardiac surgery. Unless there is a contraindication, pre- and perioperative administration of statins (see **Table 19**), regardless of LDL cholesterol levels, is recommended.

Atrial Fibrillation/Tachyarrhythmia Prophylaxis for Patients Undergoing CABG and/or Cardiac Valvular Surgery
- To reduce incidence of postoperative tachyarrhythmias, consider amiodarone po 5 mg/kg q 12 h from 6 d before surgery through 6 d after surgery. *Note:* Amiodarone potentiates warfarin; warfarin dosage should be reduced by one-third to one-half; monitor INR closely.
- To reduce incidence of postoperative AF, consider hydrocortisone 100 mg IV the evening of the operative day, followed by 100 mg IV q 8 h × 3 d, accompanied by oral metoprolol (25 mg q 12 h if HR is 60–70, 50 mg q 12 h if HR is 71–81, or 50 mg q 8 h if HR is >80) for the same time period.

Endocarditis Prophylaxis
Depends on cardiac condition and type of procedure (see pp 190–191).

DVT Prophylaxis (see p 22 and **Table 12**)

Common Problems to Monitor
- Confusion (see p 52)
- Intra- and postoperative coronary events: postoperative ECG to check
- Malnutrition (see p 139)
- Pain (see p 170)
- Polypharmacy: review medications daily
- Pulmonary complications: minimized by incentive spirometry, coughing, early ambulation
- Rehabilitation: encourage early mobility
- Skin breakdown (see p 217)

DISCHARGE PLANNING
- Ideally, all team members should participate in discharge planning, beginning early in the hospitalization.
- Physician should provide discharge summary and orders, including medications.
- Tools are available (see www.caretransitions.org) for patients and caregivers to assert care preferences, clarify discharge instructions, resolve medication discrepancies, and facilitate communication across care sites after discharge.
- Site of care after discharge should be warranted by patient's needs (see **Table 5**).

PREVENTIVE TESTS AND PROCEDURES

Table 75. Recommended Primary and Secondary Disease Prevention for People Aged 65 and Older

Preventive Strategy	Frequency
USPSTF[a] Recommendations for Primary Prevention	
Bone mineral density (women)	at least once after age 65
BP screening	yearly
Diabetes mellitus screening	at least once in people with HTN or hyperlipidemia
Influenza immunization	yearly
Lipid disorder screening	every 5 yr, more often in CAD, diabetes mellitus, PAD, prior stroke
Obesity (height and weight)	yearly
Pneumonia immunization	once at age 65[b]
Smoking cessation	at every office visit
Tetanus immunization	every 10 yr
USPSTF[a] Recommendations for Secondary Prevention	
Abdominal aortic aneurysm ultrasonography	once between age 65–75 in men who have ever smoked
Alcohol abuse screening	unspecified but should be done periodically
Depression screening	yearly
FOBT/sigmoidoscopy/colonoscopy	yearly/every 5 yr/every 10 yr
Hearing impairment screening	yearly
Mammography, clinical breast examination[c]	every 1–2 yr
Pap smear[d]	at least every 3 yr
Visual impairment screening	yearly
Other[e] Recommendations for Primary Prevention	
ASA to prevent MI	daily
Calcium (1200 mg) and vitamin D (800 IU) to prevent osteoporosis	daily
Herpes zoster immunization	once in immunocompetent people without prior zoster
Measurement of serum C-reactive protein	at least once in people with one CAD risk factor
Omega-3 fatty acids to prevent MI, stroke	at least 2 ×/wk (see MI care, p 32)
Multivitamin	1–2/d
Other[e] Recommendations for Secondary Prevention	
Skin examination	yearly
Breast self-examination	monthly
Cognitive impairment screening	yearly
Electron-beam computed tomography	at least once in people with multiple CAD risk factors
Glaucoma screening	yearly
Inquiry about falls	yearly
PSA and digital rectal examination	yearly
TSH in women	yearly

[a] US Preventive Services Task Force. See www.ahrq.gov/clinic/uspstfix.htm.
[b] Consider repeating pneumococcal vaccine every 6–7 yr.
[c] Mammograms to age 70 are almost universally recommended; many organizations, including the USPSTF, recommend that mammography should be continued in women over 70 who have a reasonable life expectancy.
[d] Pap smear testing can be stopped in most women after age 65. See p 238. Women without a cervix should not have pap smears.
[e] Not endorsed by USPSTF for all older adults, but recommended in selected patients or by other professional organizations.

The USPSTF recommends **against** screening for:
- Asymptomatic bacteriuria with urinalysis
- Bladder cancer with hematuria detection, bladder tumor antigen measurement, NMP22 urinary enzyme immunoassay, or urine cytology
- CAD with ECG, exercise treadmill test, or electron-beam computerized tomography in people with few or no CAD risk factors
- Ovarian cancer with transvaginal ultrasonography or CA-125 measurement
- Pancreatic cancer with ultrasonography or serologic markers

ENDOCARDITIS PROPHYLAXIS (AHA GUIDELINES)

Antibiotic Regimens Recommended (see Table 76)

Cardiac Conditions Requiring Prophylaxis
- Prosthetic cardiac valve
- Previous infective endocarditis
- Cardiac transplant recipients who develop cardiac valvulopathy
- Unrepaired cyanotic congenital heart disease
- Repaired congenital heart disease with residual defects at the site or adjacent to the site of a prosthetic patch or device
- Congenital heart disease completely repaired with prosthetic material or device (prophylaxis needed for only the first 6 mo after repair procedure)

Cardiac Conditions Not Requiring Prophylaxis
All cardiac conditions or procedures not listed above.

Procedures Warranting Prophylaxis (only in patients with cardiac conditions listed above)
- Dental procedures requiring manipulation of gingival tissue, manipulation of the periapical region of teeth, or perforation of the oral mucosa (includes extractions, implants, reimplants, root canals, teeth cleaning during which bleeding is expected)
- Invasive procedures of the respiratory tract involving incision or biopsy of respiratory tract mucosa
- Surgical procedures involving infected skin, skin structures, or musculoskeletal tissue

Procedures Not Warranting Prophylaxis
- All dental procedures not listed above
- All noninvasive respiratory procedures
- All GI and GU procedures

Table 76. Endocarditis Prophylaxis Regimens

Situation	Regimen (Single Dose 30-60 Min Before Procedure)*
Oral	Amoxicillin 2 g po
Unable to take oral medication	Ampicillin 2 g, cefazolin 1 g, or ceftriaxone 1 g IM or IV
Allergic to penicillins or ampicillin	Cephalexin 2 g, clindamycin 600 mg, azithromycin 500 mg, or clarithromycin 500 mg po
Allergic to penicillins or ampicillin and unable to take oral medication	Cefazolin 1 g, ceftriaxone 1 g, or clindamycin 600 mg IM or IV

* For patients undergoing invasive respiratory tract procedures to treat an infection known to be caused by *Staph aureus*, or for patients undergoing surgery for infected skin, skin structures, or musculoskeletal tissue, regimen should include an antistaphylococcal penicillin or cephalosporin.

Source: Wilson W, Taubert KA, Gewitz M et al. Prevention of infective endocarditis. Guidelines from the American Heart Association. A guideline from the American Heart Association Rheumatic Fever, Endocarditis, and Kawasaki Disease Committee, Council on Cardiovascular Disease in the Young, and the Council on Clinical Cardiology, Council on Cardiovascular Surgery and Anesthesia, and the Quality of Care and Outcomes Research Interdisciplinary Working Group. *Circulation* (online) 2007: http://circ.ahajournals.org/cgi/reprint/CIRCULATIONAHA.106.183095.

PROPHYLAXIS FOR DENTAL PATIENTS WITH TOTAL JOINT REPLACEMENTS (TJR)

Conditions Requiring: inflammatory arthropathies (eg, rheumatoid arthritis, systemic lupus erythematosus); disease-, drug-, or radiation-induced immunosuppression; HIV infection; type 1 diabetes mellitus; first 2 yr after TJR; previous prosthetic joint infection; malnourishment; hemophilia; malignancy

Conditions Not Requiring: patients >2 yr after TJR who do not have one of the above conditions; patients with pins, plates, or screws

Dental Procedures Warranting: see those listed on p 190 for endocarditis

Suggested Prophylactic Regimens: (all given 1 h before procedure)
• Not allergic to penicillin: amoxicillin, cephalexin, or cephradine 2 g po
• Not allergic to penicillin and unable to take oral medications: ampicillin 2 g or cefazolin 1 g IM or IV
• Allergic to penicillin: clindamycin 600 mg po
• Allergic to penicillin and unable to take oral medications: clindamycin 600 mg IV

Source: Modified from American Dental Association and American Academy of Orthopaedic Surgeons. Antibiotic prophylaxis for dental patients with total joint replacements. *JADA* 2003;134:895–899. Copyright © 2003 American Dental Association. All rights reserved. Adapted 2008 with permission.

EXERCISE PRESCRIPTION
Before Giving an Exercise Prescription
Screen patient for:
• Musculoskeletal problems: decreased flexibility, muscular rigidity, weakness, pain, ill-fitting shoes
• Cardiac disease: consider stress test if patient is beginning a vigorous exercise program and is sedentary with ≥2 cardiac risk factors (male gender, HTN, smoking, diabetes mellitus, dyslipidemia, obesity, family hx, sedentary lifestyle).

Individualize the Prescription

Specify short- and long-term goals; include the following components:

Flexibility: Static stretching; daily, >15 sec per muscle group

Endurance: Walking, cycling, swimming at 50%–75% of max HR (220 – age for men; 220 – [0.6 × age] for women); 3–4 ×/wk; goal of 20–30 min duration

Strength: Muscle resistance (weight training); 3 sets (8–15 repetitions) per muscle group 2–3 ×/wk

Balance: Tai Chi, dance, yoga, postural awareness; 1–3 ×/wk

Patient Information: See www.nia.nih.gov/HealthInformation/Publications

See also Assessment and Management of Falls, **Figure 3**, p 83.

BENIGN PROSTATIC HYPERPLASIA
Evaluation
Detailed medical hx focusing on physical examination of the urinary tract, including abdominal examination, digital rectal examination, and a focused neurologic examination; UA and culture if pyuria or hematuria; measurement of serum creatinine. Postvoid residual if neurologic disease or prior procedure that can affect bladder or sphincter function, urinary incontinence, or reports of incomplete emptying. Measurement of PSA is optional.

Management
Mild Symptoms: (eg, AUA score ≤7; see p 250) watchful waiting
Moderate to Severe Symptoms: (eg, AUA score ≥8) watchful waiting, medical or surgical treatment
Nonpharmacologic Treatment: Avoid fluids before bedtime, reduce mild diuretics (eg, caffeine, alcohol), double voiding to empty bladder completely.
Pharmacologic Treatment: Combining drugs from different classes may have better long-term effectiveness than single-agent therapy.

- **α_1-Blockers** (reduce dynamic component by relaxing prostatic and bladder detrusor smooth muscle). Nonselective and selective agents are equally effective.
  (*Note:* sildenafil [*Viagra*], vardenafil [*LEVITRA*], or tadalafil [*Cialis*] can cause hypotension in men receiving α_1-blockers.)
  - **Nonselective** (less expensive):
    - Terazosin (*Hytrin*) increase dosage as tolerated—days 1–3, 1 mg/d hs; days 4–7, 2 mg; days 8–14, 5 mg; day 15 and beyond, 10 mg [T: 1, 2, 5, 10]
    - Doxazosin (*Cardura*) start 0.5 mg with max of 16 mg/d [T: 1, 2, 4, 8]
    - Prazosin (*Minipress*) start 1 mg/d (first dose hs) or q 12 h with max 20 mg/d [T: 1, 2, 5]
  - **Selective** (fewer side effects):
    - Tamsulosin (*Flomax*) 0.4 mg 30 min after the same meal each day and increase to 0.8 mg if no response in 2–4 wk [T: 0.4]
    - Alfuzosin ER (*Uroxatral*) 10 mg after the same meal every day [T: 10]
- **5-α Reductase inhibitors** (reduce prostate size; treatment for 6–12 mo may be needed before symptoms improve):
  - Finasteride (*Proscar*) 5 mg/d [T: 5] (may reduce risk of developing prostate cancer by 20%–25% but increases risk of developing high-grade prostate cancer.)
  - Dutasteride (*Avodart*) 0.5 mg/d [C: 0.5]
- **Antimuscarinic agents** (bladder relaxants) may have additional benefit beyond α_1-blockers on urinary frequency and urgency
  - Tolterodine ER (*Detrol LA*) 4 mg/d

Surgical Management: Indicated if recurrent UTI, recurrent or persistent gross hematuria, bladder stones, or renal insufficiency are clearly secondary to BPH or as indicated by severe symptoms (AUA score >16), patient preference, or ineffectiveness of medical treatment.** For men with moderate symptoms (AUA scores 8–15), surgical therapy is more effective than watchful waiting, but the latter is a reasonable alternative.

** Source: McConnell JD, Barry MJ, Bruskewitz RC, et al. *Benign Prostatic Hyperplasia: Diagnosis and Treatment.* Clinical Practice Guideline No. 8. Rockville, MD: Agency for Health Care Policy and Research, Public Health Service, US Dept. of Health and Human Services, February 1994. AHCPR Publication No. 94-0582.

Surgical options are:
- Transurethral resection of the prostate (TURP)
- Transurethral incision of the prostate (TUIP), which is limited to prostates with an estimated resected tissue weight (if done by TURP) of ≤30 g
- Open prostatectomy for large glands (>50 g)
- Urethral stents may be an option for poor surgical candidates.
- For laser prostatectomy, microwave therapy, and electrovaporization, data to support effectiveness and safety are limited.
- Transurethral needle ablation (TUNA) is less effective than TURP but may be an option for men with substantial comorbidity who are poor surgical candidates.

PROSTATE CANCER
Evaluation
Predicting extent of disease:
- PSA (see **Table 75**)
- Biopsy
- Digital rectal examination
- CT abdomen and pelvis (selectively)
- Bone scan (selectively)

Histology
- Gleason score 2–6 has low 15–20 yr morbidity and mortality; watchful waiting usually appropriate.
- Gleason score ≥7, higher PSA and younger age associated with higher morbidity and mortality; best treatment strategy (surgery, radiation, androgen suppression, etc) is not known.

Treatment of Early Prostate Cancer
- Radical prostatectomy (reduced overall and disease-specific mortality, metastasis, and local progression compared with watchful waiting in men <75 yr with early disease, well or moderately well differentiated histology, and PSA <50 ng/mL)
- Radiation therapy
  ○ External beam
  ○ Brachytherapy (radioactive seed implantation)
- Watchful waiting (avoid if life expectancy >15 yr or Gleason score ≥7)
- Hormonal therapy is generally reserved for locally advanced or metastatic disease.

Therapy for Locally Advanced and Metastatic Disease
- For locally advanced (T3) disease (tumor extension beyond prostate capsule or invasion of seminal vesicles), external beam radiation is commonly used with androgen deprivation therapy (ADT).
- Use ADT (**Table 77**) in T3, T4, or metastatic disease.
- Monotherapy can be either orchiectomy or a GnRH agonist.

- Combined androgen blockade (GnRH agonist plus antiandrogen) is used to avoid "flare" phenomenon (ie, increased symptoms early in treatment), but survival benefit is uncertain and side effects are greater than with monotherapy.
- In case of relapse:
  ○ Withdrawal of antiandrogen may induce remission.
  ○ Patients often respond when changed to a second antiandrogen.
  ○ When antiandrogens no longer control disease, adrenal suppression with aminoglutethimide or ketoconazole and hydrocortisone replacement may be effective.

Therapy for Metastatic Bone Disease

In men receiving long-term ADT or hormone therapy for cancer and in those with bone metastasis, zoledronic acid reduces the proportion of patients with skeletal-related events or fracture.

Table 77. Common Medications for Prostate Cancer Therapy

Class, Medication	Dosage	Metabolism	Adverse Events/Comments
GnRH Agonists			Class adverse events: certain symptoms (urinary obstruction, spinal cord compression, bone pain) may be exacerbated early in treatment; risk is less when combined with antiandrogens
Goserelin acetate implant (*Zoladex*)	3.6 mg SC q 28 d or 10.8 mg q 3 mo	Rapid urinary and hepatic excretion, no dosage adjustment in renal impairment	Hot flushes (60%), breast swelling, libido change, impotence, nausea
Leuprolide acetate (*Lupron Depot*)	7.5 mg IM q mo or 22.5 mg q 3 mo or 30 mg q 4 mo	Unknown; active metabolites for 4–12 wk, dose-dependent	Hot flushes (60%), edema (12%), pain (7%), nausea, vomiting, impotence, dyspnea, asthenia (all 5%), thrombosis, PE, MI (all 1%); headache as high as 32%
Triptorelin (*Trelstar Depot, Trelstar LA*)	Depot: 37.5 mg q 28 d IM LA: 11.25 mg q 84 d	Hepatic metabolism and renal excretion (42% as intact peptide)	Hot flushes, ↑ glucose, ↓ Hb, ↓ RBC, ↑ alkaline phosphatase, ↑ ALT or AST, skeletal pain, ↑ BUN

(cont.)

Table 77. Common Medications for Prostate Cancer Therapy (cont.)

Class, Medication	Dosage	Metabolism	Adverse Events/Comments
Histrelin acetate (Vantas)	50-mg SC implant q 12 mo	Hepatic metabolism	Hot flushes, fatigue, headaches, nausea, mild renal impairment
Antiandrogens (most often used in combination with GnRH agonists)			Class adverse events: nausea, hot flushes, breast pain, gynecomastia, hematuria, diarrhea, liver enzyme elevations, galactorrhea
Bicalutamide (Casodex)	50 mg/d po [T: 50]	Metabolized in liver, excreted in urine; half-life 10 d at steady state	
Flutamide (Eulexin)	250 mg po q 8 h [C: 125]	Renal excretion; half-life 5–6 h	Greatest GI toxicity in the class; severe liver dysfunction reported
Nilutamide (Nilandron)	300 mg/d po for 30 d, then 150 mg/d po [T: 50]	80% protein bound; liver metabolism, renal excretion; half-life 40–60 h	Delayed light adaptation
GnRH Antagonist Abarelix (Plenaxis)	100 mg IM q 28 d	Liver metabolism, 13% renal excretion; half-life 13 d	Hypersensitivity 4%, prolonged QT interval; use limited to initial treatment of advanced cancer; restricted access in US

PROSTATITIS

Definition
Acute or chronic inflammation of the prostate secondary to bacterial and nonbacterial causes

Symptoms and Diagnosis
Acute: fever; chills; dysuria; tender, tense, or boggy on examination (examination should be minimal to avoid bacteremia); Gram stain and culture of urine
Chronic: obstructive or irritative symptoms with voiding, perineal pain, normal examination; compare first void or midstream urine with prostatic secretion or postmassage urine: bacterial if leukocytosis and bacteria in expressed sample, nonbacterial if sample sterile with leukocytosis

Treatment (see **Table 53**)

Antibiotic therapy should be based on Gram stain and culture.

Acute prostatitis
- Co-trimoxazole DS 1 po q 12 h × 2 wk, *or*
- Ciprofloxacin 500 mg po or 400 mg IV q 12 h × 10–14 d, *or*
- Ofloxacin 400 mg po once, then 300 mg q 12 h × 10 d, *or*
- 3rd-generation cephalosporin or aminoglycoside IV

Chronic prostatitis
- Co-trimoxazole DS 1 po q 12 h × 2–4 mo, *or*
- Ciprofloxacin 500 mg po q 12 h × 1 mo, *or*
- Levofloxacin 500 mg po q 24 h × 1 mo, *or*
- Ofloxacin 200 mg q 12 h × 3 mo

PSYCHOTIC DISORDERS

DIFFERENTIAL DIAGNOSIS
- Bipolar affective disorder
- Delirium
- Dementia
- Medications/drugs: eg, antiparkinsonian agents, anticholinergics, benzodiazepines or alcohol (including withdrawal), stimulants, corticosteroids, cardiac medications (eg, digitalis), opioid analgesics
- Late-life delusional (paranoid) disorder
- Major depression
- Physical disorders: hypo- or hyperglycemia, hypo- or hyperthyroidism, sodium or potassium imbalance, Cushing's syndrome, Parkinson's disease, B_{12} deficiency, sleep deprivation, AIDS
- Pain, untreated
- Schizophrenia
- Structural brain lesions: tumor or stroke
- Seizure disorder: eg, temporal lobe

Risk Factors for Psychotic Symptoms in Older Adults: chronic bed rest, cognitive impairment, female gender, sensory impairment, social isolation

MANAGEMENT
- Alleviate underlying physical causes.
- Address identifiable psychosocial triggers.
- If psychotic symptoms are severe, frightening, or may affect safety, use antipsychotic.
- Aripiprazole, olanzapine, quetiapine, risperidone are first choice because of fewer adverse events (TD extremely high in older adults taking typical antipsychotics). See **Table 80** for adverse events of atypical antipsychotics.
- First-generation (typical) antipsychotics may increase mortality more than atypical antipsychotics.

Table 78. Representative Medications for Treatment of Psychosis			
Class, Medication	Dosage*	Formulations	Comments (Metabolism)
Atypical Antipsychotics			
✔Aripiprazole (*Abilify*)	10–15 (1) initially; max 30/d	T: 10, 15, 20, 30	Wait 2 wk between dosage changes (CYP2D6, -3A4) (L)
Clozapine (*Clozaril*)	25–150 (1)	T: 25, 100	May be useful for parkinsonism and TD; significant risk of neutropenia and agranulocytosis (L)
✔Olanzapine (*Zyprexa*)	2.5–10 (1)	T: 2.5, 5, 7.5, 10, 15, 20; disintegrating tab: 5, 10, 15, 20	(L)

(cont.)

Table 78. Representative Medications for Treatment of Psychosis (cont.)

Class, Medication	Dosage*	Formulations	Comments (Metabolism)
Paliperidone (*Invega*)	3–12 (1)	T: ER 3, 6, 9	CrCl 51–80 mL/min, max 6 mg/d; CrCl ≤50 mL/min, max 3 mg/d; very limited geriatric data (K)
✔Quetiapine (*Seroquel*)	25–800 (1–2)	T: 25, 100, 200, 300	(L, K)
✔Risperidone (*Risperdal*)	0.5–1 (1–2)	T: 0.25, 0.5, 1, 2, 3, 4 scored; S: 1 mg/mL; IM long-acting: 25, 37.5, and 50 mg/2 mL	Dose-related EPS; IM not for acute treatment; do not exceed 6 mg (L, K)
Ziprasidone (*Geodon*)	20–80 (1–2)	C: 20, 40, 60, 80; IM: 20 mg/mL	May increase QT$_C$; very limited geriatric data (L)
Low Potency			
Thioridazine (eg, *Mellaril*)	25–200 (1–3)	T: 10, 15, 25, 50, 100, 150, 200; S: 30 mg/mL	Anticholinergic effects, orthostasis, QT$_C$ prolongation, sedation, TD; for acute use only (L, K)
Intermediate Potency			
Loxapine (*Loxitane*)	2.5–20 (1–3)	C: 5, 10, 25, 50; S: 25 mg/mL	Anticholinergic effects, orthostasis, sedation, TD; for acute use only (L, K)
High Potency			
Haloperidol (*Haldol*)	0.5–2 (1–3); depot 100–200 mg IM q 4 wk	T: 0.5, 1, 2, 5, 10, 20; S: conc 2 mg/mL; Inj: 5 mg/mL (lactate)	EPS, TD; for acute use only (L, K)

✔ = preferred for treating older adults but does not imply low risk; mortality may be increased in patients with dementia.
* Total mg/d (frequency/d)

Table 79. Choosing an Atypical Antipsychotic

Atypical Antipsychotic	Aripiprazole	Clozapine	Olanzapine	Quetiapine	Risperidone	Ziprasidone
Level of Evidence	CR	CR	RCT	RCT	RCT	CR
Adverse Events						
Cardiovascular						
Hypotension	?	0/+++	+	+++	+	?
QT$_C$ prolongation	?	+	+	+	+	++
Endocrine/Metabolic						
Weight gain	?	+++	+++	++	++	?
Diabetes	?	+++	+++	++	++	?
Hypertriglyceridemia	0	+	+	0	?	0
Hyperprolactinemia	?	?	?	?	+++	+
Gastrointestinal						
Nausea, vomiting, constipation	0	?	0	+	?	?

(cont.)

Table 79. Choosing an Atypical Antipsychotic (cont.)

Atypical Antipsychotic	Aripiprazole	Clozapine	Olanzapine	Quetiapine	Risperidone	Ziprasidone
Level of Evidence	CR	CR	RCT	RCT	RCT	CR
Neurologic						
Extrapyramidal symptoms	?	?	+	?	+++	+
Seizures	?	+++	?	?	ND	ND
Sedation	?	+++	+	+	+	?
Systemic						
Anticholinergic	0	+++	++	+	0	?
Neuroleptic malignant syndrome	ND	+	ND	ND	+	ND

CR = case reports; RCT = randomized clinical trials; ND = no data
? = uncertain effect
0 = no effect
+ = mild effect; ++ = moderate effect; +++ = severe effect; 0/+++ = no effect to severe effect in the case of drug interactions

Table 80. Management of Adverse Events of Antipsychotic Medications

Adverse Event	Treatment	Comment
Drug-induced parkinsonism	Reduce dosage or change drug or drug class	Often dose related; avoid anticholinergic agents
Akathisia (motor restlessness)	Consider adding β-blocker (eg, propranolol [*Inderal*] 20–40 mg/d) or low-dose benzodiazepine (eg, lorazepam 0.5 mg q 12 h)	Also seen with atypical antipsychotics; more likely with traditional agents
Hypotension	Slow titration; reduce dosage; change drug class	More common with low-potency agents
Sedation	Reduce dosage; give at bedtime; change drug class	More common with low-potency agents
TD	Stop drug (if possible); consider atypical antipsychotic (eg, aripiprazole, quetiapine) with lower potential for EPS	Increased risk in older adults; may be irreversible

Note: Periodic (q 4 mo) reevaluation of antipsychotic dosage and ongoing need is important (see CMS guidance on unnecessary drugs in the nursing home p 252). Older adults are particularly sensitive to adverse events of antipsychotic drugs. They are also at higher risk of developing TD. Periodic use of an adverse-event scale such as the AIMS is highly recommended. (see: www.geriatricsatyourfingertips.org)

COUGH

Among the most common symptoms in office practice; consider likely diagnosis based on duration of symptoms and treat the specific disorder (**Table 81**). **Table 82** also includes agents sometimes used in symptomatic management of cough.

Table 81. Diagnosis and Treatment of Cough by Duration of Symptoms

Cause	Preferred Treatment
Acute cough: duration up to 3 wk	
Common cold	Sinus irrigation or nasal ipratropium (*Atrovent*, see **Table 85**). Not recommended: sedating antihistamines (dry mouth, urinary retention, confusion); oral pseudoephedrine (hypertension, tachycardia, urinary retention)
Allergic rhinitis	See p 203.
Bacterial sinusitis	Oxymetazalone nasal spr (eg, *Afrin*) × 5 d; antibiotic against *Haemophilus influenzae* and streptococcal pneumonia × 2 wk
Pertussis	Macrolide or trimethoprim-sulfa antibiotic × 2 wk
Other: pneumonia, HF, asthma, COPD exacerbation	See pneumonia, p 113; HF, p 32; asthma, p 208; COPD, p 207.
Subacute cough: duration 3–8 wk*	
Postinfectious	Inhaled ipratropium (*Atrovent*, see **Table 89**); systemic steroids tapered over 2–3 wk; if protracted, dextromethorphan with codeine; use bronchodilators if there is bronchospasm
Subacute bacterial sinusitis	As for acute sinusitis, but treat for 3 wk
Asthma	See treatment, p 209.
Pertussis	Macrolide or trimethoprim-sulfa antibiotic × 2 wk; may need to treat as above for postinfectious cough
Chronic cough: duration >8 wk*	
Perennial rhinitis *or* vasomotor rhinitis	See p 203.
Chronic bacterial sinusitis	Oxymetazalone nasal spr (eg, *Afrin*) × 5 d; antibiotic against *Haemophilus influenzae*, streptococcal pneumonia, and mouth anaerobes × 3 wk; may need follow-up course of nasal steroids
Asthma	See treatment, p 209.
Other: ACEIs, reflux esophagitis	Stop ACEI; treat reflux for ≥3 mo using a PPI
Aspiration	See Dysphagia, p 87.

*Obtain chest radiograph, sputums to exclude malignancy, TB, etc.

Management
- Do not suppress cough in stable COPD.
- For symptomatic relief, see **Table 82**.

Table 82. Antitussives and Expectorants

Medication	Dosage and Formulations	Adverse Events (Metabolism)
Benzonatate[a] (*Tessalon Perles*)	100 mg po q 8 h (max: 600 mg/d) C: 100, 200	CNS stimulation or depression, headache, dizziness, hallucination, constipation (L)
Dextromethorphan[b] (eg, *Robitussin DM*)	10–30 mL po q 4–8 h C: 30 S: 10 mg/5 mL	Mild drowsiness, fatigue; interacts with fluoxetine, paroxetine; combination may cause serotonin syndrome (L)
Guaifenesin[b] (eg, *Robitussin*)	5–20 mL po q 4 h S: 100 mg/5 mL	None at low dosages; high dosages cause nausea, vomiting, diarrhea, drowsiness, abdominal pain (L)
Histussin HC[b]	10 mL q 4 h up to 40 mL/d S: hydrocodone 2.5 mg + phenylephrine 5 mg + chlorpheniramine 2 mg/mL	Sedation, constipation, nervousness, tachycardia, hypertension, urinary retention (L)
Hydrocodone[b] (*Hycodan*)	5 mL po q 4–6 h S: 5 mg/5 mL	Sedation, constipation, confusion (L)

[a] Antitussive and expectorant
[b] Antitussive

DYSPNEA

Definition

"A subjective experience of breathing discomfort that consists of qualitatively distinct sensations that vary in intensity" (ATS)

Characteristics

- >65 yr: occurs in 17% at rest at least occasionally; in 38% when hurrying on level ground or on slight hill.
- Hx: consider if level of dyspnea is appropriate to level of exertion (versus suggests pathology)
  - Consider age, peers, usual activities, level of fitness
  - Ask, "What activities have you stopped doing?"
- Associated symptoms: cough, sputum, wheezing, chest pain, orthopnea, paroxysmal nocturnal dyspnea

Evaluation

Hx and physical examination should suggest organ system; then evaluate for cause (**Table 83**).

Table 83. Diagnosis of Dyspnea

Suspected System	Diagnostic Strategy	Diagnosis
Cardiac	Chest radiograph, ECG, echocardiogram, radionuclide imaging	Ischemic or other form of heart disease

(cont.)

Table 83. Diagnosis of Dyspnea (cont.)		
Suspected System	**Diagnostic Strategy**	**Diagnosis**
Lung	Spirometry	Asthma or COPD
	Diffusing capacity	Emphysema or interstitial lung disease
	Echocardiogram	Pulmonary hypertension
Respiratory muscle dysfunction	Inspiratory and expiratory mouth pressures	Neuromuscular disease
Deconditioning/obesity versus psychological disorders	Cardiopulmonary exercise test	Deconditioning shows decreased maximal oxygen consumption but normal cardiorespiratory exercise responses.

Therapy
Nonpharmacologic
- Exercise reduces dyspnea and improves fitness in almost all older adults regardless of cause; physical conditioning reduces dyspnea during ADLs and exercise, and is primary treatment for deconditioning.
  - Use low-impact, indoor activity
  - Base intensity on heart rate or symptom of dyspnea
  - Recommend 20–30 min on most days
- Indications for pulmonary rehabilitation include the following:
  - Dyspnea during rest or exertion
  - Hypoxemia, hypercapnia
  - Reduced exercise tolerance or a decline in ADLs
  - Worsening dyspnea and a reduced but stable exercise tolerance level
  - Pre- or postoperative lung resection, transplantation, or volume reduction
  - Chronic respiratory failure and the need to initiate mechanical ventilation
  - Ventilator dependence
  - Increasing need for emergency department visits, hospitalization, and unscheduled office visits

Pharmacologic: See specific diseases elsewhere in this chapter.

ALLERGIC RHINITIS AND CONJUNCTIVITIS
Description
- The most common atopic disorder.
- Symptoms include rhinorrhea; sneezing; and irritated eyes, nose, and mucous membranes.
- May be seasonal, but in older adults is more often perennial.
- Postnasal drip, mainly from chronic rhinitis, is the most common cause of chronic cough.

Therapy
Nonpharmacologic: Saline and sodium bicarbonate nasal irrigation may be helpful (eg, SinuCleanse); avoid allergens, eliminate pets and their dander, dehumidify to reduce molds; reduce outdoor exposures during pollen season; reduce house dust mites by encasing pillows and mattresses. Arachnocides reduce mites.

Pharmacologic: Target therapy to symptoms and on whether symptoms are seasonal or perennial; see **Table 84** and **Table 85**.

Stepped therapy: Begin with oral second-generation antihistamine or nasal steroid; if symptoms uncontrolled, add the other agent; if still uncontrolled, add or substitute a leukotriene modifier for one of the other agents.

Table 84. Choosing Medication for Allergic Rhinitis or Conjunctivitis

Medication or Class	Rhinitis	Sneezing	Pruritus	Congestion	Eye Symptoms
Nasal steroids[a]	+++	+++	++	++	++
Ipratropium, nasal[a]	++	0	0	0	0
Antihistamines[b,c]	++	++	++	+	++
Pseudoephedrine, nasal[d]	0	0	0	++++	0
Cromolyn, nasal[c]	+	+	+	+	0
Leukotriene modifiers	+	0	0	++	++

Note: 0 = drug is not effective; the number of "+'s" grades the drug's effectiveness.
[a] Effective in seasonal, perennial, and vasomotor rhinitis.
[b] Better in seasonal than in perennial rhinitis; nasal, ocular, and oral forms; ocular form effective only for eye symptoms, and nasal form only for nasal symptoms.
[c] Start before allergy season.
[d] Topical therapy rapid in onset but results in rebound if used for more than a few days; enhances effectiveness of nasal steroids and sleep during severe attacks.

Table 85. Medications for Allergic Rhinitis or Conjunctivitis

Type, Medication	Geriatric Dosage	Formulations	Geriatric Half-life	Adverse Events/Comments
H₁-Receptor Antagonists or Antihistamines				Class adverse events: bitter taste, nasal burning, sneezing (nasal preparations), eye burning, stinging (ocular preparations)
✔Azelastine (*Astelin*)	2 spr q 12 h[a]	topical spr 0.1% (100 spr)	22–25 h	
(*Optivar*)	1 gtt OU q 6 h	ophthalmic 0.05%		
✔Cetirizine (*Zyrtec**)	5 mg/d (max)	T: 5, 10; syr 5 mg/5 mL	Prolonged	
✔Desloratadine (*Clarinex*)	5 mg/d	T: 5	27 h	
Emedastine (*Emadine*)	1 gtt OU q 6 h	0.05%		
Fexofenadine (✔*Allegra, Allegra-D*[b])	60 mg po q12 h; q 24 h if CrCl <40 mL/min	T: 30, 60, 180; C: 60	14 h	Least sedating in the class
Levocabastine (*Livostin*)	1 gtt OU q 6 h	0.05%		

* OTC

(cont.)

Table 85. Medications for Allergic Rhinitis or Conjunctivitis (cont.)

Type, Medication	Geriatric Dosage	Formulations	Geriatric Half-life	Adverse Events/Comments
Loratadine (✓ Claritin, Claritin-D,[b] generic*)	5–10 mg/d	T: 10; rapid-disintegrating tab 10 mg; syr 1 mg/mL	Metabolites >12 d; wide variation	
Chlorpheniramine (eg, ChlorTrimeton*)	8–12 mg q 12 h	T: 4, 8, 12; ChT: 2; CR: 8, 12; S: 2 mg/5 mL	20 h, longer with kidney dysfunction	Sedation, dry mouth, confusion, urinary retention; dries lung secretions
Diphenhydramine (eg, Benadryl*)	25–50 mg q 12 h	T: 25, 50; S: elixir 12.5 mg/mL	13.5 h	Same as chlorpheniramine
Hydroxyzine (eg, Atarax)	25–30 mg q 12 h	T: 10, 25, 50	30 h	Same as chlorpheniramine
Decongestant				
Pseudoephedrine (eg, Sudafed, combinations*)	60 mg po q 4–6 h	T: 30, 60; SR: 120; S: elixir 30 mg/5 mL	2–16 h; varies with urine pH	Arrhythmia, insomnia, anxiety, restlessness, elevated BP, urinary retention in men
Nasal Steroids Beclomethasone (eg, Beconase, Vancenase)	1 spr q 6–12 h[a]	topical spr 16 g (80 spr)	Rapid absorption, hepatic metabolism	Class adverse events: nasal burning, sneezing, bleeding; septal perforation (rare); fungal overgrowth (rare); no significant systemic effects
Budesonide (eg, Rhinocort)	2 spr q 12 h or 4 spr/d[a]	7 g (200 spr)		
Ciclesonide (Omnaris)	1–2 spr/d[a]	12.5 g (250 sgr)		
Dexamethasone (eg, Dexacort)	2 spr q 8–12 h[a]	25 mL (200 spr)		
Flunisolide (eg, Nasalide, Nasarel)	2–4 spr q 8–12 h[a]	25 mL (200 spr)		
Fluticasone (eg, Flonase)	2 spr/d[a]	16 g (120 spr)		
Mometasone (Nasonex)	2 spr/d[a]	17 g (120 spr)		
Triamcinolone (eg, Nasacort)	2–4 spr/d[a]	10 g (100 spr)		

* OTC

(cont.)

Table 85. Medications for Allergic Rhinitis or Conjunctivitis (cont.)

Type, Medication	Geriatric Dosage	Formulations	Geriatric Half-life	Adverse Events/Comments
Mast Cell Stabilizers				
Cromolyn (*NasalCrom*)	1 spr q 6–8 h;[a] begin 1–2 wk before exposure to allergen	2%, 4%		Nasal irritation, headache, itching of throat
Lodoxamide (*Alomide*)	1–2 gtt OU q 6 h	0.1%		Ocular irritation, burning, stinging
Nedocromil (*Alocril*)	1–2 gtt OU q 12 h	2%		Headache, ocular irritation, burning, stinging
Pemirolast (*Alamast*)	1–2 gtt OU q 6 h	0.1%		Headache, rhinitis, flu-like symptoms, ocular irritation, burning, stinging
Mast Cell Stabilizers and H₁ antagonists				
Ketotifen (*Zaditor*)	1 gtt OU q 8–12 h	0.025%		Conjunctival injection, headache, rhinitis, ocular irritation
Olopatadine (*Patanol*)	1 gtt OU q 12 h	0.1%		Cold syndrome, dysgeusia, headache, keratitis, ocular irritation
NSAID				
Ketorolac (*Acular*)	1 gtt OU q 6 h	0.5%		Ocular irritation, burning, stinging
Leukotriene Modifier (see also p 211)				
Montelukast (*Singulair*)	10 mg/d po	T: 10 mg; gran 4 mg/packet		Less effective than nasal steroids
Other				
Ipratropium (*Atrovent NS*)	2 spr q 6–12 h[a]	0.03, 0.06%[c] sol	1.6 h	Epistaxis, nasal irritation, upper respiratory infection; sore throat, nausea Caution: Do not spray in eyes.

✔ = preferred for treating older adults
[a] Spr per nares
[b] *Allegra-D* and *Claritin-D*, also available as *Allegra-D 24 Hour* and *Claritin-D 24 Hour*, are not recommended; all contain pseudoephedrine. Contraindicated in narrow angle glaucoma, urinary retention, MAOI use within 14 d, severe HTN, or CAD. May cause headache, nausea, insomnia.
[c] Use 0.06% for treatment of viral upper respiratory infection.

CHRONIC OBSTRUCTIVE PULMONARY DISEASE

Definition

A spectrum of chronic respiratory diseases characterized by:

- Airflow limitation
- Cough
- Dyspnea
- Frequent pulmonary infection
- Impaired gas exchange
- Sputum production

Therapy

Smoking Cessation: Essential at any age. See p 18.

Anxiety or Major Depression: Seen in up to 40% of patients and should be treated.

Nebulizers: Consider for patients with disabling or distressing breathlessness on maximal therapy with inhalers.

Mucolytic Therapy: Not recommended in stable COPD. Consider for patients with chronic productive cough; continue if reduced cough and sputum during a trial. Treatment with mucolytics is associated with a small reduction in acute exacerbations and a greater reduction in total number of days of disability. Example therapy: guiafenesin long-acting 600 mg po q 12 h

Rehabilitation: Patients at all stages benefit from exercise training, ie, increased exercise tolerance results in decreased dyspnea and fatigue (p 203).

Long-term Oxygen Therapy: For indications, see **Table 90**. Assess patients with FEV_1 <30%, cyanosis, edema, HF, resting O_2 sats ≤92%.

MDIs and Dry Powder Inhalers: Educate patients on use; dry powder inhalers should be used with an AeroChamber (requires separate prescription). Use a separate AeroChamber for inhaled steroids; wash AeroChamber monthly.

Stepped Approach: Add steps when symptoms inadequately controlled; D/C medication if no improvement. Assess improvement in symptoms, ADLs, exercise capacity, rapidity of symptom relief. See **Table 86** and **Table 89**.

Table 86. COPD Therapy

Stage	Treatment	
Mild COPD		
FEV_1 ≥80%	Short-acting β_2-agonist when needed	
Moderate COPD		
50% ≤FEV_1 <80%	Regular treatment with one or more bronchodilators[a] Rehabilitation	Long-acting bronchodilator if needed for added benefit or if ≥2 exacerbations/yr
Severe COPD		
30% ≤FEV_1 <50%	Regular treatment with one or more bronchodilators[a] Rehabilitation	Inhaled steroids[b] if significant symptoms and lung function response or if ≥2 exacerbations/yr
Very Severe COPD		
FEV_1 <30% or FEV_1 <50% plus chronic repiratory failure	Regular treatment with one or more bronchodilators[a] Inhaled steroids[b] if significant symptoms and lung function response or if repeated exacerbations Treatment of complications Long-term O_2 therapy if respiratory failure	

(cont.)

Table 86. COPD Therapy (cont.)	
Stage	**Treatment**
COPD Exacerbation	
(increased breathlessness, wheezing, cough, and sputum of acute onset and beyond normal day-to-day variation)	Increase dosage and/or frequency of B₂-agonists with or without anticholinergics
	Add steroid (eg, methylprednisolone 30–40 mg po q 24 h × 7–10 d)
	Add antibiotics if ↑ sputum with ↑ purulence or ↑ dyspnea (cover *Streptococcus pneumoniae, Haemophilus influenzae, Moraxella catarrhalis*)
	CBC, CXR, ECG, ABG; titrate O₂ to 90% sat and recheck ABG
	If 2 or more of severe dyspnea, respiratory rate ≥25, or PCO_2 45–60, then noninvasive positive-pressure ventilation reduces risk of ventilator use and mortality and length of hospital stay.

[a] β_2-agonists, ipratropium, slow-release theophylline (caution in older adults with other conditions and taking other medications).
[b] Consider osteoporosis prophylaxis.
Source: www.goldcopd.org

ASTHMA
Definition
Chronic inflammatory disorder of the airways; may be triggered by:
- Air pollution
- Allergens
- Chemicals
- Emotional distress
- Exercise
- Tobacco smoke
- Viruses

Characteristics
- Second peak in incidence after 65 yr; 5–10% after 65 yr are affected and account for 40% of asthma deaths.
- Cough is a common presentation, symptoms less variable and episodic than in younger people, more fixed obstruction as a chronic sequela.
- Symptoms include chest tightness, cough, shortness of breath, and wheezing.
- Symptoms may be confused with those of HF, COPD; PEF often not reliable.

Therapy
Nonpharmacologic
Avoid triggers; educate patients on disease management, use of MDIs and dry powder inhalers, and peak flow meters (document severity and response to therapy).
Pharmacologic
Stepped approach:
- Based on level of symptom control (see **Table 87**).
- When symptoms controlled for 3 mo, try stepwise reduction, eg, step down from twice-daily steroid to once daily plus long-acting, once-daily $\beta_2$agonist.
- If control not achieved, step up, but first review medication technique, adherence, and avoidance of triggers (see **Table 87** and **Table 88**).

MDIs should be used with an AeroChamber (requires separate prescription). Use separate AeroChamber for steroids; wash AeroChamber monthly.

Table 87. Levels of Asthma Control

Characteristic	Controlled (all of the following)	Partly Controlled (any measure present in any week)	Uncontrolled
Daytime symptoms	0–2 times/wk	>2 times/wk	
Limitations of activities	None	Any	Three or more features of partly controlled asthma present in any week
Nighttime symptoms/awakening	None	Any	
Need for reliever/rescue treatment	0–2 times/wk	>2 times/wk	
Lung function (PEF or FEV₁)	Normal	<80% predicted or personal best (if known)	
Exacerbations	None	≥1/yr[a]	One in any week[b]

[a] Any exacerbation should prompt review of maintenance treatment to ensure that it is adequate.
[b] By definition, an exacerbation in any week makes that an uncontrolled asthma week.
Source: www.ginasthma.com

Table 88. Asthma Therapy for Older Adults

Step*	Treatment Options	Comments
Step 1	Inhaled β-agonist prn	
Step 2	Low-dose inhaled glucocorticoid (IGC) *or* leukotriene modifier	Leukotriene modifiers have not been studied in older adults.
Step 3	Low-dose IGC + long-acting β-agonist *or* medium- to high-dose IGC *or* low-dose IGC + leukotriene modifier *or* low-dose IGC + SR-theophylline	Many older people have fixed obstruction, and ipratropium is helpful and well tolerated; many drug interactions with theophylline.
Step 4	**Add**: medium- to high-dose IGC + long-acting β-agonist *and/or* leukotriene modifier *and/or* SR-theophylline	Inhaled steroids are associated with bone loss.
Step 5	**Add**: oral glucocorticoid (lowest dose) and/or anti-IgE treatment	Oral steroids are associated with bone loss.

* Go to next step if symptoms not controlled.
Adapted from: www.ginasthma.com (2006); and NAEPP *Working Group Report: Considerations for Diagnosing and Managing Asthma in the Elderly*. National Heart, Lung and Blood Institute; Feb 1996. NIH Publication No. 96;3662.

Table 89. Asthma and COPD Medications

Packaging Color (Body/Cap)[a]	Dosage	Adverse Events (Metabolism, Excretion)
Anticholinergics		
✔ Ipratropium (*Atrovent*, generic) (silver/green)	2–6 puffs q 6 h or 0.5 mg by nebulizer q 6 h	Dry mouth, bitter taste (lung, poorly absorbed; F)
Tiotropium (*Spiriva*) (gray/green)	1 inhalation cap (18 mcg) daily	Same as ipratropium (14% K, 86% F)

(cont.)

Table 89. Asthma and COPD Medications (cont.)

Packaging Color (Body/Cap)[a]	Dosage	Adverse Events (Metabolism, Excretion)
Short-acting β₂-Agonists[b]		Class adverse events: tremor, nervousness, headache, palpitations, tachycardia, cough, hypokalemia. Caution: use half-doses in patients with known or suspected coronary disease (L)
✔ Albuterol (*Proventil, Ventolin*) (yellow/orange)	2–6 puffs q 4–6 h or 2.5 mg by nebulizer q 6 h; ER tabs 4–8 mg po q 12 h	Adverse events more common with oral formulation
(*Ventolin Rotacaps*) (light blue/dark blue)	1–2 caps q 4–6 h; dry powder inhaler 200 mcg/inhalation	
✔ Bitolterol (*Tornalate*)	1–3 puffs q 4–6 h	
Levalbuterol (*Xopenex*)	0.31, 0.63, 1.25 mg q 6–8 h by nebulizer; inhaler 2 puffs q 4–6 h	Expensive; no advantage over racemic albuterol (intestine, L)
Pirbuterol (*Maxair*) (blue/white)	2–3 puffs q 4–6 h	Mechanism may be difficult for older adults to trigger (L, K)
Long-acting β-Agonists Arformoterol (*Brovana*) ✔ Salmeterol (*Serevent Diskus*) (teal/light teal)	2 mL q 12 h by nebulizer 1 cap q 12 h; dry powdered inhaler 50 mcg/inhalation	Class adverse events: tremor, nervousness, headache, palpitations, tachycardia, cough, hypokalemia. Caution: use half-doses in patients with known or suspected coronary disease; not for acute exacerbation (L)
✔ Formoterol (*Foradil*) (white/light blue)	1 puff q 12 h; 20 mcg/2 mL q 12 h per nebulizer	Onset of action 1–3 min (L, K)
Corticosteroids: Inhaled ✔ Beclomethasone (*Beclovent*) (white/brown) (*Vanceril*) (pink/dark pink)	2–4 puffs q 6–12 h [42, 84 mcg/puff, max 840 mcg/d]	Class adverse events: nausea, vomiting, diarrhea, abdominal pain; oropharyngeal thrush; dosages >1 mg/d may cause adrenal suppression, reduce calcium absorption and bone density, and cause bruising (L)
✔ Budesonide (eg, *Pulmicort*) (white/brown)	1–2 puffs q 6–12 h [100, 200, 400 mcg/puff]	
✔ Dexamethasone (eg, *Dexacort*)	3 puffs q 6–8 h [100 mcg/puff]	
✔ Flunisolide (eg, *AeroBid*) (gray/purple or green)	2–4 puffs q 12 h [250 mcg/puff]	
✔ Fluticasone (eg, *Flovent*) (orange/light orange)	1 puff q 12 h [44, 110, 220 mcg/puff]	
Mometasone (*Asmanex*)	1 inhalation/d [220 mcg]	
✔ Triamcinolone (eg, *Azmacort*) (white/white)	2 puffs q 6–8 h or 4 puffs q 12 h [100 mcg/puff]	

(cont.)

Table 89. **Asthma and COPD Medications** (cont.)

Packaging Color (Body/Cap)[a]	Dosage	Adverse Events (Metabolism, Excretion)
Corticosteroids: Oral		
Prednisone (eg, *Deltasone, Orasone*)	20 mg po q 12 h [T: 1, 2.5, 5, 10, 20, 50; elixir 5 mg/5 mL]	Leukocytosis, thrombocytosis, sodium retention, euphoria, depression, hallucination, cognitive dysfunction; other effects with long-term use (L)
Methylxanthines Long-acting theophyllines (eg, *Quibron-T/SR*)	300–400 mg/d [T: 300 bisect, trisect tabs]	Class adverse events: atrial arrhythmias, seizures, increased gastric acid secretion, ulcer, reflux, diuresis; clearance ↓ by 30% after 65 yr; initial dosage ≤400 mg/d, titrate using blood levels (L)
(eg, *Theo-Dur, Slo-Bid*)	100–200 mg po q 12 h [T: 100, 200, 300, 450]	
(eg, *Uniphyl, Theo-24*)	400 mg/d po [T: 100, 200, 300, 400]	
Leukotriene Modifiers Montelukast (*Singulair*)	10 mg po in AM [T: 10; ChT: 4, 5]	Headache, drowsiness, fatigue, dyspepsia; minimal data in older adults; leukotriene-receptor antagonist (L)
Zafirlukast (*Accolate*)	20 mg po q 12 h 1 h before or 2 h after meals [T: 10, 20]	Headache, somnolence, dizziness, nausea, diarrhea, abdominal pain, fever; monitor LFTs; monitor coumarin anticoagulants; leukotriene-receptor antagonist (L, reduced by 50% if >65 yr)
Zileuton (*Zyflo*)	600 mg po q 6 h [T: 600]	Dizziness, insomnia, nausea, abdominal pain, abnormal LFTs, myalgia; monitor coumarin anticoagulants; other drug interactions; inhibits synthesis of leukotrienes (L)
Other Medications ✔ Albuterol-Ipratropium (*Combivent*) (silver/orange)	0.09/0.018 mg/puff, 2-3 puffs q 6 h; 3 mg/0.5 mg by nebulizer q 6 h	Same as individual agents (L, K)
Budesonide-Formoterol (*Symbicort*) (red/gray)	2 puffs q 12 h (80 mcg/4.5 mcg or 160 mcg/4.5 mcg)	Same as individual agents (L, K)
Cromolyn sodium (eg, *Intal*) (white/blue)	2–4 puffs or 20-mg caps q 6 h	Because of propellant, use MDI with caution in coronary disease or arrhythmia (L, K)

(cont.)

Table 89. Asthma and COPD Medications (cont.)

Packaging Color (Body/Cap)[a]	Dosage	Adverse Events (Metabolism, Excretion)
Nedocromil (*Tilade*) (white/white)	2 puffs q 6 h	Bitter taste, headache, dizziness, sore throat, cough, chest tightness (K, F)
Omalizumab (*Xolair*)	150–375 mg SC q 2–4 wk based on body weight and pretreatment IgE level	Malignancy, anaphylaxis; half-life 26 d (L, bile); expensive (6,000–$25,000/yr)
✔Salmeterol-Fluticasone combination (*Advair Diskus*) (purple/light purple)	1 puff q 12 h (50 mcg/100, 250, or 500 mcg/inhalation)	

✔ = preferred for treating older adults
[a] Generics may have different color on body and cap.
[b] Older nonselective β_2-agonists such as isoproterenol, metoproterenol, or epinephrine are not recommended and are more toxic.

Table 90. Indications for Long-term Oxygen Therapy[a]

PaO₂ Level	SaO₂ Level	Other
≤55 mmHg	≤88%	>15 h/d for benefit[a], greater if 20 h/d[b]
55–59 mmHg	≥89%	Signs of tissue hypoxia (eg, cor pulmonale by ECG, HF, hematocrit >55%); or nocturnal desaturation, sats <90% for >30% of the time
≥60 mmHg	≥90%	Desaturation with exercise Desaturation with sleep apnea not corrected by CPAP

[a] Titrate O_2 saturation to approximately 90%.
[b] Improves survival, hemodynamics, polycythemia, exercise capacity, lung mechanics, and cognition.
Source: www.goldcopd.org

PULMONARY EMBOLISM (PE)

Prevalence triples between 65–90 yr; age >70 yr associated with missed antemortem diagnosis.

Symptoms

Classic triad—dyspnea, chest pain, hemoptysis—seen in ≤20% of cases.
Consider PE with any of the following:

- Chest pain
- Hemoptysis
- Hypotension
- Hypoxia
- Shortness of breath
- Syncope
- Tachycardia

Diagnosis

Calculate clinical probability of PE using clinical decision rule (**Table 91**), then follow evaluation of PE algorithm (**Figure 9**). Clinical probability of PE unlikely: total ≤4 points; clinical probability of PE likely: total >4 points.

Table 91. Clinical Decision Rule

Variable	Points
Clinical signs and symptoms of DVT (minimal leg swelling and pain with palpation of the deep veins)	3
Alternative diagnosis less likely than PE	3
Heart rate >100/min	1.5
Immobilization (>3 d) or surgery in the previous 4 wk	1.5
Previous PE or DVT	1.5
Hemoptysis	1
Malignancy (receiving treatment, treated in last 6 mo, or palliative)	1
Total	

Source: Wells PS, Anderson DR, Rodger M, et al. Derivation of a simple clinical model to categorize patients' probability of pulmonary embolism: increasing the model's utility with the SimpliRED D-dimer. *Thromb Haemost* 2000;83(3):416–420. Reprinted with permission.

Figure 9. Evaluation of Suspected Pulmonary Embolism

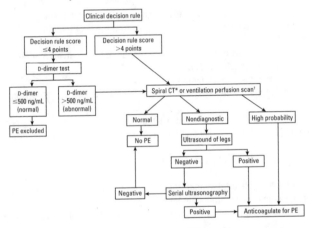

* Multidetector-row CT more sensitive than single-detector CT. Patient must be able to hold breath for 10 sec.
† When unable to use contrast (eg, renal dysfunction), need to avoid ionizing radiation.

Pharmacologic Therapy
- Low-molecular-weight heparin (LMWH) (see **Table 12**) is preferred to unfractionated heparin (UFH) in most patients due to lower risk of hemorrhage and mortality. Reduce dose when CrCl <30 mL/min.
- Warfarin may be started on the same day as heparin (see p 21 and **Table 10**)
- Continue heparin for at least 5 d and 1–3 d after INR is therapeutic.
- Acute massive PE (filling defects in 2 or more lobar arteries, or the equivalent, by angiogram) associated with hypotension or severe hypoxia or high pulmonary pressures on echocardiogram should usually be treated with thrombolytic therapy within 48 h of onset (see **Table 12**).

SEXUAL DYSFUNCTION

IMPOTENCE (ERECTILE DYSFUNCTION)

Definition
Inability to achieve sufficient erection for intercourse. Prevalence nearly 70% by age 70.

Causes
Often multifactorial; >50% of cases arterial, venous, or mixed vascular cause. Also:
- Chronic high-dose opioids
- Diabetes mellitus
- Drug adverse events
- Hyperprolactinemia
- Hypogonadism
- Neurologic: eg, disorders of the CNS, spinal cord, or PNS; autonomic neuropathy; temporal lobe epilepsy
- Psychologic: eg, depression, anxiety, bereavement
- Thyroid or adrenal disorders

Low testosterone is associated more with decreased libido than with erectile dysfunction.

Evaluation
History: Type and duration of problem; relation to surgery, trauma, medication. Problems with orgasm, libido, or penile detumescence are not erectile dysfunction.

Physical Findings:
- Neuropathy: orthostatic hypotension, impaired response to Valsalva's maneuver, absent bulbocavernosus or cremasteric reflexes
- Peyronie's disease: penile bands, plaques
- Hypogonadism: diminished male pattern hair, gynecomastia, small (<20–25 mm long) testes

Assessment:
- Reduced penile-to-brachial pressure index suggests vascular disease.
- Cavernosometry used for diagnosing venous leak syndrome; reserved for surgical candidates.
- Test dose of prostaglandin E or papaverine can exclude vascular disease or confirm venous leak syndrome.
- For libido problems check total testosterone, luteinizing hormone, TSH, and prolactin. Most late-life hypogonadism is hypothalamic failure.
- Diagnose testosterone deficiency only in men with consistent symptoms and unequivocally low testosterone levels.
- Morning total testosterone level <300 ng/dL that remains <300 ng/dL on repeat testing using a reliable assay such as LC-MS/MS suggests deficiency.
- Because sex hormone binding globulin increases with age, bioavailable testosterone should be a better test in older men. If total testosterone <300 ng/dL, can use free or bioavailable testosterone as the second confirming test if a reliable assay is used.

Therapy

Table 92. Management of Male Sexual Dysfunction

Cause	Therapy	Comments
Hypogonadism, poor libido	Testosterone: scrotal transdermal (*Testoderm*) [4, 5, 6] 4–6 mg/d; *or* skin transdermal (*Androderm*) [2.5, 5] 5 mg/d; *or* testosterone cypionate or enanthate 200 mg IM q 2–4 wk; *or* testosterone gel 1% (*AndroGel*) [5 g (50 mg/24 h), 7.5 g (75 mg), 10 g (100 mg)] begin with 5-g pk qam; (*Testim*) [5 g (50 mg/24 h)] begin with 5-g pk qam	Not recommended with breast or prostate cancer, prostate nodule or induration or PSA >3 ng/dL, hematocrit >50%, untreated sleep apnea, HF, significant prostate obstructive symptoms. Probably effective in the treatment of opioid-induced androgen deficiency. Check serum testosterone concentration and adjust dose to achieve concentration in midrange of normal. Monitor adverse events and response q 3 mo. Adverse events: polycythemia, fluid retention, liver dysfunction. Review cautions for individual preparations.
Neuropathic, vascular, or mixed	Vacuum tumescence devices (*Osbon-Erec Aid, Catalyst Vacuum Device, Pos-T-Vac, Rejoyn*)	Rare: ecchymosis, reduced ejaculation, coolness of penile tip. Good acceptance in older population; intercourse successful in 70%–90% of cases.
	Intracavernosal [5, 10, 20, 40 mcg] *or* intraurethral [125, 250, 500, 1000 mcg] prostaglandin E (*Alprostadil*)	Risks: hypotension, bruising, bleeding, priapism; erection >4 h requires emergency treatment; intraurethral safer and more acceptable.
	Penile prosthesis	Complications: infection, mechanical failure, penile fibrosis
Organic, psychogenic, or mixed	PDE5 inhibitors	All agents: contraindicated with use of nitrates; caution in vascular disease, least effective in vascular impotence. Caution with use of α-blockers; hypotension may occur with higher dosages of PDE5 inhibitors. Metabolism reduced in liver, kidney disease. Adverse events: headache, flushing, dyspepsia, dizziness, rhinitis. Nonarteritic ischemic optic neuropathy has been reported, but cause and effect have not been proved.
	Sildenafil (*Viagra*) [25, 50, 100]: start 25 mg 1 h before sexual activity	Other adverse events: color tinge in vision, increased sensitivity to light, blurred vision
	Vardenafil (*LEVITRA*) [2.5, 5, 10, 20]: start 2.5 mg 1 h before sexual activity	Caution with CYP3A4 inhibitors. Avoid using in congenital or acquired QT prolongation and in patients taking class IA or III antiarrhythmics.
	Tadalafil (*Cialis*) [5, 10, 20]: start 5 mg 30–60 min before sexual activity; lasts 24 h	Caution with CYP3A4 inhibitors. Other adverse events: back pain, myalgia, pain in limbs

DYSPAREUNIA

Definition
Pain with intercourse

Aggravating Factors
- Gynecologic tumors
- Interstitial cystitis
- Myalgia from overexertion during Kegel's exercises
- Osteoarthritis
- Pelvic fractures
- Retroverted uterus
- Sacral nerve root compression
- Vaginal atrophy from estrogen deprivation
- Vulvar or vaginal infection

Evaluation
- Ask about sexual problems (eg, changes in libido, partner's function, and health issues).
- Screen for depression.
- Perform pelvic examination for vulvovaginitis, vaginal atrophy, conization (decreased distensibility and narrowing of the vaginal canal), scarring, pelvic inflammatory disease, cystocele, and rectocele.

Management
- Identify and treat clinical pathology.
- Educate and counsel patients.
- Water-soluble lubricants (eg, *Replens*) are highly effective as monotherapy for those who cannot or will not use hormones, or as a supplement to estrogen.
- For vaginismus (vaginal muscle spasm), trial cessation of intercourse and gradual vaginal dilation may help.
- For diminished libido, short-term use of androgens (which used long-term adversely affect health) may help; refer for counseling or sex therapy.
- Topical estrogens (**Table 93**) treat symptoms and complications of estrogen deficiency such as dyspareunia and recurrent urinary tract infections with minimal systemic absorption.

Table 93. Topical Estrogens Without Systemic Effects

Estrogen	Dosage
Estrogen cream (*Premarin, Ogen, Estrace*)	Use min dose (0.5 g for *Premarin*, 2 g for *Ogen* and *Estrace*) daily × 2 wk, then 1–3 times/wk thereafter
Estradiol vaginal ring (*Estring*)	Insert intravaginally and change q 90 d
Estradiol vaginal tablets (*Vagifem*)	Insert 25 mcg intravaginally daily × 2 wk, then twice/wk

SSRI-INDUCED SEXUAL DYSFUNCTION
- Incidence varies widely, from 1% to 20% of patients making spontaneous reports to 75% when patients are systematically questioned.
- Symptoms include anorgasmia, decreased libido, and ejaculatory dysfunction.
- Wait for tolerance to develop (12 wk of treatment may be needed).
- Pharmacologic management:
  - For sertraline and citalopram (not other SSRIs), reducing dosage or "drug holidays" (skip or reduce weekend dose) may help.
  - Adjuvant medications reported as effective in case reports include PDE5 inhibitors 1 h before intercourse
  - Controlled trials of mirtazapine, yohimbine, olanzapine, and bupropion did not show a benefit different from that of placebo, although most trials were small.

CHRONIC WOUND ASSESSMENT AND TREATMENT

Wound Assessment

Evaluation of chronic wounds should include the following (see **Table 94** for wound characteristics specific to ulcer type):

- Location
- Wound size and shape: length, width, depth, stage (pressure ulcer), grade (diabetic foot ulcer)
- Wound bed: color, presence of slough, necrotic tissue, granulation tissue, epithelial tissue, undermining or tunneling
- Exudate: purulent versus nonpurulent (serous, serosanguineous)
- Wound edges: distinct, diffuse, rolled under
- Periwound surface: erythema, edema, induration, temperature
- Presence of pain
- Signs of wound infection
  - Increased necrotic tissue
  - Foul odor of exudates
  - Purulent exudates
  - Faint halo of erythema at wound edges
  - Wound breakdown
  - Increasing pain
  - Edema
  - Granulation tissue that bleeds easily
  - Serous exudates with inflammation
  - Nonhealing or enlarging wound
- Swab culture is of limited value in diagnosing infection due to contaminated wound bed.

Wound Treatment

- Remove debris from wound surface
  - Cleanse with normal saline
  - Avoid antiseptics because of cytotoxicity
  - Irrigate with 4–15 psi to cleanse adherent debris
- Remove necrotic tissue; more than one method may be indicated.
  - Sharp debridement
  - Autolytic methods (eg, moisture-retaining dressings or hydrogels)
  - Mechanical (eg, wet-to-dry dressings)
  - Chemical (eg, topical enzymes such as *Accuzyme, Santyl*)
- Control bacterial burden/infection
  - Monitor for signs of infection
  - Debride all necrotic tissue (*except* when wound is ischemic)
  - If infection suspected in debrided ulcer (absence of contraction and epithelialization from wound edge within 2 wk of debridement and pressure relief), obtain tissue biopsy or validated quantitative swab to determine type and level of infection.
  - For ulcers with ≥ 1 million CFU/g of tissue or any tissue level of β-hemolytic streptococci, use a topical antimicrobial (eg, *Silvadene* or silver-containing dressing). Limit duration of use of topical antimicrobials to avoid cytotoxicity or bacterial resistance.
  - Use systemic antibiotics only in presence of spreading cellulitis, sepsis, or osteomyelitis
- Provide moist wound environment and control exudates
  - Dressings (see **Table 95** and **Table 96**)
- Adjunctive therapies to support wound healing process
  - Negative-pressure wound therapy (ie, vacuum-assisted closure [*VAC*])

- Indications: Stage III and IV pressure ulcers, neuropathic ulcers, venous ulcers, dehisced incisions with trapping of third-space fluid around wound
- Contraindications: Presence of *any* nonviable, necrotic tissue in wound; untreated osteomyelitis; malignancy in or surrounding wound
- Precautions: unstable hemostasis, anticoagulant therapy
- Guidelines for use:
  - Negative pressure = 75–125 mm Hg depending on wound characteristics
  - Dressing change regimen: 48 hr after placement, then every other day
  - Cycle: continuous for initial 48 hr, then intermittent (5 min negative pressure followed by 2 min of no pressure) for remainder of treatment
  - Specialized training in application and monitoring of therapy essential to successful outcome
- Electrical stimulation
  - Indications: Stage III and IV pressure ulcers, arterial ulcers, diabetic foot ulcers, and venous ulcers if no evidence of measurable improvement after ≥30 d of standard wound care
  - Contraindications: presence of cardiac pacemaker, malignancy, osteomyelitis
  - Precautions: avoid placement of electrodes over topical substances containing metal ions, tangential to the heart, or over the carotid sinus
  - Guidelines for use:
    - Predominant type of current used is pulsed current (either low- or high-voltage)
    - Electrode placement—two options:
      - One electrode placed directly in contact with saline-moistened gauze on wound surface and second electrode 15–30 cm from wound edge
      - Electrodes placed on skin at wound edges on opposite sides of wound
    - Pulse frequency: 100 pulses/sec with current sufficient to produce tingling sensation
    - Treatment administered for 1 h, 5–7 days/wk, continued as long as wound is progressing toward closure
- Prevent further injury
  - Use pressure-reducing mattresses and chair cushions
  - Position patient to avoid any pressure on the wound
- Support repair process
  - Protein (1.25–1.5 g/kg/d) and calories (30–35/kg/d)
  - Vitamin and mineral supplements if deficiencies suspected
  - Avoid exposure to cold; vasoconstriction reduces blood flow to wound

Table 94. Wound Characteristics by Ulcer Type

	Arterial	Diabetic	Pressure	Venous
Location	Tips of toes or between toes, on pressure points of foot (eg, heel or lateral foot), or in areas of trauma	Plantar surface of foot, especially over metatarsal heads, toes, and heel	Over bony prominences (eg, trochanter, coccyx, ankle)	Gaiter area, particularly medial malleolus
Size and shape	Small craters with well-defined borders	Even wound margins with callus	Variable length, width, depth depending on stage (see staging system, p 223)	Edges may be irregular with depth limited to dermis or shallow subcutaneous tissue
Wound bed	Pale or necrotic	Granular tissue unless PAD present	Varies from bright red, shallow crater to deeper crater with slough and necrotic tissue; tunneling and undermining	Ruddy red; yellow slough may be present; undermining or tunneling uncommon
Exudate	Minimal amount due to poor blood flow	Variable amount; serous unless infection present	Purulent, becoming serous as healing progresses; foul odor with infection	Copious; serous unless infection present
Surrounding skin	Halo of erythema or slight fluctuance indicates infection	Normal	May be distinct, diffuse, rolled under; erythema, edema, induration if infected	May appear macerated, crusted, or scaly
Pain	Cramping or constant deep aching	None, because of neuropathy	Painful, unless sensory function impaired	Variable; may be severe, dull, aching, or bursting in character

ARTERIAL ULCERS
Definition
Any lesion caused by severe tissue ischemia secondary to atherosclerosis and progressive arterial occlusion.

Management (see also PAD, p 47, and Diabetes, p 76)
Protect from Injury
• Avoid friction and pressure by using lamb's wool or foam between toes
• Use positioning devices to avoid pressure on feet (eg, heel protectors)
Wound Assessment
• See Chronic Wound Assessment (p 217).
• Assess ankle-brachial index (ABI): If ABI <0.5, wound healing unlikely without revascularization.
Local Wound Care
Treatment dictated by adequacy of perfusion and status of wound bed:
• Avoid debridement of necrotic tissue until perfusion status is determined.

- If wound is infected, revascularization procedures, surgical removal of necrotic tissue, and systemic antibiotics are treatments of choice.
- Topical antibiotics should not be used solely to treat infected ischemic wounds and may cause sensitivity reactions.
- If wound is uninfected and dry eschar is present, maintain dry intact eschar as a barrier to bacteria. Application of an antiseptic may decrease bacterial burden on wound surface.
- If wound is uninfected and soft slough and necrotic tissue are present, apply moisture-retaining dressings that allow frequent inspection of wound for signs of infection.
- Assess vascular perfusion and refer for surgical intervention if consistent with overall goals of care.

DIABETIC FOOT ULCERS
Definition
Any lesion on the plantar surface of the foot caused by neuropathy and repetitive pressure on foot.

Management (see also Diabetes, p 76)
Wound Assessment
- See Chronic Wound Assessment (p 217).
- Assess for specific diabetes-related signs of infection:
  - Sudden increase in blood glucose
  - Wound can be probed to the bone—highly sensitive indicator of osteomyelitis
  - Exclude gross arterial disease by assessment for palpable pedal pulses, toe:brachial index >0.7 (or ankle:brachial index >0.9), a transcutaneous oxygen pressure of >30 mmHg, or normal Doppler-derived wave form.
- Determine grade of ulcer (Wagner Classification)
  - Grade 0: Preulcerative lesions; healed ulcers present; bony deformity present
  - Grade 1: Superficial ulcer without subcutaneous tissue involvement
  - Grade 2: Penetration through subcutaneous tissue
  - Grade 3: Osteitis, abscess, or osteomyelitis
  - Grade 4: Gangrene of digit
  - Grade 5: Gangrene of foot requiring disarticulation

Local Wound Care
In addition to recommendations under Chronic Wound Treatment (see p 217):
- Debride devitalized tissue and callus: surgical debridement is method of choice for effective, rapid removal of nonviable tissue
- Avoid occlusive dressings to reduce risk of wound infection
- Offload pressure and stress from foot
  - Avoidance of pressure on foot essential to management of diabetic foot ulcer
  - Use orthotic that redistributes weight on plantar surface of foot when ambulating (eg, total contact cast, *DH Pressure Relief Walker*)
- If ulcer does not reduce in size by ≥50% after 4 wk of therapy, reassess treatment and consider alternative options (eg, negative-pressure wound therapy, growth factor therapy, hyperbaric oxygen therapy).

Growth Factor Therapy

Regranex, a recombinant platelet-derived growth factor, applied topically in thin layer to a clean wound bed for 12 h followed by 12 h of saline-moistened gauze dressing:

- Must be used in conjunction with offloading of pressure on foot, regular sharp debridement, and maintenance of uninfected status.
- If wound closure is not ≥30% in 10 wk or complete in 20 wk, reevaluate treatment plan and consider surgical intervention (especially if osteomyelitis is present).

Assessment and Treatment of Infection

- If infection is suspected, assess type and quantity of bacteria by validated quantitative swab or tissue biopsy. Suspect infection if epithelialization from margin is not progressing within 2 wk of debridement and initiation of offloading (use of cast, splint, or special shoe to shift pressure from wound to surrounding support structure).
- Use topical antimicrobial agent to treat a high bacterial level confined to granulating tissue (systemic antibiotics ineffective in granulating wounds). D/C once bacterial level has decreased (confirmed by culture or clinical evidence of epithelialization progressing) to minimize risk of bacterial resistance.
- Use systemic antibiotics to treat acute diabetic foot infections not limited to granulating tissue.
- Treat cellulitis surrounding ulcer with a systemic gram-positive bactericidal antibiotic (see cellulitis, p 67).
- If osteomyelitis is suspected, evaluate with radiographs, MRI, CT, or radionuclide scan.
- Referral for surgical evaluation is warranted.
- Optimize blood glucose control.

PRESSURE ULCERS

Definition

Any lesion caused by unrelieved pressure resulting in damage of underlying tissue; usually develops over bony prominence.

Table 95. Wound and Pressure Ulcer Products, by Drainage and Stage

Product	Drainage			Wound Stage			
	Light	Moderate	Heavy	I	II	III	IV
Transparent film	•			•	•		
Foam island	•	•			•	•	
Hydrocolloids	•	•			•	•	
Petroleum-based nonadherent	•				•	•	
Alginate		•	•			•	•
Hydrogel	•				•	•	•
Gauze packing (moistened with saline)		•	•			•	•

Table 96. Common Dressings for Pressure Ulcer Treatment

Dressing	Indications/Use	Contraindications
Transparent film (eg, *Bioclusive*, *Tegaderm*, *Op-site*)	Stage I, II Protection from friction Superficial scrape Autolytic debridement of slough Apply skin prep to intact skin to protect from adhesive	Draining ulcers Suspicion of skin infection or fungus
Foam island (eg, *Allevyn*, *Lyofoam*)	Stage II, III Low to moderate exudate Can apply as window to secure transparent film	Excessive exudate Dry, crusted wound
Hydrocolloids (eg, *DuoDERM*, *Extra thin film DuoDERM*, *Tegasorb*, *RepliCare*, *Comfeel*, *Nu-derm*)	Stage II, III Low to moderate drainage Good periwound skin integrity Autolytic debridement of slough Leave in place 3–5 d Can apply as window to secure transparent film Can apply over alginate to control drainage Must control maceration Apply skin prep to intact skin to protect from adhesive	Poor skin integrity Infected ulcers Wound needs packing
Alginate (eg, *Sorbsan*, *Kaltostat*, *Algosteril*, *AlgiDERM*)	Stage III, IV Excessive drainage Apply dressing within wound borders Requires secondary dressing Must use skin prep Must control maceration	Dry or minimally draining wound Superficial wounds with maceration
Hydrogel (amorphous gels) (eg, *IntraSite gel*, *SoloSite gel*, *Restore gel*)	Stage II, III, IV Needs to be combined with gauze dressing Stays moist longer than saline gauze Changed 1–2 times/d Used as alternative to saline gauze for packing deep wounds with tunnels, undermining Reduces adherence of gauze to wound Must control maceration	Macerated areas Wounds with excess exudate
(gel sheet) (eg, *Vigilon*, *Restore Impregnated Gauze*)	Stage II Needs to be held in place with topper dressing	Macerated areas Wounds with moderate to heavy exudate

(cont.)

Table 96. Common Dressings for Pressure Ulcer Treatment (cont.)

Dressing	Indications/Use	Contraindications
Gauze packing (moistened with saline) (eg, square 2 × 2s/ 4 × 4s, *Fluffed Kerlix, Plain NuGauze*)	Stage III, IV Wounds with depth, especially those with tunnels, undermining Must be remoistened often to maintain moist wound environment	
Silver dressings (silver with alginates, gels, charcoal) (eg, *Silvercel, Silvadene, Aquacel Ag, Acticoat*)	Malodorous wounds High level of exudates Wound highly suspicious for critical bacterial load Periwound with signs of inflammation Slow-healing wound	Systemic infection Cellulitis Signs of systemic side effects, especially erythema multiforme Fungal proliferation Sensitivity of skin to sun Interstitial nephritis Leukopenia Skin necrosis Concurrent use with proteolytic enzymes

Source: Copyright © 2008 by Rita Frantz. Used with permission.

Management
Wound Assessment
- See Chronic Wound Assessment (see p 217).
- Determine level of tissue injury by using Pressure Ulcer Staging System:
  - **Stage I:** An observable pressure-related alteration of intact skin that, as compared with an adjacent or opposite area on the body, may include changes in one or more of the following: skin temperature (warmth or coolness), tissue consistency (firm or boggy feel), and/or sensation (pain, itching). The ulcer appears as a defined area of persistent redness in lightly pigmented skin, whereas in darker skin tones, it may appear with persistent red, blue, or purple hues.
  - **Stage II:** Partial-thickness skin loss involving epidermis and/or dermis; presents as abrasion, blister, or shallow crater.
  - **Stage III:** Full-thickness skin loss involving damage or necrosis of subcutaneous tissue that may extend down to, but not through, underlying fascia; presents as deep crater with or without undermining of adjacent tissue.
  - **Stage IV:** Full-thickness skin loss with extensive destruction; tissue necrosis; or damage to muscle, bone, or supporting structures. May have associated undermining of sinus tracts. *Note:* eschar-covered ulcers cannot be staged until eschar is removed.

Local Wound Care
In addition to recommendations under Chronic Wound Treatment (see p 217):
- Consider combining autolytic or typical enzyme debridement methods with sharp debridement to facilitate more rapid removal of necrotic tissue.
- Cleanse using normal saline with each dressing change. Irrigate using 8 mmHg pressure (19-gauge catheter and 35-mL syringe) when wound is deep, tunneled, or undermined.

- Pack dead space (tunnels, undermining) with moistened gauze dressings or strips of calcium alginate.
- If ulcer does not show signs of healing over 2-wk period of optimal therapy, reevaluate wound management strategies and factors affecting healing.

Protect Wound from Pressure/Trauma
- Avoid positioning directly on ulcer.
- Use pressure-reduction strategies:
  - Reposition q 2 h.
  - Use pressure-reducing cushions, mattresses, and heel protectors.

Treatment of Infection
- Ensure that necrotic tissue has been debrided completely from wound bed.
- Consider 2-wk trial of topical antibiotic for clean ulcers that are not healing after 2–4 wk optimal care; antibiotic spectrum should include gram-negative, gram-positive, and anaerobic organisms.
- Avoid using systemic antibiotics in the absence of advancing cellulitis or systemic infection.

Support Healing Systemically
- Provide nutritional support (see p 140).
- Provide adequate hydration with oral or parenteral fluids.

Surgical Repair
Surgical referral is warranted for Stage IV pressure ulcers and for severely undermined or tunneled wounds.

VENOUS ULCERS
Definition
Any lesion caused by venous insufficiency precipitated by venous hypertension

Management
Wound Assessment
- See Chronic Wound Assessment (see p 217).
- Assess lower-extremity edema.

Compression Therapy
- Essential component of venous ulcer treatment
- Provides externally applied pressure to lower extremity to facilitate normal venous return
- Therapeutic level of compression is 30–40 mmHg at ankle, decreasing toward knee
- Avoid compression therapy when ABI ≥0.8
- Types of compression therapy:
  - Static compression device
    - Layered compression wraps (*Profore, ProGuide, Dynapress*)
    - Short-stretch wraps (*Comprilan*)
    - Paste-containing bandages (*Unna's boot, Duke boot*)
      - Preferable for actively ambulating patient; support compression of calf muscle "pump"
  - Dynamic compression devices (indicated when static compression not feasible)
    - Pneumatic compression device (intermittent pneumatic pumps)
    - Powered devices that propel venous blood upward when applied to lower leg

◦ Compression therapy for long-term maintenance

▪ Therapeutic compression stockings (*Jobst, Juzo, Sig-Varis, Medi-Strumpf, Therapress Duo*)

Local Wound Care

In addition to recommendations under Chronic Wound Treatment (see p 217):

- Use exudate-absorbing dressings (eg, calcium alginate dressings, foam dressings)
- Use skin sealant to protect skin around wound from exudates
- Infected venous ulcers should be treated with systemic antibiotics because of development of resistant organisms with topical antibiotics.
- Monitor healing progress; if no signs of healing over 2-wk period, reevaluate wound management strategies and factors affecting healing.

Surgical Intervention

If manifestations of chronic venous insufficiency and ulceration are resistant to more conservative therapies or if venous obstruction is present, surgical repair (eg, skin graft) is treatment of choice.

CLASSIFICATION
- Disturbance of the sleep-wake cycle
- Hypersomnolence
- Insomnia (difficulty initiating or maintaining sleep)
- Parasomnias (disorders of arousal, partial arousal, and sleep stage transition)
- Sleep apnea

SLEEP DISORDERS OTHER THAN SLEEP APNEA
Risk Factors and Aggravating Factors
Treatable Associated Medical and Psychiatric Conditions: adjustment disorders, anxiety, bereavement, cough, depression, dyspnea (cardiac or pulmonary), GERD, nocturia, pain, paresthesias, stress

Medications That Cause or Aggravate Sleep Problems: alcohol, antidepressants, β-blockers, bronchodilators, caffeine, clonidine, cortisone, diuretics, levodopa, methyldopa, nicotine, phenytoin, progesterone, quinidine, reserpine, sedatives, sympathomimetics including decongestants

Management
Sleep improvements are better sustained over time with behavioral treatment.
Nonpharmacologic
- Stimulus control

  Measures recommended to improve sleep hygiene:
  - During the daytime:
    - Get out of bed at the same time each morning regardless of how much you slept the night before.
    - Exercise daily but not immediately before bedtime.
    - Get adequate exposure to bright light during the day.
    - Decrease or eliminate naps, unless necessary part of sleeping schedule.
    - Limit or eliminate alcohol, caffeine, and nicotine, especially before bedtime.
  - At bedtime:
    - Maintain a regular sleeping time, but don't go to bed unless sleepy.
    - If hungry, have a light snack before bed (unless there are symptoms of GERD or it is otherwise medically contraindicated), but avoid heavy meals at bedtime.
    - Don't read or watch television in bed.
    - Relax mentally before going to sleep; don't use bedtime as worry time.
    - Relax before bedtime, and maintain a routine period of preparation for bed (eg, washing up and going to the bathroom).
    - Control nighttime environment, ie, comfortable temperature, quiet, dark.
    - Wear comfortable bedclothes.
    - If it helps, use soothing noise, eg, a fan or other appliance or a "white noise" machine.
    - If unable to fall asleep within 15–20 min, get out of bed and perform soothing activity, such as listening to soft music or reading (but avoid exposure to bright light).

- Cognitive-behavioral therapy
- Sleep restriction: reduce time in bed to estimated total sleep time (min 5 h) and increase by 15 min/wk when ratio of time asleep to time in bed is ≥90%.
- Relaxation techniques—physical (progressive muscle relaxation, biofeedback); mental (imagery training, meditation, hypnosis)
- Bright light: 2,500 lux for 2 h/d to 10,000 lux for 30 min/d

Pharmacologic—Principles of Prescribing Medications for Sleep Disorders:
- Use lowest effective dose.
- Use intermittent dosing (2–4 times/wk).
- Prescribe medications for short-term use (no more than 3–4 wk).
- Discontinue medication gradually.
- Be alert for rebound insomnia after discontinuation.

Table 97. Useful Medications for Sleep Disorders in Older Adults

Class, Medication	Usual Dose	Formulations	Half-life	Comments (Metabolism, Excretion)
Antidepressant, sedating				
✔ Trazodone (*Desyrel*)	25–150 mg	T: 50, 100, 150, 300	12 h	Moderate orthostatic effects; effective for insomnia with or without depression (L)
Mirtazapine (*Remeron*)	7.5–15 mg	T: 15, 30, 45	31–39 h	May increase appetite, daytime carry over
Benzodiazepine, intermediate-acting[a]				
Estazolam (*ProSom*)	0.5–1 mg	T: 1, 2	12–18 h	Rapidly absorbed, effective in initiating sleep; slightly active metabolites that may accumulate (K)
Lorazepam (*Ativan*)	0.25–2 mg	T: 0.5, 1, 2	8–12 h	Effective in initiating and maintaining sleep; associated with falls, memory loss, rebound insomnia (K)
Temazepam (*Restoril*)	7.5–15 mg	C: 7.5, 15, 30	8–10 h[b]	Daytime drowsiness may occur with repeated use; effective for sleep maintenance; delayed onset of effect (K)
Nonbenzodiazepine, short-acting[a]				
Eszopiclone (*Lunesta*)	1–2 mg	T: 1, 2, 3	5–6 h	CYP3A4 interactions; avoid administration with high-fat meal; not for treatment of anxiety (L)
Zaleplon (*Sonata*)	5 mg	C: 5, 10	1 h	Avoid taking with alcohol or food (L)
Zolpidem (*Ambien*)	5 mg	T: 5, 10	1.5–4.5 h[c]	Confusion and agitation may occur but are rare (L)
(*Ambien CR*)	6.25 mg	T: 6.25, 12.5	1.6–5.5 h	Do not divide, crush or chew

(cont.)

Table 97. Useful Medications for Sleep Disorders in Older Adults (cont.)

Class, Medication	Usual Dose	Formulations	Half-life	Comments (Metabolism, Excretion)
CNS depressant, nonbarbiturate and nonbenzodiazepine				
Chloral hydrate (*Aquachloral, Supprettes*)	500–1000 mg (not to exceed 2 g as single dose or total daily dose)	C: 500; syr 500 mg/5 mL; Sp: 324, 500, 648	8 h (active metabolite)	Hypnotic effect lost after 2 wk of continual use; contraindicated in marked cardiac, hepatic, or renal impairment (K, L)
Hormone and Hormone Receptor Agonist				
Melatonin	0.3–5 mg	various	1 h	Not regulated by FDA
Ramelteon (*Rozerem*)	8 mg within 30 min of bedtime	T: 8	Ramelteon: 1–2.6 h; active metabolite: 2–5 h	Do not administer with or immediately after high-fat meal (L, K)

✔ = preferred for treating older adults
[a] May cause severe allergic reactions and complex sleep-related behavioral disturbances
[b] Can be as long as 30 h in older adults
[c] 3 h in older adults; 10 h in those with hepatic cirrhosis

SLEEP APNEA
Definition
Repeated episodes of apnea (cessation of airflow for ≥10 sec) or hypopnea (transient reduction [≥30% decrease in thoracoabdominal movement or airflow and with ≥4% oxygen desaturation, or an arousal] of airflow for ≥10 sec) during sleep with excessive daytime sleepiness or altered cardiopulmonary function.

Classification
Obstructive (90% of cases): Airflow cessation as a result of upper airway closure in spite of adequate respiratory muscle effort
Central: Cessation of respiratory effort
Mixed: Features of both obstructive and central

Associated Risk Factors, Clinical Features
Family hx, HTN, increased neck circumference, male gender, obesity, smoking, snoring, upper airway structural abnormalities (eg, soft palate, tonsils)

Evaluation
• Full night's sleep study (polysomnography) in sleep laboratory is indicated for those who habitually snore and either report daytime sleepiness or have observed apnea.
• Results are reported as the apnea-hypopnea index (AHI), which is the number of episodes of apneas and hypopneas per hour of sleep.

- Medicare reimbursement threshold for CPAP based on a min of 2 h sleep by polysomnography is AHI (1) $\geq$15 or (2) $\geq$5 and $\leq$14 with documented symptoms of excessive daytime sleepiness, impaired cognition, mood disorders, or insomnia, or documented HTN, ischemic heart disease, or hx of stroke.

Management
Nonpharmacologic
- Use CPAP by nasal mask, nasal prongs, or mask that covers the nose and mouth (considered initial treatment for clinically important sleep apnea).
- Use oral appliances that keep the tongue in an anterior position during sleep or keep the mandible forward; less effective than CPAP in reducing daytime sleepiness but may be better tolerated.
- Avoid use of alcohol or sedatives.
- Lie in lateral rather than supine position; may be facilitated by soft foam ball in a backpack.
- Lose weight (obese patients).

Pharmacologic
- Modafinil (*Provigil*) 200 mg qam for excessive daytime sleepiness (CYP3A4 inducer and CYP2C19 inhibitor) [T: 100, 200]; use in addition to (not instead of) CPAP
- Fluoxetine (*Prozac*) 10–20 mg [T: 10, 20, 40; S: 20 mg/5 mL]

Surgical
- Tracheostomy (indicated for patients with severe apnea who cannot tolerate positive pressure or when other interventions are ineffective)
- Uvulopalatopharyngoplasty (curative in fewer than 50% of cases)
- Maxillofacial surgery (rare cases)

OTHER CONDITIONS ASSOCIATED WITH SLEEP DISORDERS
Nocturnal Leg Cramps
Stretching exercises or use of heating pad 10 min before bedtime may be helpful. Quinine is not recommended for nocturnal leg cramps.

Restless Legs Syndrome
Diagnostic Criteria
- A compelling urge to move the limbs, usually associated with paresthesias or dysesthesias
- Motor restlessness (eg, floor pacing, tossing and turning in bed, rubbing legs)
- Vague discomfort, usually bilateral, most commonly in calves
- Symptoms occur while awake and are exacerbated by rest, especially at night
- Symptoms relieved by movement—jerking, stretching, or shaking of limbs; pacing

Secondary Causes: Iron deficiency, spinal cord and peripheral nerve lesions, uremia, diabetes, Parkinson's disease, venous insufficiency, medications/drugs (eg, TCAs, SSRIs, lithium, dopamine antagonists, caffeine)

Nonpharmacologic Treatment
- Sleep hygiene measures (see p 226).
- Avoid alcohol, caffeine, nicotine.
- Rub limbs.
- Use hot or cold baths, whirlpools.

Pharmacologic Treatment
- Exclude or treat iron deficiency, peripheral neuropathy.
- If possible, avoid SSRIs, TCAs, lithium, and dopamine antagonists.

Start at low dosage, increase as needed:
- First line: dopamine agonists (preferred for daily symptoms) (see **Table 63**) or carbidopa-levodopa (preferred for intermittent symptoms) (*Sinemet*) 25/100 mg, 1–2 h before bedtime. Symptom augmentation may develop earlier in the day (eg, afternoon instead of evening) and may be more severe with carbidopa-levodopa; treatment may require reducing dosage or switching to dopamine agonist.
- Second-line agents include carbamazepine and gabapentin (see **Table 64**).
- For refractory cases, benzodiazepines or opioids can be tried.

Periodic Limb Movement Disorder
Diagnostic Criteria
- Insomnia or excessive sleepiness
- Repetitive, highly stereotyped limb muscle movements (eg, extension of big toes with partial flexion of ankle, knee, and sometimes hip) that occur during nonREM sleep
- Polysomnographic monitoring showing repetitive episodes of muscle contractions and associated arousals or awakenings
- No evidence of a medical, mental, or other sleep disorder that can account for symptoms

Treatment: Indicated for clinically significant sleep disruption or frequent arousals documented on a sleep study.
- Nonpharmacologic: sleep hygiene measures (see p 226).
- Pharmacologic: See restless legs syndrome, p 229.

VISUAL IMPAIRMENT

DEFINITION
Visual acuity 20/40 or worse; severe visual impairment (legal blindness) 20/200 or worse

EVALUATION
- Acuity testing
  - Near vision: check each eye independently with glasses using handheld Rosenbaum card at 14" or Lighthouse Near Acuity Test at 16". *Note:* Distance must be accurate.
  - Far vision: Snellen wall chart at 20'
- Visual fields (by confrontation)
- Ophthalmoscopy
- Emergent referral for acute change in vision.

Causes of Visual Impairment in Decreasing Order of Frequency
Refractive Error: Most common cause of impairment

Cataracts: Lens opacity on ophthalmoscopic examination. Risk factors: age, sun exposure, smoking, corticosteroids, diabetes mellitus, alcohol, low vitamin intake.

Age-related Macular Degeneration (AMD): Atrophy of cells in the central macular region of retinal pigmented epithelium; on ophthalmoscopic examination, white-yellow patches (drusen) or hemorrhage and scars in advanced stages. Risk factors: age, smoking, sun exposure, family hx, white race.

Diabetic Retinopathy: Microaneurysms, dot and blot hemorrhages on ophthalmoscopy with proliferative retinopathy ischemia and vitreous hemorrhage. Risk factors: chronic hyperglycemia, smoking.

Glaucoma: Characteristic optic cupping and nerve damage and loss of peripheral visual fields. Risk factors: black race, age, family hx, elevated ocular pressures. Most common cause of blindness in black Americans. Primary open-angle glaucoma is most common, a chronic disease of older adults. Angle-closure glaucoma is an acute disease requiring emergent management.

MANAGEMENT
Prevention
Biennial full eye examinations for people >65 yr old, annually for people with diabetes.

Nonpharmacologic Treatment
Cataract
- Reduce UV light exposure.
- Surgery (AHRQ guidelines [AHCPR Publication No. 93-0542]):
  - if acuity 20/50 or worse with symptoms of poor functional acuity
  - if 20/40 or better with disabling glare or frequent exposure to low light situations, diplopia, disparity between eyes, or occupational need
  - when cataract removal will treat another lens-induced disease (eg, glaucoma)
  - when cataract coexists with retinal disease requiring unrestricted monitoring (eg, diabetic retinopathy)

AMD: Laser or photodynamic therapy (when laser would damage fovea) for some wet forms: monitor for conversion to wet form using Amsler grid daily. Patients with large drusen most at risk of conversion to wet AMD.

Diabetic Retinopathy: Laser treatment of proliferative retinopathy or macular edema

Glaucoma Surgery:
- Open angle—laser trabeculoplasty, surgical trabeculectomy, drainage devices, aqueous shunt
- Angle closure—laser iridotomy
- Used primarily when pressures or optic nerve damage are poorly controlled by topicals.

Low-vision Services
- Address the full range of functional visual impairment from blindness to partial sight. Refer patients with uncompensated visual loss that reduces function.
- Recommend optical aids:
  - Magnifiers with lights
  - Wearable telescopes for distance vision
  - Closed-circuit television to enlarge text
  - A variety of high-technology devices are available (see www.lighthouse.org).
  - Optical aids (like the above) may improve mood unlike traditional aids such as talking books, Braille watches, etc, which do not.
- Environmental modifications that improve function include color contrast, floor lamps to reduce glare, and motion sensors to turn on lights.
- Many states have "Services for the Visually Impaired" through the health department.

Pharmacologic Treatment

Wet AMD: Pagaptanib *(Macugen),* a vascular endothelial growth factor antagonist, at 0.3 mg intravitreal q 6 wk for up to 2 yr; ranibizumab (*Lucentis*) at 0.5 mL intravitreal monthly for up to 2 yr.

Dry AMD: In intermediate or more advanced stages, zinc oxide 80 mg, cupric oxide 2 mg, β-carotene 15 mg, vitamin C 500 mg, and vitamin E 400 IU taken in divided doses q 12 h reduces risk of progression (eg, *Ocuvite PreserVision* 2 tabs po q 12 h). Not recommended for smokers (β-carotene) or for people with CAD (vitamin E).

Diabetic Retinopathy: Glycemic control HbA_{1c} approx 7%; BP <130/80; lipid control not well studied (see p 35)

Glaucoma: Treat when there is optic nerve damage or visual field loss (see **Table 98**). Therapy reduces intraocular pressure. Instill one drop under lower lid, close eye for at least 1 min to reduce systemic absorption; repeat if a second drop is needed. Wait 5 min before instilling a second type of drop.

Table 98. Medications for Treating Glaucoma

Medication	Strength	Dosage	Comments (Metabolism)
Adrenergic Agonists (bottles with purple caps)			
Apraclonidine (*Iopidine*)	0.5%, 1%	1–2 drops q 8 h	Low BP, fatigue, drowsiness, dry mouth, dry nose (unknown)
Brimonidine (*Alphagan*)	0.2%	1 drop q 8 h	Low BP, fatigue, drowsiness, dry mouth, dry nose (L)
(*Alphagan P*)	0.15%	1 drop q 8 h	Benzalkonium-chloride free (L)
Dipivefrin (*AKPro, Propine*)	0.1%	1 drop q 12 h	HTN, headache, tachycardia, arrhythmia (eye, L)
Epinephrine (*Epifrin, Glaucon*)	0.1%–2%	1 drop q 12–24 h	HTN, headache, tachycardia, arrhythmia (L)
Epinephrine borate (*Epinal*)	0.25%–0.5%	1 drop q 12 h	HTN, headache, tachycardia, arrhythmia (L)
β-Blockers (bottles with blue or yellow caps)			Class adverse events:
✔Betaxolol (*Betoptic, Betoptic-S*)	0.25%, 0.5%	1–2 drops q 12 h	hypotension, bradycardia, HF, bronchospasm, anxiety, confusion, hallucination, diarrhea, nausea, cramps, lethargy, weakness, masking of hypoglycemia, impotence (L)
✔Carteolol (*Ocupress*)	1%	1 drop q 12 h	
✔Levobunolol (*AKBeta, Betagan*)	0.25%, 0.5%	1 drop q 12 h	
✔Metipranolol (*OptiPranolol*)	0.3%	1 drop q 12 h	
✔Timolol drops (*Betimol, Timoptic*)	0.25%, 0.5%	1 drop q 12 h	
Miotics, Direct-acting (bottles with green caps)			
Pilocarpine gel (*Pilopine HS*) (*Ocusert*)	4% 20, 40 mcg/h	1/2" qhs weekly	Systemic cholinergic effects (tissues, K)
Pilocarpine (*Adsorbocarpine, Akarpine, Isopto Carpine, Pilagan, Pilocar, Piloptic, Pilostat*)	0.25%–10%	1 drop q 6 h	Systemic cholinergic effects are rare (K)

(cont.)

Table 98. Medications for Treating Glaucoma (cont.)

Medication	Strength	Dosage	Comments (Metabolism)
Miotics, Cholinesterase Inhibitors (bottles with green caps)			Class adverse events: cholinomimetic effects
Demecarium (*Humorsol*)	0.125%, 0.25%	1–2 drops q 12 h	(sweating, tremor, headache, salivation), confusion, high or low BP, bradycardia, bronchoconstriction, urinary frequency, cramps, diarrhea, nausea, deterioration of mental status in people with AD
Echothiophate (*Phospholine*)	0.03%–0.25%	1 drop q 12 h	
Isoflurophate (*Floropryl*)	0.025% oint	0.25" strip q 8–72 h	
Physostigmine (*Eserine, Fisostin, Isopto Eserine*)	0.25% oint	1" q 8 h	(L)
Carbonic Anhydrase Inhibitors (bottles with orange caps)			
Topical			Caution in kidney failure (K)
✔Brinzolamide (*Azopt*)	1%	1 drop q 8 h	
✔Dorzolamide (*Trusopt*)	2%	1 drop q 8 h	
Oral			Class adverse events: fatigue, weight loss, paresthesias, depression, COPD exacerbation, cramps, diarrhea, kidney failure, blood dyscrasias, hypokalemia, acidosis; not recommended in kidney failure (K)
Acetazolamide (eg, *Diamox*)	125–500 mg, SR 500 mg	250–500 mg q 6–12 h, SR 500 mg q 12 h	
Dichlorphenamide (*Daranide*)	50 mg	25–50 mg q 8–24 h	
Methazolamide (eg, *Neptazane*)	25–50 mg	50–100 mg q 8–12 h	(L, K)
Prostaglandin Analogs			Class adverse events: change in eye color and periorbital tissues, hyperemia, itching; expensive
✔Bimatoprost (*Lumigan*)	0.03%	1 drop qhs	(L, K, F)
✔Latanoprost (*Xalatan*)	0.005%	1 drop qhs	(L)
✔Travoprost (*Travatan*)	0.004%	1 drop qhs	(L)
✔Unoprostone (*Rescula*)	0.15%	1 drop qhs	(L)

(cont.)

Table 98. Medications for Treating Glaucoma (cont.)			
Medication	**Strength**	**Dosage**	**Comments (Metabolism)**
Other Topical			
Dorzolamide/timolol (*Cosopt*)	0.05%, 0.2%	1 drop q 12 h	Unusual taste, ocular itching, burning (K, L)

✔ = preferred for treating older adults
Note: Patients may not know names of drugs but instead refer to them by the color of the bottle cap. The usual colors are listed above.

ACUTE CONJUNCTIVITIS

Symptoms: Red eye, foreign body sensation, discharge, photophobia
Signs: Conjunctival hyperemia and discharge.
Etiology: Viral, bacterial, chlamydial
Viral Versus Bacterial:
Viral—profuse tearing, minimal exudation, preauricular adenopathy common, monocytes in stained scrapings and exudates
Bacterial—moderate tearing, profuse exudation, preauricular adenopathy uncommon, bacteria and polymorphonuclear cells in stained scrapings and exudates
Both—minimal itching, generalized hyperemia, occasional sore throat and fever
Treatment: Majority are viral; treat symptoms with artificial tears and cool compresses. If purulent discharge, suspect bacterial; start broad-spectrum topical antibiotics (see **Table 99**). If severe, obtain culture and Gram's stain, then start treatment. If signs and symptoms do not improve in 24–48 h, refer to ophthalmologist.
Other: Wash hands frequently and use separate towels to avoid spread.

Table 99. Treatment for Acute Bacterial Conjunctivitis[a]		
Medication	**Formulations[b]**	**Comments**
Ciprofloxacin (*Ciloxan*)	0.3% sol, 0.3% oint	Very broad spectrum, well tolerated, a first choice in severe cases, expensive
Erythromycin ophthalmic (*AK-Mycin, Ilotycin*)	5 mg/g oint	Good if staphylococcal blepharitis is present
Gatifloxacin (*Tequin*)	0.3% sol	See ciprofloxacin
Moxifloxacin (*Avelox*)	0.5% sol	See ciprofloxacin
Norfloxacin (*Chibroxin*)	0.3% sol	See ciprofloxacin
Ofloxacin (*Floxin, Ocuflox*)	0.3% sol, 0.3% oint	See ciprofloxacin
Sulfacetamide sodium (*Sodium Sulamyd*)	10%, 30% drops, 10% oint	Well tolerated
Tobramycin (*AKTob, Tobrex*)	3 mg/g oint, 3 mg/mL sol	Well tolerated but more corneal toxicity
Trimethoprim and polymyxin (*Polytrim*)	1 mg/mL, 10,000 IU/mL sol	Well tolerated but some gaps in coverage

[a] Do not use steroid or steroid-antibiotic preparations in initial treatment.
[b] In mild cases, solution is applied q 6 h and gel or ointment q 12 h for 5–7 d. In more severe cases, solution is applied q 2–3 h and ointment q 6 h; as the eye improves, solution is applied q 6 h and ointment q 12 h.

RED EYE

The "red eye" is an eye with vascular congestion: some conditions that cause this pose a threat to vision and warrant prompt ophthalmologic referral. See **Fig 10**.

Fig 10. Red Eye Decision Tree

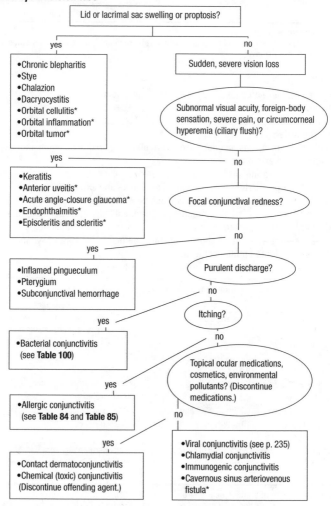

* Potentially dangerous; requires prompt referral to ophthalmology.

Source: Trobe JD. *Physician's Guide to Eye Care, 2nd ed.* American Academy of Ophthalmology, 2001. Reprinted with permission.

DRY EYE SYNDROME

Symptoms: Itchy or sandy eyes (foreign body sensation)

Etiology: Many; consider autoimmune (Sjögren's syndrome), drug-induced causes; refer to ophthalmology for diagnostic assistance.

Therapy:

- Artificial tear formulations (eg, *HypoTears*); formulations containing either chondroitin sulfate or hyaluronic acid are not better.
- Cyclosporine ophthalmic emulsion 0.05% (*Restasis*) 1 gtt OU q 12 h. Indicated when tear production is suppressed by inflammation. Does not increase tears in people using topical anti-inflammatories or punctal plugs. Adverse events: burning, hyperemia, discharge, pain, blurring.
- Temporary or permanent punctual plugs

SYSTEMIC MEDICATIONS WITH OCULAR ADVERSE EVENTS (SYMPTOMS, SIGNS)

- Amiodarone: halos, blurred vision, corneal changes, optic neuropathy
- Anticholinergics: blurry near vision, angle-closure glaucoma (rare)
- Cisplatin: optic neuritis, papilledema, retrobulbar neuritis, cortical blindness
- Corticosteroids: cataracts, glaucoma
- Digoxin: yellowish orange vision; snowy, flickering vision
- Ethambutol or INH: loss of color vision, visual acuity, visual field
- Hydroxychloroquine or chloroquine: loss of color vision, visual acuity, visual field
- Niacin: decreased visual field, maculopathy
- Sildenafil: color tinge in vision, increased sensitivity to light, blurred vision. Nonarteritic ischemic optic neuropathy has been reported in association with PDE5 inhibitors.

PREVENTION

(See also **Table 75**.)

- Annual breast and pelvic and perineal examination
- Annual mammography if life expectancy >4 yr
- Discuss HT risks and benefits with patients on and considering treatment.
- Only one negative Pap smear needed after 65 yr if low risk (ie, one established sexual partner, good prior screening, no hx of abnormal Pap smear)
- Osteoporosis evaluation (see p 166)
- Heart disease
  - The leading cause of death in older women.
  - Assess risk based on Framingham criteria using the online calculator that uses age, smoking, systolic BP, total and HDL cholesterol at www.nhlbi.nih.gov/guidelines/cholesterol/index.htm.
  - Encourage all women to make lifestyle changes, including smoking cessation, regular exercise, weight management, and heart-healthy diet. Other recommendations are based on whether patient is at high, intermediate, or low risk. See **Table 19** for cholesterol treatment recommendations.
  - ASA (75–162 mg/d) is recommended in older women.

COMMON DISORDERS

Breast Cancer

Prevention: See also **Table 75**. Tamoxifen 20 mg/d po reduces breast cancer risk by 49% in women at high risk but increases risk of endometrial cancer. Raloxifene (60 mg/d) reduces risk of invasive breast cancer (but not noninvasive disease) and of endometrial cancer. Both tamoxifen and raloxifene increase risk of venous thromboembolism (VTE), but rates of VTE are lower for raloxifene (see also Osteoporosis, p 166). For risk assessment, see www.cancer.gov/cancerinfo/pdq/prevention/breast/healthprofessional.

Monitoring:

- History, physical
- LFTs, calcium q 4–6 mo for 5 yr, then yearly
- Annual mammography, pelvic examination, and FOBT

Oral Hormone Adjuvant Therapy: Postmenopausal women with estrogen-receptor- or progesterone-receptor-positive tumors at high risk of recurrence (tumors >1 cm, or positive nodes) should be treated with oral adjuvant therapy. Therapy should include an aromatase inhibitor, which may be the initial treatment. Options include an aromatase inhibitor for 5 yr, or sequential treatment with tamoxifen (for 2–5 yr) followed by an aromatase inhibitor for 2–5 yr. See **Table 100**.

Adjuvant Chemotherapy: Reduces risk of recurrence for receptor-negative tumors. Recurrence is reduced by an additional 5%–10% in estrogen-receptor- or progesterone-receptor-positive tumors treated with both oral hormone adjuvant and chemotherapy.

Therapy for Metastatic Bone Disease: Pamidronate or zoledronic acid reduces morbidity and delays time to onset of bone symptoms. Consult oncology.

Table 100. Oral Agents for Breast Cancer Treatment

Class, Medication	Dosage and Formulations	Monitoring	Adverse Events (Metabolism)
Antiestrogen Drugs			
Fulvestrant (*Faslodex*)	250 mg/mo IM in 1 or 2 injections Inj: 250 mg/5 mL; 125 mg/2.5 mL	Blood chemistry, lipids	Has potent CYP3A4 inhibitors; GI reactions, anesthesia, pain (back, pelvic, headache), hot flushes (L)
Tamoxifen* (*Nolvadex*)	20 mg/d po T: 10, 20	Annual eye examination; endometrial cancer screening	Drug interactions: erythromycin, calcium channel blockers; ↑ risk of thrombosis (L)
Toremifene (*Fareston*)	60 mg/d po T: 60	CBC, Ca, LFTs, BUN, Cr	Drug interactions with CYP3A4–6 inhibitors and inducers (see **Table 8**); ↑ warfarin effect (L)
Aromatase Inhibitors			
Anastrozole (*Arimidex*)	1 mg/d po T: 1	Periodic CBC, lipids, serum chemistry profile	Common: arthritis, arthralgia, bone pain, asthenia, cough, dyspnea, pharyngitis, depression, headache, nausea, rash, edema. Less common: anemia, leukopenia, thromboembolism, thrombophlebitis, hypercholesterolemia, fractures, vaginal hemorrhage (L)
Exemestane (*Aromasin*)	25 mg/d po T: 25	Periodic WBC count with differential, lipids, serum chemistry profile	Common: anxiety, depression, fatigue, insomnia, dyspnea, hot flushes, weight gain, nausea, pain at tumor site. Rare: myocardial infarction (L)
Letrozole (*Femara*)	2.5 mg/d po T: 2.5	Periodic CBC, LFTs, TSH	Common: arthralgia, back pain, bone pain, dyspnea, hot flushes, nausea. Less common: fracture, myocardial infarction or ischemia, pancytopenia, thromboembolism, pleural effusion, pulmonary embolism. Metabolized by CYP3A4, CYP2A6; strongly inhibits CYP2A6 and moderately inhibits CYP2C19 (L)

*Reduce dosage if CrCl <10 mL/min

Vulvar Diseases
Non-neoplastic:

- Lichen sclerosus—Common on vulva of middle-aged and older women; causes 1/3 of benign vulvar lesions, extends to perirectal areas (classic hourglass appearance); lesions are white to pink macules or papules, may coalesce; asymptomatic or itching, soreness, or dyspareunia. Must biopsy for diagnosis: associated with squamous cell cancer in 4%–5%. Treatment: clobetasol propionate 0.05% q 12–24 h for 8–12 wk; then taper gradually to zero. Long-term follow-up advised.

- Squamous hyperplasia—Raised white keratinized lesions difficult to distinguish from VIN; must biopsy to exclude malignancy. Treatment: betamethasone dipropionate 0.05% for 6–8 wk, then 1% hydrocortisone if symptoms persist. Long-term follow-up advised.

Neoplastic:
- VIN—Most often seen in postmenopausal women; asymptomatic or may cause pruritus; hypo- or hyperpigmented keratinized lesions; often multifocal; inspection $\pm$ colposcopy of the entire vulva with biopsy of most worrisome lesions; lesions graded on degree of atypia. Treatment: surgical or other ablative therapy.
- Vulvar malignancy—Half of cases are in women >70 yr old; 80% are squamous cell, with melanoma, sarcoma, basal cell, and adenocarcinoma <20%; biopsy any suspicious lesion. Treatment: radical surgery is preferred treatment.

Postmenopausal Bleeding
Bleeding after 1 yr of amenorrhea:
- Exclude malignancy, identify source, treat symptoms.
- Examine genitalia, perineum, rectum.
- If endometrial source, use endometrial biopsy or vaginal probe ultrasound to assess endometrial thickness (<5 mm virtually excludes malignancy).
- D&C when endometrium not otherwise adequately assessed.
- Evaluation is needed for:
  ○ Women on combination continual estrogen and progesterone who bleed after 12 mo.
  ○ Women on cyclic replacement with bleeding at unexpected times (ie, bleeding other than during the second week of progesterone therapy).
  ○ Women on unopposed estrogen who bleed at any time.

Vaginal Prolapse
- Child-bearing and other causes of increased intra-abdominal pressure weaken connective tissue and muscles supporting the genital organs, leading to prolapse.
- Symptoms include pelvic pressure, back pain, fecal or urinary incontinence, difficulty evacuating the rectum. Symptoms may be present even with mild prolapse.
- The degree of prolapse and organs involved dictate therapy; no therapy if asymptomatic.
- Estrogen and Kegel's exercises may help in mild cases.
- Pessary or surgery indicated with increase in symptoms. Surgery needed for fourth-degree symptomatic prolapse.
- Precise anatomic defect(s) dictates the surgical approach. Surgical closure of the vagina is a simple option for frail patients who are not sexually active.
- A common classification (ACOG) for degrees of prolapse:
  ○ First degree—extension to mid-vagina
  ○ Second degree—approaching hymenal ring
  ○ Third degree—at hymenal ring
  ○ Fourth degree—beyond hymenal ring

HORMONE THERAPY
Symptoms Associated with the Postmenopausal State
- Hot flushes and night sweats
- Sleep disturbances
- Vaginal dryness and dyspareunia
- Depression

- Insufficient evidence exists to link the following commonly reported symptoms to the postmenopausal state: cognitive disturbances, fatigue, sexual dysfunction.

Therapy for Menopausal Symptoms
- Vasomotor and vaginal symptoms respond to estrogen (see **Table 102**) in dose-response fashion; start at low dosage, titrate to effect. Dyspareunia and vaginal dryness respond to topical estrogen (see **Table 93**).

Estrogen Therapy
- For current understanding of risks for women >65 yr old on HT, see **Table 101**.
- If the woman has a uterus, estrogen combined with progesterone reduces risk of endometrial cancer.
- Some women prefer unopposed estrogen and annual endometrial biopsy.
- For common regimens, see **Table 101**.
- Older women can get hot flushes if estrogen is discontinued suddenly. Tapering (eg, q 48 h for 1–2 mo and then q 72 h for a few months) is better tolerated.

Table 101. Risks and Benefits of Systemic Hormone Therapy After Age 65		
Systemic Outcome[a]	Estrogen	Estrogen/Progesterone
MI	none	↑
Thromboembolic disease	↑ DVT	↑ DVT, PE
Stroke	↑	↑
Breast cancer	possibly ↓	↑
Hip fracture	↓	↓
Colon cancer	none	uncertain
Endometrial cancer	↑	no change or ↓
Gallbladder disease	↑	↑
Urogenital disease[b]	↓	↓
Dementia	possibly ↑	↑
Ovarian cancer	↑	unknown
Global	risk = benefit	risk exceeds benefit

Note: ↑ = increased risk; ↓ = decreased risk
[a] Global outcome: CAD; stroke; hip fracture; PE; breast, colon, endometrial cancer; and death from other causes
[b] Dyspareunia, UTI, and vaginal dryness; oral HT worsens urinary incontinence

Contraindications to Hormone Therapy
- Undiagnosed vaginal bleeding
- Thromboembolic disease
- Breast cancer
- Prior stroke or TIA
- Endometrial cancer more advanced than Stage 1
- Possibly gallbladder disease
- CHD

Intolerable Vasomotor Symptoms
- 25% of women continue with vasomotor symptoms 5 yr after menopause and a smaller percentage have even longer-term symptoms.
- Note contraindications above.

- Assess risk of venous thromboembolism (VTE) and cardiovascular disease:
  - VTE risk increased by history of VTE, malignancy/myeloproliferative disorder, leg immobilization, or both smoking and obesity.
  - Cardiovascular disease risk increased by known CAD, PAD, abdominal aortic aneurysm, carotid artery disease, diabetes mellitus, or risk factors that confer a 10-yr risk of coronary disease >20% (http://hp2010.nhlbihin.net/atpiii/calculator.asp?usertype=prof)
- If increased cardiovascular or VTE risk, then oral standard dosage estrogen-progestin should not be used.
- If increased cardiovascular risk (but not VTE risk), attempt to control symptoms with transdermal estrogen.
- If risk of VTE is increased and risk of cardiovascular disease is usual and patient has no uterus, transdermal estrogen may be appropriate; if patient has uterus, adding a progestin raises additional concerns.
- If neither VTE nor cardiovascular disease risk is increased, estrogen or estrogen-progestin may be appropriate given orally or transdermally at lowest dosage to control symptoms.
- Continue to advocate tapering (as described above) at 2-yr intervals.
- If estrogen cannot be taken or if risks exceed benefits, try one of the less effective alternatives for vasomotor symptoms:
  - Venlafaxine (*Effexor*) 75–150 mg/d
  - Fluoxetine (*Prozac*) 20 mg/d
  - Paroxetine (*Paxil*) 12.5–25 mg/d
  - Gabapentin (*Neurontin*) [C: 100, 300, 400; T: 600, 800; S: 250/5 mL] usually 300–600 mg q 8 h
  - Clonidine (*Catapres, Duraclon*): [T: 0.1, 0.2, 0.3] 0.1–0.3 mg/d; use lowest effective dosage, watch for orthostatic hypotension and rebound increase in BP if used intermittently.
  - Megestrol (*Megace*): [T: 20, 40] 20 mg q 12–24 h; increases risk of DVT

Table 102. Common Regimens for Systemic Hormone Therapy

Preparation	Starting Dosage (mg/d)	Cyclic Dosing	Continual Dosing	Formulations
Oral				
Conjugated equine estrogen (*Premarin*)*	0.3–0.625	—	Daily	T: 0.3, 0.625, 0.9, 1.25, 2.5
Conjugated synthetic estrogen (*Cenestin*)	0.625	—	Daily	T: 0.625, 0.9, 1.25
Esterified estrogen (eg, *Estratab, Menest*)*	0.3–0.625	—	Daily	T: 0.3, 0.625, 1.25, 2.5
Estradiol acetate (*Femtrace*)	0.45	—	Daily	T: 0.45, 0.9, 1.8
Estropipate (*Ogen, Ortho-Est*)*	0.625	—	Daily	T: 0.625, 1.25, 2.5
Micronized 17-β estradiol (*Estrace*)*	0.5–1	—	Daily	T: 0.5, 1, 2
Synthetic conjugated estrogens, B (*Enjuvia*)	0.625	—	Daily	T: 0.625, 1.25

(cont.)

Table 102. Common Regimens for Systemic Hormone Therapy (cont.)

Preparation	Starting Dosage (mg/d)	Cyclic Dosing	Continual Dosing	Formulations
Oral Combinations				
Conjugated estrogen *and* medroxyprogesterone (*Prempro*)	0.625, 0.45 1.5, 2.5, 5	—	Daily	Fixed dose 0.625/2.5 or 0.625/5 or 0.45/1.5
Conjugated estrogen *and* medroxyprogesterone (*Premphase*)	0.625 5	Days 1–28 Days 15–28	—	Fixed dose 0.625 days 1–14, 0.625/5 days 15–28
Estradiol *and* norethindrone (*FEMHRT 1/5*)	1 5	—	Daily	Fixed dose 1/5
Transdermal				
Estradiol				
(*Alora*)	0.05	—	Biweekly	Pch: 0.05, 0.075, 0.1
(*Climara*)	0.025–0.05	—	Weekly	Pch: 0.025, 0.05, 0.06, 0.075, 0.1
(*Divigel*)	0.25	—	Daily	Gel: 0.25, 0.5, 1
(*Elestrin*)	0.52	—	Daily	Gel: 0.06%
(*Estraderm*)	0.05	—	Biweekly	Pch: 0.05, 0.1
(*Estrogel*)	0.75	—	Daily	Gel: 0.06%
(*Evamist*)	1–3 sprays	—	Daily (applied to inside of forearm)	1.7% sol (1.53 mg estradiol per spray)
(*Fempatch*)	0.025	—	Weekly	Pch: 0.025
(*Vivelle*)	0.025	—	Biweekly	Pch: 0.025, 0.0375, 0.05, 0.075, 0.1
Estradiol *and* norethindrone (*CombiPatch*)	0.05/0.14		Biweekly	Pch: 0.05/0.14, 0.05/0.25
Other				
Femring	0.05	—	Vaginal ring, change q 90 d	0.05, 0.10
Medroxyprogesterone (*Cycrin, Provera*)	2.5–10	5–10 mg, days 1–14	2.5–5 mg/d	T: 2.5, 5, 10

Note: See also **Table 93** for topical estrogens without systemic effects.
* FDA approved for long-term use to prevent osteoporosis.

Some assessment instuments commonly used in geriatrics practice are included on the following pages. These instruments, as well as some additional ones, are available on the *Geriatrics At Your Fingertips* Web site, where they can be printed for use in clinical practice. For a list of all instruments, with direct links to each, see www.geriatricsatyourfingertips.org.

MINI-COG™ SCREEN FOR DEMENTIA

The Mini-Cog™ screen combines an uncued 3-item recall test with a clock-drawing test (CDT) that serves as a recall distractor. The Mini-Cog™ can be administered in about 3 min, requires no special equipment, and is less influenced by level of education or language differences.

Administration

1. Make sure you have the patient's attention. Instruct the patient to listen carefully to and remember 3 unrelated words and then to repeat the words back to you (to be sure the patient heard them).
2. Instruct the patient to draw the face of a clock, either on a blank sheet of paper, or on a sheet with the clock circle already drawn on the page. After the patient puts the numbers on the clock face, ask him or her to draw the hands of the clock to read a specific time (11:10 or 8:20 are most commonly used and more sensitive than some others). These instructions can be repeated, but no additional instructions should be given. If the patient cannot complete the CDT in 3 min or less, move on to the next step.
3. Ask the patient to repeat the 3 previously presented words.

Scoring

Give 1 point for each recalled word after the CDT distractor. Score 0–3 for recall.
Give 2 points for a normal CDT, and 0 points for an abnormal CDT. The CDT is considered normal if all numbers are depicted, once each, in the correct sequence and position, and the hands readably display the requested time. Add the recall and CDT scores together to get the Mini-Cog score:
- 0–2   positive screen for dementia.
- 3–5   negative screen for dementia.

Source: Adapted from Borson S, Scanlan J, Brush M, Vitaliano P, Dokmak A. The Mini-Cog: a cognitive "vital signs" measure for dementia screening in multi-lingual elderly. *Int J Geriatr Psychiatry* 2000; 15(11):1021–1027, and Borson S, Scanlan JM, Watanabe J, Tu SP, Lessig M. Improving identification of cognitive impairment in primary care. *Int J Geriatr Psychiatry*, 2006;21(4):349–355.

Mini-Cog™ Copyright 2000, 2004, 2006. All rights reserved. Described here under license from the University of Washington, solely for use as a clinical aid. Any other use is strictly prohibited. To obtain information on the Mini-Cog™ contact Soo Borson at soob@u.washington.edu.

PHYSICAL SELF-MAINTENANCE SCALE (ACTIVITIES OF DAILY LIVING, OR ADLS)

In each category, circle the item that most closely describes the person's highest level of functioning and record the score assigned to that level (either 1 or 0) in the blank at the beginning of the category.

A. Toilet _____
1. Care for self at toilet completely; no incontinence 1
2. Needs to be reminded, or needs help in cleaning self, or has rare (weekly at most) accidents...0
3. Soiling or wetting while asleep more than once a week.......................................0
4. Soiling or wetting while awake more than once a week.......................................0
5. No control of bowels or bladder 0

B. Feeding _____
1. Eats without assistance..1
2. Eats with minor assistance at meal times and/or with special preparation of food, or help in cleaning up after meals..0
3. Feeds self with moderate assistance and is untidy..0
4. Requires extensive assistance for all meals 0
5. Does not feed self at all and resists efforts of others to feed him or her.....................0

C. Dressing _____
1. Dresses, undresses, and selects clothes from own wardrobe 1
2. Dresses and undresses self with minor assistance 0
3. Needs moderate assistance in dressing and selection of clothes...........................0
4. Needs major assistance in dressing but cooperates with efforts of others to help............0
5. Completely unable to dress self and resists efforts of others to help 0

D. Grooming (neatness, hair, nails, face, clothing) _____
1. Always neatly dressed and well-groomed without assistance 1
2. Grooms self adequately with occasional minor assistance, eg, with shaving...................0
3. Needs moderate and regular assistance or supervision with grooming.......................0
4. Needs total grooming care but can remain well-groomed after help from others...............0
5. Actively negates all efforts of others to maintain grooming 0

E. Physical Ambulation _____
1. Goes about grounds or city..1
2. Ambulates within residence on or about one block distant...................................0
3. Ambulates with assistance of (check one)
   a ( ) another person, b ( ) railing, c ( ) cane, d ( ) walker, e ( ) wheelchair 0
   1.___Gets in and out without help. 2.___Needs help getting in and out
4. Sits unsupported in chair or wheelchair but cannot propel self without help...................0
5. Bedridden more than half the time 0

F. Bathing _____
1. Bathes self (tub, shower, sponge bath) without help...1
2. Bathes self with help getting in and out of tub..0
3. Washes face and hands only but cannot bathe rest of body...................................0
4. Does not wash self but is cooperative with those who bathe him or her......................0
5. Does not try to wash self and resists efforts to keep him or her clean........................0

For scoring interpretation and source, see note after the next instrument.

INSTRUMENTAL ACTIVITIES OF DAILY LIVING SCALE (IADLS)

In each category, circle the item that most closely describes the person's highest level of functioning and record the score assigned to that level (either 1 or 0) in the blank at the beginning of the category.

A. Ability to Use Telephone _____
1. Operates telephone on own initiative; looks up and dials numbers. 1
2. Dials a few well-known numbers. 1
3. Answers telephone but does not dial. 1
4. Does not use telephone at all. 0

B. Shopping _____
1. Takes care of all shopping needs independently. 1
2. Shops independently for small purchases. 0
3. Needs to be accompanied on any shopping trip. 0
4. Completely unable to shop. 0

C. Food Preparation _____
1. Plans, prepares, and serves adequate meals independently. 1
2. Prepares adequate meals if supplied with ingredients.. 0
3. Heats and serves prepared meals or prepares meals but does not maintain adequate diet. 0
4. Needs to have meals prepared and served. 0

D. Housekeeping _____
1. Maintains house alone or with occasional assistance (eg, domestic help for heavy work). 1
2. Performs light daily tasks such as dishwashing, bedmaking. 1
3. Performs light daily tasks but cannot maintain acceptable level of cleanliness.. 1
4. Needs help with all home maintenance tasks. 1
5. Does not participate in any housekeeping tasks. 0

E. Laundry _____
1. Does personal laundry completely. 1
2. Launders small items; rinses socks, stockings, etc. 1
3. All laundry must be done by others. 0

F. Mode of Transportation _____
1. Travels independently on public transportation or drives own car. 1
2. Arranges own travel via taxi but does not otherwise use public transportation.. 1
3. Travels on public transportation when assisted or accompanied by another.. 1
4. Travel limited to taxi or automobile with assistance of another. 0
5. Does not travel at all.. 0

G. Responsibility for Own Medications _____
1. Is responsible for taking medication in correct dosages at correct time. 1
2. Takes responsibility if medication is prepared in advance in separate dosages. 0
3. Is not capable of dispensing own medication. 0

H. Ability to Handle Finances ___

    1. Manages financial matters independently (budgets, writes checks, pays rent and bills,
       goes to bank); collects and keeps track of income... 1
    2. Manages day-to-day purchases but needs help with banking, major purchases, etc............ 1
    3. Incapable of handling money.. 0

Scoring Interpretation: For ADLs, the total score ranges from 0 to 6, and for IADLs, from 0 to 8. In some categories, only the highest level of function receives a 1; in others, two or more levels have scores of 1 because each describes competence at some minimal level of function. These screens are useful for indicating specifically how a person is performing at the present time. When they are also used over time, they serve as documentation of a person's functional improvement or deterioration.
Source: Lawton MP, Brody EM. Assessment of older people: self-maintaining and instrumental activities of daily living. *Gerontologist* 1969, 9:179–186. Copyright by the Gerontological Society of America. Reproduced by permission of the publisher.

GERIATRIC DEPRESSION SCALE (GDS, SHORT FORM)

Choose the best answer for how you felt over the past week.

1. Are you basically satisfied with your life?	yes/**no**
2. Have you dropped many of your activities and interests?	**yes**/no
3. Do you feel that your life is empty?	**yes**/no
4. Do you often get bored?	**yes**/no
5. Are you in good spirits most of the time?	yes/**no**
6. Are you afraid that something bad is going to happen to you?	**yes**/no
7. Do you feel happy most of the time?	yes/**no**
8. Do you often feel helpless?	**yes**/no
9. Do you prefer to stay at home, rather than going out and doing new things?	**yes**/no
10. Do you feel you have more problems with memory than most?	**yes**/no
11. Do you think it is wonderful to be alive now?	yes/**no**
12. Do you feel pretty worthless the way you are now?	**yes**/no
13. Do you feel full of energy?	yes/**no**
14. Do you feel that your situation is hopeless?	**yes**/no
15. Do you think that most people are better off than you are?	**yes**/no

Score 1 point for each bolded answer. Cut-off: normal 0–5; above 5 suggests depression.

Source: Courtesy of Jerome A. Yesavage, MD. For 30 translations of the GDS, see www.stanford.edu/~yesavage/GDS.html
For additional information on administration and scoring, refer to the following references:
Sheikh JI, Yesavage JA. Geriatric Depression Scale: recent evidence and development of a shorter version. *Clin Gerontol* 1986;5:165–172.
Feher EP, Larrabee GJ, Crook TH 3rd. Factors attenuating the validity of the Geriatric Depression Scale in a dementia population. *J Am Geriatr Soc* 1992;40:906–909.
Yesavage JA, Brink TL, Rose TL et al. Development and validation of a geriatric depression rating scale: a preliminary report. *J Psychiatr Res* 1983;17:27.

KARNOFSKY SCALE

This 10-point scale is a quick and easy way to indicate how a person is feeling on a given day, without going through several multiple-choice questions or symptom surveys.

Score	Description
100	Able to work; normal, no complaints, no evidence of disease
90	Able to work; able to carry on normal activity, minor symptoms
80	Able to work; normal activity with effort, some symptoms
70	Unable to work or carry on normal activity, cares for self independently
60	Mildly disabled, dependent; requires occasional assistance, cares for most needs
50	Moderately disabled, dependent; requires considerable assistance and frequent care
40	Severely disabled, dependent; requires special care and assistance
30	Severely disabled; hospitalized, death not imminent
20	Very sick; active supportive treatment needed
10	Moribund; fatal processes rapidly progressing

Source: Karnofsky DA, Burchenal JH. The clinical evaluation of chemotherapeutic agents in cancer. In: MacLeon CM, ed. *Evaluation of Chemotherapeutic Agents*. Columbia University Press; 1949:196.

PALLIATIVE PERFORMANCE SCALE, VERSION 2 (PPSv2)

PPS Level (%)	Ambulation	Activity and Evidence of Disease	Self-care	Intake	Conscious Level
100	Full	Normal activity and work, no evidence of disease	Full	Normal	Full
90	Full	Normal activity and work, some evidence of disease	Full	Normal	Full
80	Full	Normal activity with effort, some evidence of disease	Full	Normal or reduced	Full
70	Reduced	Unable to do normal job or work, significant disease	Full	Normal or reduced	Full
60	Reduced	Unable to do hobby or housework, significant disease	Occasional assistance required	Normal or reduced	Full or confusion
50	Mainly sit/lie	Unable to do any work, extensive disease	Considerable assistance required	Normal or reduced	Full or confusion
40	Mainly in bed	Unable to do most activity, extensive disease	Mainly assistance	Normal or reduced	Full or drowsy, ± confusion
30	Totally bed bound	Unable to do any activity, extensive disease	Total care	Normal or reduced	Full or drowsy, ± confusion

(cont.)

PPS Level (%)	Ambulation	Activity and Evidence of Disease	Self-care	Intake	Conscious Level
20	Totally bed bound	Unable to do any activity, extensive disease	Total care	Minimal to sips	Full or drowsy, ± confusion
10	Totally bed bound	Unable to do any activity, extensive disease	Total care	Mouth care only	Drowsy or coma, ± confusion
0	Death	—	—	—	—

Instructions: PPS level is determined by reading left to right to find a 'best horizontal fit.' Begin at left column reading downwards until current ambulation is determined, then, read across to next and downwards until each column is determined. Thus, 'leftward' columns take precedence over 'rightward' columns. Also, see 'definitions of terms' for interpretation of PPSv2 and complete instructions at www.victoriahospice.org. Victoria Hospice Society©

Palliative Performance Scale, Version 2 (PPSv2). *Medical Care of the Dying, 4th ed.* Victoria, BC, Canada: Victoria Hospice Society; 2006: 120-121. Reprinted with permission.

REISBERG FUNCTIONAL ASSESSMENT STAGING (FAST) SCALE

This 16-item scale is designed to parallel the progressive activity limitations associated with AD. Stage 7 identifies the threshold of activity limitation that would support a prognosis of ≤6 mo remaining life expectancy.

FAST Scale Item	Activity Limitation Associated with AD
Stage 1	No difficulty, either subjectively or objectively
Stage 2	Complains of forgetting location of objects; subjective work difficulties
Stage 3	Decreased job functioning evident to coworkers; difficulty in traveling to new locations
Stage 4	Decreased ability to perform complex tasks (eg, planning dinner for guests, handling finances)
Stage 5	Requires assistance in choosing proper clothing
Stage 6	Decreased ability to dress, bathe, and toilet independently
Substage 6a	Difficulty putting clothing on properly
Substage 6b	Unable to bathe properly, may develop fear of bathing
Substage 6c	Inability to handle mechanics of toileting (ie, forgets to flush, does not wipe properly)
Substage 6d	Urinary incontinence
Substage 6e	Fecal incontinence
Stage 7	Loss of speech, locomotion, and consciousness
Substage 7a	Ability to speak limited (1–5 words a day)
Substage 7b	All intelligible vocabulary lost
Substage 7c	Nonambulatory
Substage 7d	Unable to smile
Substage 7e	Unable to hold head up

Source: Reisberg, B. Functional assessment staging (FAST), *Psychopharmacol Bull* 1988;24(4):653–659. Copyright MedWorks Media LLC. Reprinted with permission.

Questions to be answered (circle one number on each line)	Not at all	Less than 1 time in 5	Less than half the time	About half the time	More than half the time	Almost always
1. Over the past month or so, how often have you had a sensation of not emptying your bladder completely after you finished urinating?	0	1	2	3	4	5
2. Over the past month or so, how often have you had to urinate again less than 2 hours after you finished urinating?	0	1	2	3	4	5
3. Over the past month or so, how often have you found you stopped and started again several times when you urinated?	0	1	2	3	4	5
4. Over the past month or so, how often have you found it difficult to postpone urination?	0	1	2	3	4	5
5. Over the past month or so, how often have you had a weak urinary stream?	0	1	2	3	4	5
6. Over the past month or so, how often have you had to push or strain to begin urination?	0	1	2	3	4	5
7. Over the last month, how many times did you most typically get up to urinate from the time you went to bed at night until the time you got up in the morning?	none	1 time	2 times	3 times	4 times	>5 times

AUA Symptom Score = sum of responses to questions 1–7 =____. For interpretation, see p 193.

Source: Barry MJ, Fowler FJ Jr, O'Leary MP et al. The American Urological Association symptom index for benign prostatic hyperplasia. *J Urol* 1992;148(5):1549–1557. Reprinted with permission.

MEDICATIONS RECENTLY AVAILABLE AS GENERIC FORMULATIONS

Medication	Formulations
Carvedilol	T: 3.125, 6.25, 12.5 mg
Famciclovir	T: 125, 250, 500 mg
Metopropolol succinate	T ER: 50, 100, 200 mg
Nimodipine	C: 30 mg
Oxcarbazepine	T: 150, 300, 600 mg
Propranolol	C ER: 60, 80, 120, 160 mg
Zolpidem	T (immediate release): 5, 10 mg

CMS GUIDANCE ON UNNECESSARY DRUGS IN THE NURSING HOME

For greater detail than can be provided in this overview, see the complete guidance at www.cms.hhs.gov/transmittals/downloads/R22SOMA.pdf or Appendix PP of the CMS State Operations Manual.

In December 2006, CMS released updated surveyor guidance for unnecessary drugs (greatly expanded from earlier OBRA guidelines), focusing on the resident's entire medication regimen and the components of medication management:
• Indication
• Monitoring, dosage
• Duration
• Attempts to discontinue or reduce dosage
• Prevention, identification, and response to adverse consequences

In general, each resident's medication regimen must be free of unnecessary drugs. An unnecessary drug is any drug used under any of the following conditions:
• In excessive dosage (including duplicate therapy)
• For excessive duration
• Without adequate monitoring
• Without adequate indications for use
• In the presence of adverse consequences that indicate the dosage should be reduced or discontinued
• Any combination of the above

Indications for Use of Medication
Circumstances that warrant evaluation of the resident and medication(s) may include:
• Admission or readmission
• A clinically significant change in condition/status
• A new, persistent, or recurrent clinically significant symptom or problem
• A worsening of an existing problem or condition
• An unexplained decline in function or cognition
• A new medication order or renewal of orders
• An irregularity identified in the pharmacist's monthly medication regimen review

Monitoring for Efficacy and Adverse Consequences
The information gathered during the initial and ongoing evaluations must be incorporated into a comprehensive care plan that reflects appropriate medication-related goals and parameters for monitoring the resident's condition. Monitoring involves several steps, including the following:

- Identifying the essential information and how it will be obtained and reported
- Determining the frequency of monitoring
- Defining the methods for communicating, analyzing, and acting on relevant information
- Reevaluating and updating monitoring approaches

Dosage (Including Duplicate Therapy)
Factors influencing the appropriateness of any dosage include:
- The resident's clinical response
- Possible adverse consequences
- Other resident and medication-related variables
- Laboratory test results, such as serum concentrations of medication(s)

Duplicate therapy is generally not indicated, unless current clinical standards of practice and documented clinical rationale confirm the benefits of multiple medications from the same class or with similar therapeutic effects.

Duration
Periodic reevaluation of the medication regimen is necessary to determine whether prolonged or indefinite use of a medication is indicated. The clinical rationale for continued use of a medication(s) may have been demonstrated in the clinical record, or the staff and prescriber may present pertinent clinical reasons for the duration of use.

Tapering of a Medication Dose/Gradual Dose Reduction (GDR)
The purpose of tapering a medication is to find an optimal dose or to determine whether continued use of the medication is benefiting the resident. A GDR may be indicated when the resident's clinical condition has improved or stabilized, the underlying causes of the original target symptoms have resolved, and/or nonpharmacologic interventions (including behavioral interventions) have been effective in reducing the symptoms.

Adverse Consequences
When reviewing medications used for a resident, it is important to be aware of the medication's recognized safety profile, tolerability, dosing, and potential medication interactions.

ANTIPSYCHOTIC MEDICATIONS
- Residents who have not used antipsychotic medications should not be given these drugs unless antipsychotic medication is necessary to treat a specific condition as diagnosed and documented in the clinical record.
- Residents who use antipsychotic medications should receive GDRs and behavioral interventions, unless clinically contraindicated, in an effort to discontinue these drugs.

- Indications for appropriate use of antipsychotic medications as outlined in the guidance include conditions/diagnoses as documented in the resident's medical record and as meets the definition(s) in the *Diagnostic and Statistical Manual of Mental Disorders, Fourth Edition, Training Revision (DSM-IV TR)* or subsequent editions:
  - Schizoaffective disorder
  - Mood disorders (eg, mania, bipolar disorder, depression with psychotic features, major depression refractory to treatment)
  - Psychosis not otherwise specified
  - Brief psychotic disorder
  - Schizophrenia
  - Delusional disorder
  - Schizophreniform disorder
  - Atypical psychosis
  - Dementing illnesses with associated behavioral symptoms
  - Medical illnesses or delirium with manic or psychotic symptoms and/or treatment-related psychosis or mania (eg, thyrotoxicosis, neoplasms, high-dose steroids)
- A diagnosis alone is not sufficient to begin use of antipsychotic medication; at least one of the additional criteria must also be met:
  - Symptoms are caused by mania or psychosis.
  - Behavioral symptoms present a danger to resident or others.
  - Symptoms are severe enough that resident is experiencing inconsolable or persistent distress, significant decline in function, and/or substantial difficulty receiving necessary care.
- Inadequate indications include wandering, poor self-care, restlessness, impaired memory, mild anxiety, insomnia, unsociability, inattention or indifference to surroundings, fidgeting, nervousness, uncooperativeness, or verbal expressions or behavior not listed above and that do not constitute a danger to the resident or others.
- Treatment of acute psychiatric emergencies:
  - The treatment period is to be limited to ≤7 d, *and*
  - The resident is evaluated within 7 days to identify any contributing or underlying causes and to verify the need to continue the antipsychotic medication, *and*
  - Unless contraindicated, nonpharmacologic interventions must be attempted and documented after the acute episode has resolved.
- Within the first year after admission of a resident on an antipsychotic medication or after the facility has initiated an antipsychotic medication, a GDR must be attempted in two separate quarters (with ≥1 mo between the attempts), unless clinically contraindicated. After the first year, a GDR must be attempted annually, unless clinically contraindicated.

Table 103. Daily Dose Thresholds for Antipsychotic Medications Used to Manage Behavioral Symptoms Related to Dementing Illnesses

Antipsychotic	Dose (mg)
Chlorpromazine	75
Fluphenazine	4
Haloperidol	2
Loxapine	10
Molindone	10
Perphenazine	8
Thioridazine	75
Thiothixene	7
Trifluoperazine	8
Aripiprazole	10
Clozapine	50
Olanzapine	7.5
Quetiapine	150
Risperidone	2
Ziprasidone	Not routinely used

SEDATIVE/HYPNOTIC MEDICATIONS

Before initiating a medication to treat insomnia, other causes should be excluded and nonpharmacologic interventions tried. Causes to exclude include the following:
- Environmental problems (eg, light, noise)
- Inadequate physical activity
- Pain and discomfort
- Caffeine or medications that disrupt sleep
- Underlying comorbidities (eg, HF, COPD, depression)

When a sedative/hypnotic is used routinely during the previous quarter, a GDR should be attempted at least quarterly. Before it can be concluded that a GDR is clinically contraindicated for the remainder of that year, a GDR must have been attempted during the previous three quarters. For the use of sedative/hypnotics, clinically contraindicated means that the physician has documented the clinical rationale for why any additional attempted tapering at that time would be likely to impair the resident's function or cause psychiatric instability by exacerbating an underlying medical or psychiatric disorder.

Table 104. Daily Dose Thresholds for Sedative/Hypnotic Medications

Sedative/Hypnotic	Dose (mg)
Chloral hydrate*	500
Diphenhydramine*	25
Estazolam	0.5
Eszopiclone	1
Flurazepam*	15
Hydroxyzine*	50
Lorazepam	1
Oxazepam	15
Quazepam*	7.5
Ramelteon	8
Temazepam	15
Triazolam*	0.125
Zaleplon	5
Zolpidem	5

*Not considered a medication of choice

CONSIDERATIONS SPECIFIC TO PSYCHOPHARMACOLOGIC MEDICATIONS

During the first year after admission of a resident on a psychopharmacologic medication (other than an antipsychotic or a sedative/hypnotic), or after the facility has initiated such medication, a GDR should be attempted during at least two separate quarters (with ≥1 mo between attempts) unless clinically contraindicated. After the first year, a GDR should be attempted annually unless clinically contraindicated.

MEDICARE PART D PRESCRIPTION DRUG PLAN 2008

- Deductible: Once an individual has spent $275 for eligible medications (monthly premium does not count toward the deductible), coinsurance begins.
- Coinsurance: The individual is responsible for 25% of the medication cost or a copay depending on the plan, and the plan pays 75% until the combined total equals $510.
- The "gap" or "doughnut hole" is the time when there is no plan contribution once the $510 annual threshold has been reached until a total of $4050 has been spent out-of-pocket for the year. Monthly premiums do not count toward the $4050.
- Catastrophic coverage begins once an individual has spent $4050 out-of-pocket for the year on medications. Once the threshold has been crossed, participants pay a small percentage or flat copayment for each prescription and the plan pays the rest. There is no ceiling for this part of the program.
- A new enrollment period begins every November 15 through December 31.
- A new cycle begins on January 1 of each year.

Table 105. Medicare Part D Coverage Levels*

Total Yearly Prescription Medication Costs	$0–$275	$276–$2510	$2511–$5726	>$5726
Covered by patient	TC	$275 + 25%(TC − $275)	TC − $1676	$4050 + 5%(TC − $5726)
Covered by Medicare Part D Plan	$0	75%(TC − $275)	$1676	$1676 + 95%(TC − $5726)

* Does not include Part D premium, another patient out-of-pocket cost, which averaged $41/mo in 2007.
Note: TC = total prescription medication cost

Table 106. Patient Out-of-Pocket Expenses Under Part D Plan

Yearly Total Medication Cost	Yearly Patient Out-of-Pocket Expenses*
$500	$823
$1,000	$948
$2,000	$1,198
$4,000	$2,816
$6,000	$4,556
$10,000	$4,756

* Includes Part D premium (assuming average of $41/mo in 2007), deductible ($275), and coinsurance (see **Table 105** for coverage levels).

Medications Excluded from Part D Plans
• Medications for weight loss, weight gain, and anorexia
• Fertility agents
• Cosmetic agents (eg, for hair loss)
• Medications intended for the symptomatic relief of cough or colds
• Vitamin and mineral products (excluding prenatal and fluoride preparations)
• Nonprescription medications
• Inpatient medications
• Barbiturates (including phenobarbital)
• Benzodiazepines
• Medications for erectile dysfunction

For more (and updated) information, contact Medicare at www.medicare.gov or
1-800-MEDICARE (1-800-633-4227).

General Information on Aging

AGS Foundation for Health in Aging	www.healthinaging.org	800-563-4916
Administration on Aging	www.aoa.gov	202-619-0724
American Association of Retired Persons	www.aarp.org	888-OUR-AARP (888-687-2277)
American Geriatrics Society	www.americangeriatrics.org	800-247-4779
American Medical Directors Association	www.amda.com	800-876-2632
American Society of Consultant Pharmacists	www.ascp.com	800-355-2727
Assisted Living Federation of America	www.alfa.org	703-894-1805
Children of Aging Parents	www.caps4caregivers.org	800-227-7294
CDC National Prevention Information Network	www.cdcnpin.org	800-458-5231
Family Caregiver Alliance	www.caregiver.org	800-445-8106
Medicare Hotline	www.medicare.gov	800-MEDICARE (800-633-4227)
National Adult Day Services Association	www.nadsa.org	877-745-1440
National Council on the Aging	www.ncoa.org	202-479-1200
National Institute on Aging	www.nia.nih.gov	301-496-1752 TTY: 800-222-4225

Elder Mistreatment

National Center on Elder Abuse	www.ncea.aoa.gov	302-831-3525 800-677-1116 (help hotline)

End-of-Life

National Hospice and Palliative Care Organization	www.nhpco.org	800-658-8898

Smoking Cessation

American Cancer Society	www.cancer.org	800-ACS-2345 (800-227-2345) TTY: 866-228-4327
American Lung Association	www.lungusa.org	800-LUNG-USA (800-586-4872)
CDC National Center for Chronic Disease Prevention and Health Promotion	www.cdc.gov/tobacco/how2quit.htm	800-CDC-INFO (800-232-4636)
National Cancer Institute	www.smokefree.gov	800-QUITNOW (800-784-8669) TTY: 800-332-8615

Specific Health Problems

Alzheimer's Association	www.alz.org	800-272-3900 TDD: 866-403-3073
Alzheimer's Disease Education and Referral Center	www.alzheimers.org	800-438-4380

American Academy of Ophthalmology	www.aao.org	800-222-3937
American Association for Geriatric Psychiatry	www.aagponline.org	301-654-7850
American Cancer Society	www.cancer.org	800-ACS-2345 (800-227-2345)
American College of Obstetricians and Gynecologists	www.acog.org	800-673-8444
American Diabetes Association	www.diabetes.org	800-DIABETES (800-342-2383)
American Foundation for the Blind	www.afb.org	800-AFB-LINE (800-232-5463)
American Heart Association	www.americanheart.org	800-AHA-USA1 (800-242-8721)
American Lung Association	www.lungusa.org	800-LUNG-USA (800-586-4872)
American Pain Society	www.ampainsoc.org	847-375-4715
American Parkinson Disease Association	www.apdaparkinson.org	800-223-2732
American Stroke Association	www.strokeassociation.org	888-4-STROKE (888-478-7653)
American Urological Association	www.auanet.org	866-746-4282
Arthritis Foundation	www.arthritis.org	800-283-7800
Better Hearing Institute	www.betterhearing.org	800-EAR-WELL (800-327-9355)
Endocrine Society and Hormone Foundation (obesity)	www.obesityinamerica.com	301-941-0255
Geriatric Mental Health Foundation	www.gmhfonline.org	301-654-7850
Hearing Loss Association of America	www.hearingloss.org	301-657-2248 (V-TTY)
Lighthouse International	www.lighthouse.org	800-829-0500 TTY: 212-821-9713
Meals On Wheels Association of America	www.mowaa.org	703-548-5558
National Association for Continence	www.nafc.org	800-BLADDER (800-252-3337)
National Diabetes Information Clearinghouse	www.diabetes.niddk.nih.gov	800-860-8747
National Digestive Disease Information Clearinghouse	www.digestive.niddk.nih.gov	800-891-5389
National Eye Institute	www.nei.nih.gov	301-496-5248
National Heart, Lung, and Blood Institute	www.nhlbi.nih.gov	301-592-8573 TTY: 240-629-3255
National Institute of Arthritis and Musculoskeletal and Skin Diseases	www.niams.nih.gov	877-22-NIAMS (877-226-4267) TTY: 301-565-2966
National Institute of Mental Health	www.nimh.nih.gov	866-615-NIMH (866-615-6464) TTY: 866-415-8051

National Institute of Neurological Disorders and Stroke	www.ninds.nih.gov	800-352-9424 TTY: 301-468-5981
National Institute on Deafness and Other Communication Disorders	www.nidcd.nih.gov	800-241-1044 TTY: 800-241-1055
National Kidney and Urologic Diseases Information Clearinghouse	www.kidney.niddk.nih.gov	800-891-5390
National Osteoporosis Foundation	www.nof.org	800-231-4222
National Parkinson Foundation	www.parkinson.org	800-327-4545
Sexuality Information and Education Council of the US	www.siecus.org	212-819-9770
The Simon Foundation for Continence	www.simonfoundation.org	800-23-SIMON (800-237-4666)

INDEX

Page references followed by *t* and *f* indicate tables and figures, respectively.
Trade names are in *italics*.

B

Back pain, 144–145
Baclofen *(Lioresal),* 178*t*
Bacterial conjunctivitis, acute, 235, 235*t*
Bacterial sinusitis, 201*t*
Bacteriuria, 110, 115–116
Bactocill (oxacillin), 121*t*
Bactrim, 126*t. See also* Co-trimoxazole
Bactroban (mupirocin), 67
Balance assessment, 84
Balance exercises, 85, 85*t,* 192
Balance impairment, 85*t*
Barbiturates, 21
Barium swallow, 87
Basal cell carcinoma, 66, 240
Basic energy (caloric) requirements, 140
Beclomethasone *(Beclovent, Beconase,*
        Vancenase, Vanceril), 205*t,* 210*t*
Beclovent, 210*t. See also* Beclomethasone
Beconase, 205*t. See also* Beclomethasone
Behavioral therapy
    for anxiety, 26
    for dementia, 57
    for DHIC, 108
    for dizziness, 157*t*
    for drop attacks, 158*t*
    for IBS, 91
    for sleep disorders, 226
    for smoking cessation, 19
    for UI, 109
Benadryl, 205*t. See also* Diphenhydramine
Benazepril *(Lotensin),* 34*t,* 42*t,* 44*t*
Bendroflumethiazide with nadolol *(Corzide),*
        44*t*
Benecol, 35
Benemid (probenecid), 155*t*
Ben-Gay (methylsalicylate and menthol),
        149*f,* 178*t*
Benicar, 43*t. See also* Olmesartan
Benicar HCT (olmesartan with HCTZ), 44*t*
Benign paroxysmal positional vertigo, 158*t*
Benign prostatic hyperplasia (BPH), 43*t,*
        193–194, 250
Bentyl (dicyclomine), 91

Benzodiazepines
    for akathisia, 200*t*
    for anxiety, 27, 27*t*
    for delirium, 54
    fall risks, 84
    for pain at end of life, 183
    preventing falls with, 85*t*
    for restless legs syndrome, 230
    for sleep disorders, 227*t*
Benzonatate *(Tessalon Perles),* 202*t*
Benztropine *(Cogentin),* 57, 162*t*
β-Adrenergic agonists
    for asthma, 209*t,* 210*t*
    for COPD, 207*t,* 208*t,* 210*t*
    for pneumonia, 114
β-Blockers (β-adrenergic inhibitors)
    for ACS, 30
    for akathisia, 200*t*
    for anxiety disorders, 27
    for chronic angina, 32
    and coexisting conditions, 43*t*
    combined α- and β-blockers, 41*t,* 43*t*
    for glaucoma, 233*t*
    for HF, 33, 34, 35*t*
    for HTN, 38, 40*t*–41*t,* 44*t*
    for hyperthyroidism, 75
    perioperative use, 188
    and sleep problems, 226
    for tremors, 157*t*
β-Carotene, 232
Betagan (levobunolol), 233*t*
β-Lactams, 114*t,* 115, 121*t*–124*t*
Betamethasone *(Celestone),* 74*t*
Betamethasone dipropionate *(Diprolene,*
        Diprolene AF, Diprosone), 71*t,* 72*t,* 240
Betamethasone valerate *(Valisone),* 71*t,* 72*t*
Betapace (sotalol), 46*t*
Betapace AF (sotalol), 46*t*
Betaxolol *(Betoptic, Betoptic-S, Kerlone),*
        40*t,* 233*t*
Bethanechol *(Urecholine),* 89*t*
Betimol (timolol drops), 233*t*
Betoptic, 233*t. See also* Betaxolol
Betoptic-S, 233*t. See also* Betaxolol
Biaxin, 90, 124*t. See also* Clarithromycin
Biaxin XL, 124*t. See also* Clarithromycin

O

Oatmeal baths, 69, 70

Obesity
  management of HTN, 38
  post MI, 32
  resources for, 260
  screening, 189*t*

Obsessive-compulsive disorder (OCD), 26, 27

Obstruction
  bladder outlet, 107, 108
  bowel, 184
  renal, 131*t*

Obstructive pulmonary disease, chronic (COPD), 207
  medications for, 209*t*–212*t*
  preoperative risk assessment, 187
  resources for, 259, 260
  therapy for, 207*t*–208*t*

Obstructive sleep apnea, 228

Occipital inflammation, 169*t*

Occupational therapy (OT)
  for falls prevention, 84
  for osteoarthritis, 148
  for pain management, 174
  for rheumatoid arthritis, 153

OCD (obsessive-compulsive disorder), 26, 27

Octreotide *(Sandostatin)*, 184

Ocuflox, 235*t*. *See also* Ofloxacin

Ocupress, 233*t*. *See also* Carteolol

Ocusert (pilocarpine gel), 233*t*

Ocuvite PreserVision, 232

Ofloxacin *(Floxin, Ocuflox, Roxin)*, 125*t*, 197, 235*t*

Ogen (estropipate), 216*t*, 242*t*

Olanzapine *(Zyprexa, Zydis)*
  for acute mania, 64
  adverse events, 199*t*–200*t*
  for agitation, 59, 59*t*
  for bipolar disorders, 64*t*
  daily dose thresholds, 255*t*
  drug and metabolic interactions, 12*t*
  for psychotic disorders, 198, 198*t*
  for SSRI-induced sexual dysfunction, 216

Olanzapine IM *(Zyprexa Intramuscular)*, 54, 59*t*

Olmesartan *(Benicar)*, 35*t*, 43*t*, 44*t*

Olopatadine *(Patanol)*, 206*t*

Omacor, 36*t*. *See also* Omega-3 fatty acids

Omalizumab *(Xolair)*, 212*t*

Omega-3 fatty acids *(Omacor)*, 32, 36*t*, 189*t*

Omeprazole *(Prilosec)*
  drug and metabolic interactions, 12*t*, 13*t*, 14*t*
  enteral nutrition interactions, 142
  for GERD, 89*t*
  for *H pylori*-induced ulcerations, 90*t*

Omnaris (ciclesonide), 205*t*

Omnicef (cefdinir), 123*t*

OMS Concentrate, 176*t*. *See also* Morphine

Ondansetron *(Zofran)*, 13*t*, 94*t*, 184

Onychomycosis, 68, 70*t*

Opana (oxymorphone), 176*t*

Opioids
  with acetaminophen, 149*f*
  for acute pain, 173
  analgesic drugs, 176*t*
  dosage, 175
  for dyspnea, 184
  management of adverse events, 175
  for opioid-tolerant patients, 177*t*
  for osteoarthritis, 148
  for pain, 173, 174, 176*t*, 183
  for painful neuropathy, 165
  for persistent pain, 170*t*
  for restless legs syndrome, 230
  risk of addiction, 171

Op-site, 222*t*. *See also* Transparent film

Optical aids, 232

OptiPranolol (metipranolol), 233*t*

Optivar (azelastine), 204*t*

Oral nutrition, 140, 141*t*

Oral procedures: endocarditis prophylaxis for, 190, 191, 191*t*

Oral statements, 181

Oramorph SR (morphine), 177*t*

Orasone, 74*t*, 211*t*. *See also* Prednisone

Orchiectomy, 194

Orencia (abatacept), 153

Oretic (HCTZ), 39*t*

Orgaran (danaparoid), 23*t*

Ortho-Est, 242*t*. *See also* Estropipate

About the American Geriatrics Society

Founded in 1942, the American Geriatrics Society (AGS) is the leading clinical society devoted to the care of older adults. The AGS promotes high quality, comprehensive, and accessible care for America's older population, including those who are chronically ill and disabled. The organization provides leadership to health care professionals, policy makers, and the public by developing, implementing, and advocating programs in patient care, research, professional and public education, and public policy.

Its members include primary care physicians, geriatricians, geropsychiatrists, nurse practitioners, social workers, physician assistants, physical therapists, pharmacists, and others from the United States and around the world who are dedicated to improving the health, independence, and quality of life of the older population.

The AGS has long championed efforts to expand the national work force of clinicians with the specialized knowledge and skills to care for our aging population. Since the early 1990s, with funding from the John A. Hartford Foundation of New York City, the AGS has worked effectively to increase geriatrics expertise among subspecialists in internal medicine, practicing primary care physicians, and surgical and related medical specialists.

Current Major Publications and Programs of the AGS

Journal of the American Geriatrics Society—*JAGS* is consistently ranked as one of the top resources for researchers and clinicians with an interest in aging.

Annals of Long-Term Care: Clinical Care and Aging—*Annals* offers clinical reviews, analysis, and opinions focused on long-term care, and is the premier source of information for long-term care professionals.

Clinical Geriatrics—This journal focuses on both the clinical and practical issues related to the treatment and management of older persons.

Doorway Thoughts: Cross-Cultural Health Care for Older Adults—Developed by the AGS Ethnogeriatrics Committee, *Doorway Thoughts* uses illustrative case studies to discuss the unique cultural perspectives of different ethnic groups, focusing on issues such as preferred terms for cultural identity, nonverbal communication norms, differing expectations of the clinician-patient relationship, and views of end-of-life issues.

Geriatrics At Your Fingertips®—This annually updated, comprehensive pocket-sized reference to clinical geriatrics provides practical information on the evaluation and management of diseases and disorders most common to older adults. Versions for Pocket PC- and Palm-based PDAs are also available for download at www.geriatricsatyourfingertips.org.

Geriatrics Review Syllabus: A Core Curriculum in Geriatric Medicine—The newly revised 6th (2006) edition of this ground-breaking self-assessment, continuing education program for primary care providers is a premier source of clinically relevant information in geriatric medicine.

Geriatrics Nursing Review Syllabus—Now in its second edition, the core curriculum in advanced practice geriatric nursing (*GNRS*) is a concise, up-to-date, and comprehensive text developed by the AGS in collaboration with the John A. Hartford Foundation Institute of Geriatric Nursing at New York University.

Geriatrics Review Syllabus Teaching Slides—Found at www.frycomm.com/ags/teachingslides/, this series of one-hour PowerPoint® presentations is perfect for educational sessions focused on the care of older adults. Available for an annual subscription fee, the series covers topics such as osteoporosis, delirium, palliative care, dementia, and preventive care and is based on the *Geriatrics Review Syllabus*. Each slide set includes case materials and can be modified to meet the specific learning objectives for a session.

New Frontiers in Geriatrics Research: An Agenda for Surgical and Related Medical Specialties—Found at www.frycomm.com/ags/rasp/, New Frontiers presents a research agenda specifically aimed at enhancing the quality of care for older patients who are cared for by surgical and related medical specialists. Updated in 2008, this free Web-based resource is a useful source of ideas for researchers who are interested in contributing to the evidence base in support of geriatrics practice in their respective disciplines.

AGS Web site and **AGS Week In Review**—The AGS Web site provides information on AGS activities and programs, noteworthy news, public policy issues, career opportunities in geriatrics, and much more. *AGS Week in Review* offers weekly updates on AGS activities, grant opportunities and other items of interest to those working in the field - subscribe now at www.americangeriatrics.org.

Learn more about the following at www.americangeriatrics.org:

The AGS Annual Scientific Meeting—This is the premier forum for learning the latest information in clinical geriatrics, research on aging and health, health problems of older adults, and innovative models in health care delivery as well as teaching in geriatrics.

The Geriatrics Recognition Award—This award recognizes physicians and nurses who are committed to advancing their geriatrics knowledge to provide better care for older adults.

AGS Awards and Grants Programs—In conjunction with the annual meeting, AGS recognizes individuals for their contributions to improved care of older adults through its Edward Henderson Award and State-of-the-Art Lecture, and Clinician of the Year, Dennis W. Jahnigen Memorial, Nasher Manning, New Investigator, and Edward Henderson Student Awards. In collaboration with the Hartford Foundation and Atlantic Philanthropies, AGS also offers the Jahnigen Career Development Scholars Awards for young investigators in the surgical and related medical specialties and Geriatrics for Specialists Residents Program awards.

About the AGS Foundation for Health in Aging

In 1999, the AGS reached beyond its traditional role as a professional medical society and launched the **AGS Foundation for Health in Aging (FHA)**. The FHA aims to build a bridge between the research and practice of geriatrics health care professionals and the public, and to advocate on behalf of older adults regarding issues of wellness and preventive care, self-responsibility and independence, and connections to family and community. For more information about FHA initiatives and its public education resources, please visit the Foundation website at www.healthinaging.org.

Current Major FHA Publications and Programs

Aging in the Know: Your Gateway to Health and Aging Resources on the Web—This new comprehensive Web site features information on over 50 health topics related to aging, a *What to Ask Series* designed to help older adults safely navigate the health care systems, and topic-specific linkages to additional credible information on the Web. This free new resource can be found on www.healthinaging.org/agingintheknow/.

Eldercare at Home—Now in its 2ⁿᵈ edition, this is an extensive guide for families involved in providing care for older relatives who want to remain at home. In addition to the free online edition of *Eldercare at Home*, the FHA has created a fully illustrated Workbook for individuals to use at home, and a PowerPoint® presentation package that can be used in community settings to teach family caregivers how to solve problems often faced when caring for an older person at home. Information on these and other public education programs is available on the Foundation Web site.

FHA Awards Program—This program includes the Student Researcher Fund, the Hartford Geriatrics Health Outcomes Research Scholars Awards Program, and the T. Franklin Williams Research Scholars Award Program.

If you would like further information about the AGS or FHA, please visit www.americangeriatrics.org

Or contact us at:
The American Geriatrics Society
The Empire State Building
350 5th Avenue, Suite 801
New York, NY 10118 USA

Call toll-free: (800) 247-4779
Outside the US call: (212) 308-1414
E-mail: info.amger@mericangeriatrics.org

From the American Geriatrics Society
GERIATRICS *At Your* FINGERTIPS®
2008–2009, 10th Edition
(ISSN 1553-152X) (ISBN 978-1-886775-21-3)

A guide to the evaluation and management of the diseases and disorders that most commonly affect older persons.

Portable, Practical, Fully Indexed, and Up-to-Date!

Send completed order form with payment to:

Fry Communications, Inc.
American Geriatrics Society
800 West Church Road
Mechanicsburg, PA 17055

For fast service
Call: 1-800-334-1429 ext. 2529
Order online at www.geriatricsatyourfingertips.org

Please send me _____ copies of *Geriatrics At Your Fingertips*, 2008–2009, 10th Edition
@ $13.95 each ($11.95 for AGS Members)
Subtotal   _____

Shipping & Handling   _____
North America: $2.75 + $1.00 ea additional
Overseas: please call 1-717-766-0211 ext. 2529 for rates

TOTAL   _____

To order quantities of 500 or greater please contact Elvy Ickowicz at 1-212-308-1414.

Method of Payment:_____ Check or money order payable to Fry Communications
_____ MasterCard   _____VISA
Card Number _____ Exp.Date _____
Signature _____

Shipping Instructions (must be complete)

Name: _____
Address: _____
City: _____State: _____ Zip: _____
Phone: _____
E-mail Address: _____

GAYF 2008–2009

Your request places you on the AGS e-alert electronic mailing list. You will be among the first in your discipline to find out about new releases, special offers, and program announcements from AGS. After you receive your first e-alert, you have the option of canceling the service at any time. Prices subject to change without notice.